THE
STORY
of
PERFUME

For all perfume lovers and for my family

First published in Great Britain in 2024 by

Laurence King
An imprint of Quercus Editions Ltd
Carmelite House
50 Victoria Embankment
London EC4Y 0DZ

An Hachette UK company

A CIP catalogue record for this book is available from the British Library

ISBN 978-1-529432299

10 9 8 7 6 5 4 3 2 1

English translation by Alison Hughes

Cover art: (front) Parfums de Silvy advert, 1921. © Archives Larousse; (back. top) *L'habit du parfumeur,* 1965 ©akg-images; (back, bottom) *Narkiss* bottle, René Lalique for Roger&Gallet, 1920 ©Patrimoine Roger&Gallet.

Publication Directors: Sophie Descours / Carine Girac-Marinier
Editors: Françoise Mathay / Véronique Tahon
Design: Florence Le Maux
Picture research: Valérie Perrin assisted by Flore Arce Ross

For the English edition
Acquisition editor: Sophie Wise
Typesetting: The Urban Ant

Printed and bound in China
Papers used by Quercus are from well-managed forests and other responsible sources.

Élisabeth de Feydeau

THE
HISTORY
of
PERFUME

LAURENCE KING

Contents

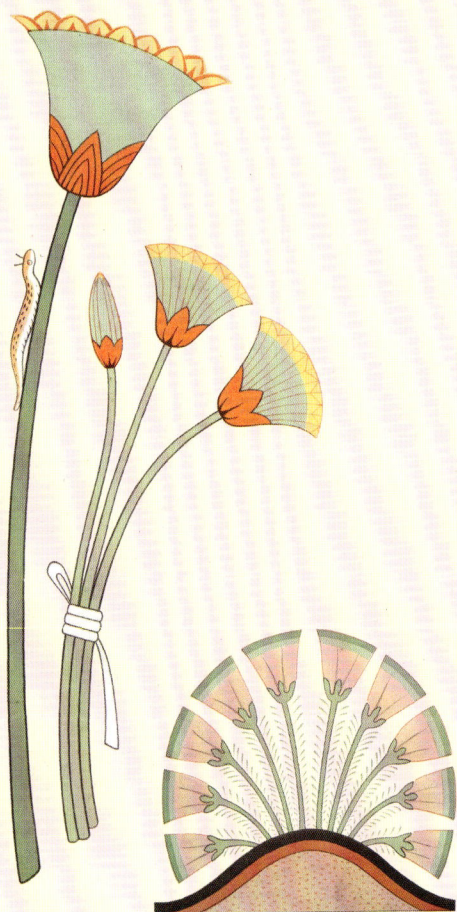

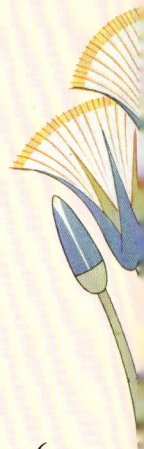

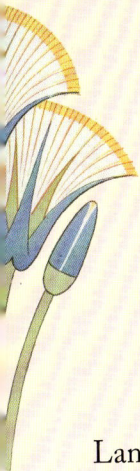

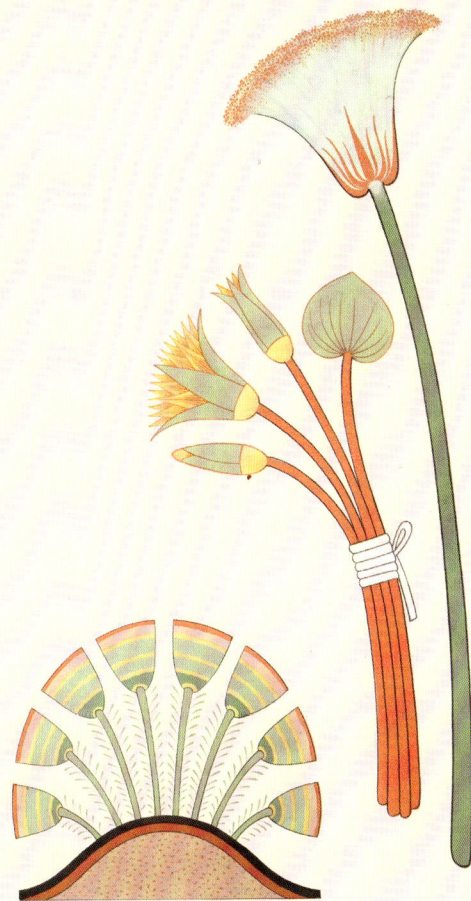

INTRODUCTION

FROM ANCIENT TIMES, AND THROUGH CENTURIES OF
SEDUCTION, WEARING PERFUME HAS BEEN A PART OF WHAT
MAKES US HUMAN. PERFUME ALWAYS TELLS A STORY –
THE STORY OF HUMAN BEINGS AND THEIR TIME. IT
APPEALS TO THE EMOTIONS AND UNITES CULTURES.
IT MAKES HEARTS SING AND RECONCILES SOULS.

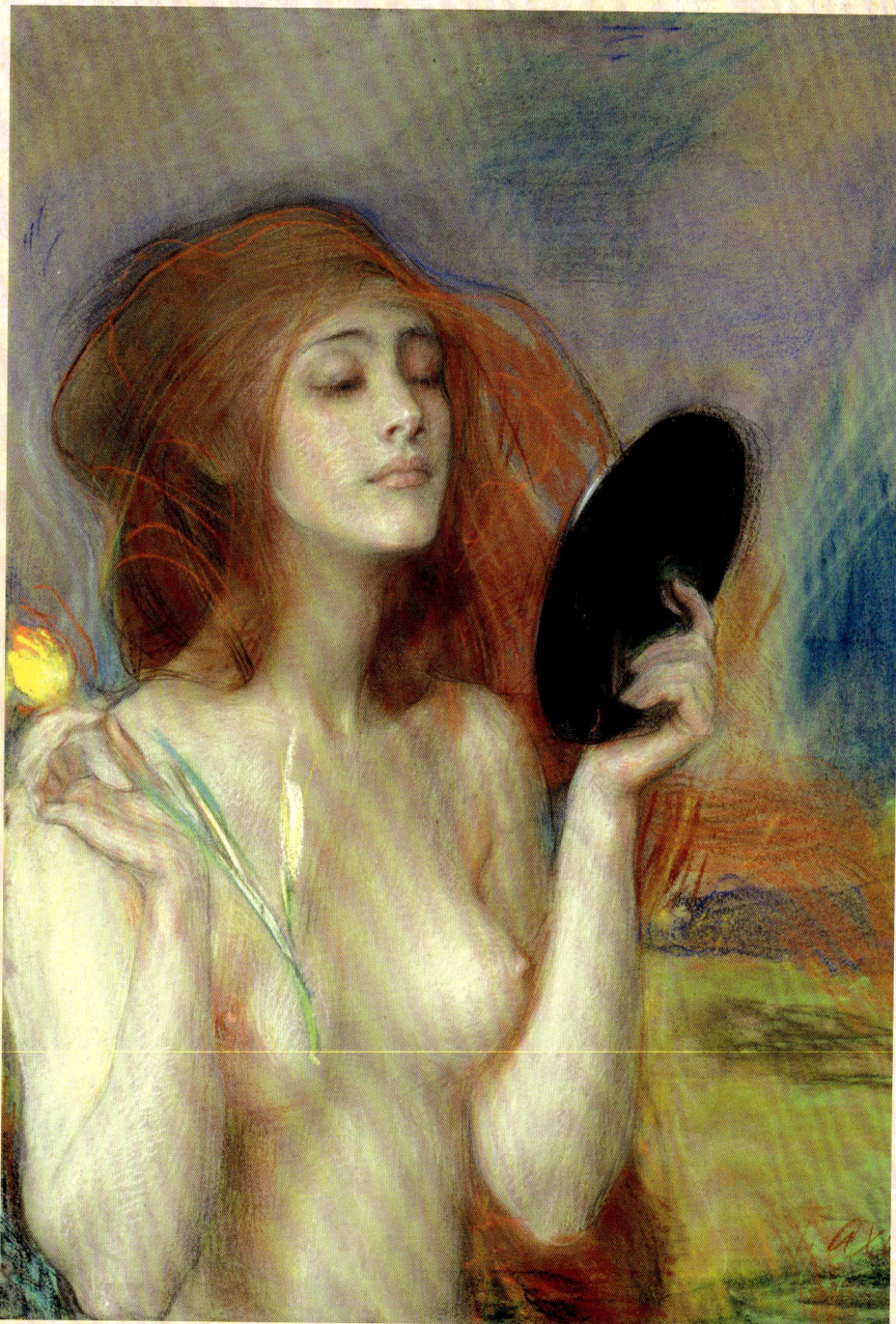

Spring by the Polish painter Teodor Axentowicz (1859–1938).

THE THREE FUNCTIONS OF PERFUME

Since time immemorial people have burned various substances as a means of communicating with and praying to the gods, hence the Latin expression *per fumum*, meaning 'through the smoke', which gives us the English word 'perfume'. Perfume plays its part in rituals, legends and beliefs. It floats from our very selves to far beyond, from believers to the gods, from humans to the cosmos. Initially it was sacred and the preserve of the gods before it became a personal-care and medicinal product for combatting epidemics. Above all, it is intimately connected with seduction. It expresses attraction and enhances our love lives.

A MIRROR TO THE WORLD

Perfume is very closely associated with personal care and therapy, which has facilitated its shift from sacred to secular over the centuries. Once freed from matters of mere survival, people could find their place in society, create an image, decide what they wished to reveal about themselves to others and enhance their social standing. Perfume became their aura, the robe of light that gave them an invisible, yet powerful, hold on others. Little by little it came to express a person's individuality, just like their facial features and body shape. It accompanies us in our daily lives, almost like our own personal mirror. It reflects our moods and we are soothed and comforted by its familiar notes. Perfume comes into its own on the skin; the scent it exudes is the most accurate reflection of our innermost being and the expression of our sensitivities. We can choose our perfume with care or without a second thought, like falling head over heels and instinctively and impulsively knowing it is 'the one'.

SCENT IS PERVASIVE

Works of literature are testament to the fact that our daily lives are bathed in scents; those of trees, flowers, earth and water, and also of objects that have taken on mysterious odours as they have aged. Think of the yellowing pages of old books, the faded silk of a dress and worn, forgotten gloves. These materials are imbued with the smell of the past. In Guy de Maupassant's novel *Strong as Death*, scent triggers passion in the mature man: 'How many times a woman's draperies had thrown to him in passing, with the evaporating breath of some essence, a host of forgotten events. At the bottom of old perfume bottles he had often found bits of his former existence; and all wandering odours – of streets, fields, houses, furniture, sweet or unsavoury, the warm odours of summer evenings, the cold breath of winter nights, revived within him far-off reminiscences, as if odours kept embalmed within him these dead-and-gone memories, as aromatics preserve mummies.'

CREATING OLFACTORY MEMORIES

Whether it awakens mystical notions or triggers sensuous thoughts, perfume digs deep into the memory to find the intensity of the emotions it arouses. Today, we acknowledge smell as one of our vital five senses – and that perfume enriches our daily lives. Every one of us knows that scents have the power to stir desire and transport us through time and space, to take us back decades or conjure up known or unknown destinations. Marcel Proust's madeleine (in his 1913 *In Search of Lost Time*) was able to erase the years. Perfumers have understood this better than anyone. They are both artists and technicians, sorcerers and alchemists, who harbour within them every source of inspiration. Unlike an apothecary, who reproduces the very same formula day after day, a perfumer creates for the inner being of every one of us. Describing his craft in the eighteenth century, Jean-Louis Fargeon, Marie-Antoinette's perfumer, said: 'Of all the arts associated with luxury and wealth, none produces such sensual emotions as that of the perfumer.'

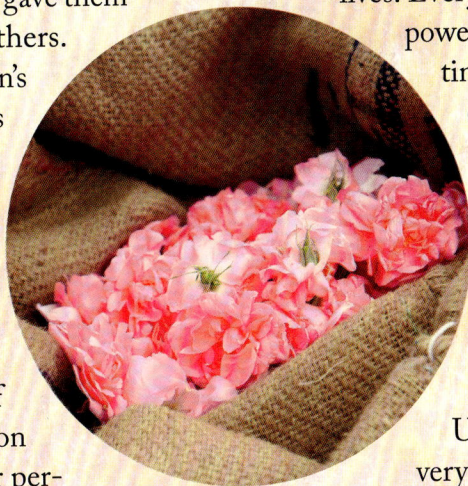

'PERFUME IS SCENT PLUS MAN'

Creating and developing a perfume is a profession which has truly unique connections with art and time. In the art of composition, there is no *creatio ex nihilo*; nothing is created from a void. The history of perfume shows us that it is a process, and that the present is built on the past. Perfume is not just a simple commodity. It is so much more. 'Perfume is scent plus man,' Provençal author of the twetntieth century Jean Giono told us, emphasizing the vital encounter of skin and fragrance, the fact that a perfume comes alive through the person who wears it. An individual, dead or alive, lives on in its intense powers of evocation and emotion. To ensure that the beautiful scent of perfume never evaporates, in 2018 UNESCO included the skills related to perfume in the Grasse area, France, on its List of Intangible Cultural Heritage.

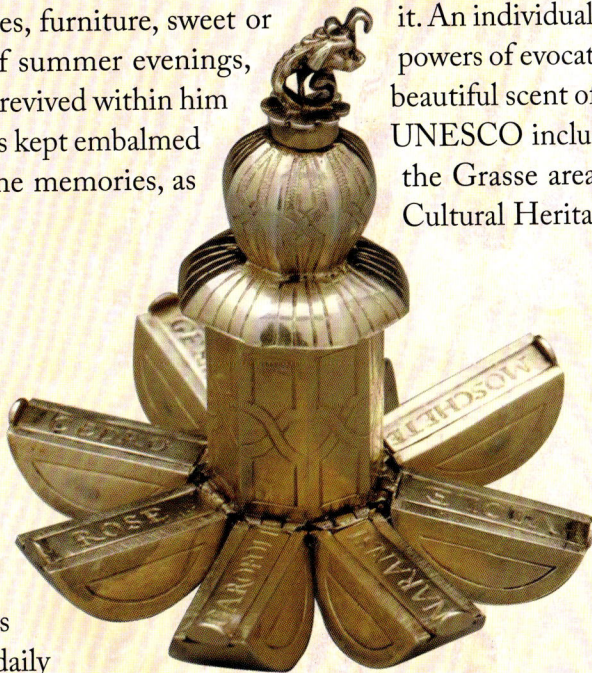

Above: Provence roses (*Rosa x centifolia*) from the Domaine de Manon, Grasse, France.

Left: English silver-gilt pomander, circa 1580. It bears the inscriptions Rose, Cedro, Gesmini, Ambra, Moschete, Viole, Naransi and Garofoli (rose, cedar, jasmine, ambergris, musk, violet, orange and clove).

THE BIRTHPLACE OF PERFUME

THE EARLIEST EVIDENCE OF PERFUME USE DATES BACK TO THE BRONZE AGE, IN MESOPOTAMIA AND THE LEVANT. THERE ARE EVEN SIGNS THAT ITS HISTORY GOES AS FAR BACK AS THE NEOLITHIC PERIOD. STONE AND POTTERY CONTAINERS DATING BACK TO THE FOURTH MILLENNIUM BCE WERE UNCOVERED DURING ARCHAEOLOGICAL EXCAVATIONS IN IRAN, AND IT IS BELIEVED THAT PERFUME WAS INVENTED IN THE EAST, THEN MIGRATED TO ANCIENT EGYPT, WHICH HELPED TO ESTABLISH PERFUME AS A MUCH-LOVED COMMODITY.

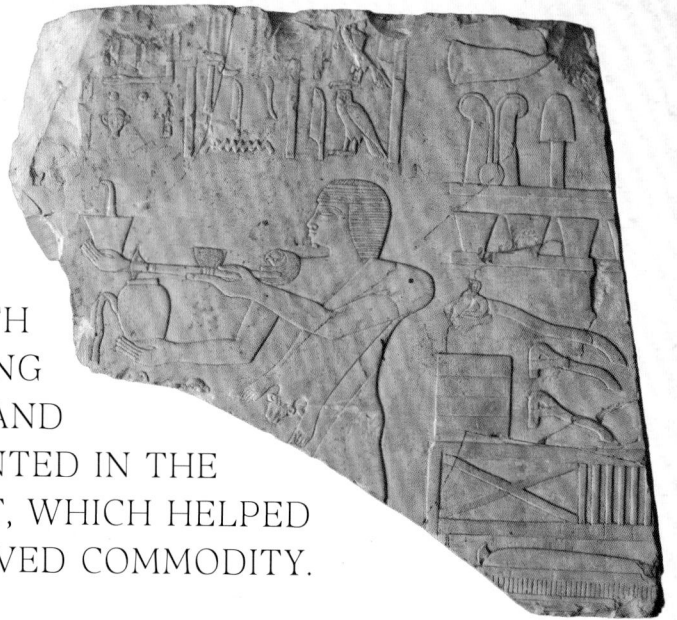

THE ORIGINS OF THE FIRST PERFUMES

The first containers of fragrant substances were discovered in Iran and date back to the fourth millennium BCE. We might conclude from this that perfume was invented in the East, and written evidence and objects have been found which indicate that it was prominent in the day-to-day lives of ancient civilizations. It is thought that from southern Arabia perfume infiltrated Mesopotamia (most of which is now present-day Iraq) and then headed north to the Levant coast, or was shipped to the Persian Gulf and then across the Indian Ocean, from the first millennium BCE onwards. By the Bronze Age, perfume could be found in the eastern Mediterranean, Levant, Egypt and in and around Mesopotamia. Scented substances – mainly resins – were used in censers and perfume burners during fumigation rituals. They were considered to be rare and bear a divine imprint, so were reserved for the gods, while perfume had associations with power. Because it elevated humans and linked them to an immutable, superior order, and because fumigation was also part of funeral rituals, perfume had cult status in all the ancient religions.

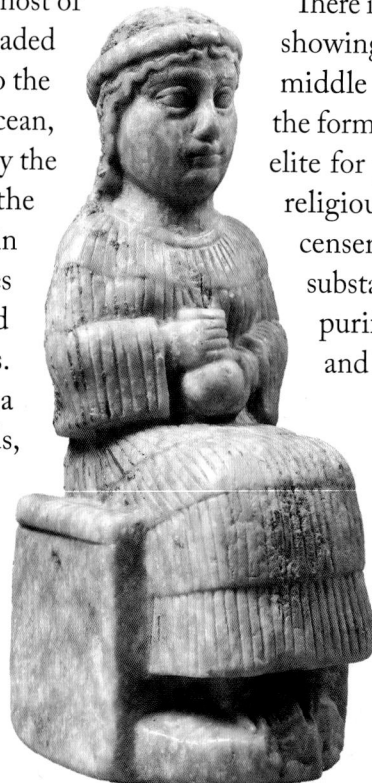

COMMUNICATING WITH THE GODS

As far back as Neanderthal man, flowers and perfumes were associated with death and burial. Cremations, which were common in Europe's Bronze Age around 1800 BCE, ended with the burning of resinous wood to release fragrant smells. In the late Bronze Age, the use of incense became commonplace.

There is documentary evidence from Mesopotamia showing that perfume made an appearance in the middle of the third millennium BCE, always in the form of scented oil. It was used by kings and the elite for personal grooming, and by priests during religious ceremonies. The perfume burners and censers found in temples and palaces tell us that substances were burned to tantalize the gods and purify the air, thereby eradicating bad smells and the emanations of evil spirits.

Above: Fragment of an Egyptian relief depicting a funeral ceremony during which censers were used extensively, 26th Dynasty (circa 664–610 BCE).

Left: Statuette of a woman known as 'Woman holding the aryballos' (a flask used to store perfumed oil), Mesopotamia, third millennium BCE.

THE IMPORTANT ROLE OF ANCIENT EGYPT

It was mainly in ancient Egypt, where many fragrant plants flourished on the banks of the Nile, that the first perfume blends were found. This country became a supplier of various essences and ben oil, extracted from the seeds of *Moringa peregrina*, a shrub found in Asia and North Africa. Initially intended for the gods, perfume was burned on holy altars. It was also part of embalming and mummification rituals. The Egyptians were fascinated by what happened to the soul after death. They preserved the remains of pharaohs and carefully mummified their bodies, perfecting the art of perfuming and deepening their devotion to the monarch. No ritual was complete without censers and incense. Most of the perfumes and other ceremonial oils were prepared in laboratories within the temples, because it was mainly priests who had perfume-making skills – so we might think of them as the first perfumers. This does not, however, mean that perfume was the sole preserve of the religious. Secular society had discovered its aphrodisiac and therapeutic properties.

In ancient Egypt, the perfumer's art was a very specific skill. In his *Natural History* (Book XII, 7), Pliny the Elder mentions the two components of a perfume: the liquid part (*sucus*) and the essence (*corpus*). The perfumers of Alexandria, ideally situated at the intersection of Eastern and African traditions, were experts in the manufacture of perfumes and balms.

Papyrus showing three priests carrying out the purification rites over the mummy of the deceased scribe Hunefer, using implements including a censer and a pot of perfumed oil. Anubis, Master of Necropolises, circa 1290–1190 BCE, illustration from the Book of the Dead.

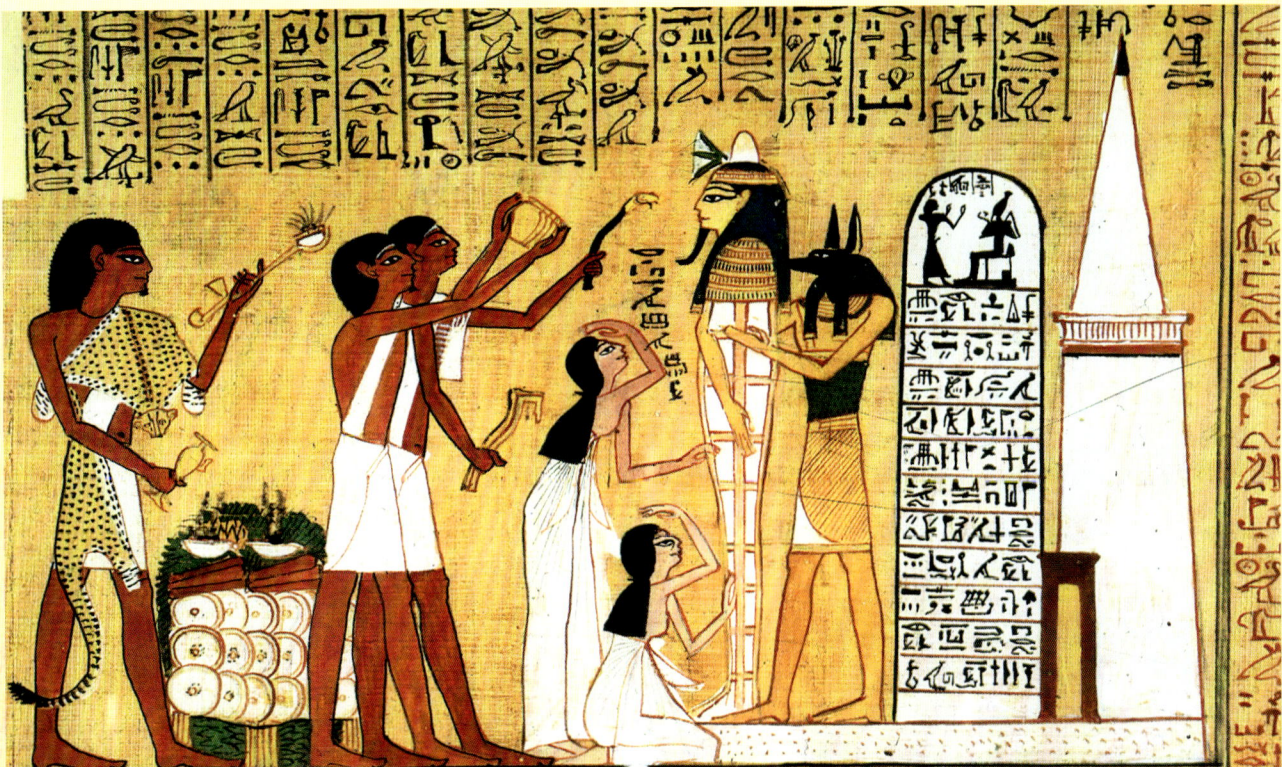

GREEK AND LATIN CIVILIZATIONS

EGYPT MAY BE THE BIRTHPLACE OF PERFUME, BUT IT PASSED ON ITS KNOWLEDGE TO THE GREEKS, CRETANS AND PHOENICIANS. A GOLDEN AGE OF ANCIENT PERFUME, SHARED BY ALL THREE CULTURES, EXTENDED FROM THE TIME OF THE INVENTION OF WRITING, CIRCA 3500 BCE, UNTIL THE END OF THE WESTERN ROMAN EMPIRE IN THE FIFTH CENTURY CE.

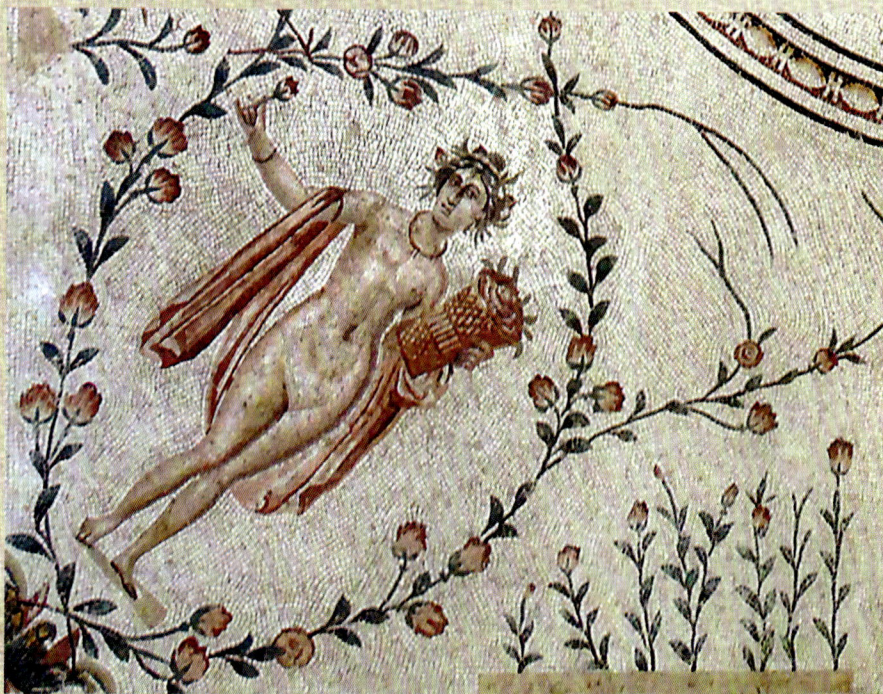

The Triumph of Neptune and the Four Seasons, detail of a mosaic, Tunis, second century CE.

THE 'ORIENTALIZING' REVOLUTION

In Archaic Greece, a period lasting from the eighth century until the early fifth century BCE, the Mediterranean became a vast area of exchange where its own cultures came into contact with the ancient civilizations of the Near and Middle East. Archaeologists call this widespread phenomenon, which affected the cultures, techniques and economies in which perfume featured prominently, the 'orientalizing revolution'. According to the ancient Greeks, southern Arabia (modern-day Yemen) was fortunate because of its abundant natural resources of scented products, gums and resins such as frankincense and myrrh.

The new Greek, Latin, Etruscan and Iberian cities imported raw materials and finished products, as well as exotic animals and enslaved people, from the eastern Mediterranean, Africa and the Far East. From the Bronze Age, Mesopotamian and Egyptian perfume was distributed and then made in the eastern Mediterranean. Tablets found in Mycenaean palaces tell us about how the use of perfume flourished in this period, with information about where it was made, the raw materials used and the craft of the perfumer. We know from the painted pottery perfume vessels produced in Corinth and on the islands of the eastern Aegean from the eighth century onwards that perfume remained the preserve of the gods and the elite.

Aromatics: a gift from nature

The Greeks believed that aromatics were the result of a special conjunction of the Earth and the Sun. They were a gift from wild nature and the practices associated with them were intended to bring together the near with the far and link the high with the low. Although many aromatics were used in cooking, some, such as incense and myrrh, were earmarked for balms and perfumes or for the sacrificial rituals required for the worship of the gods.

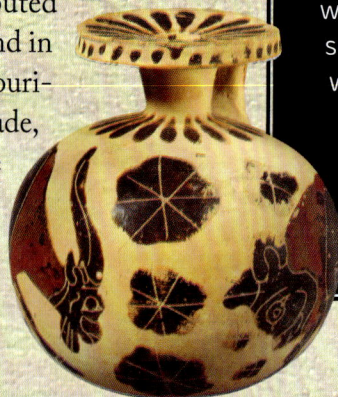

Corinthian vessel for storing perfumed oil, circa 620–590 BCE.

DIVINE PERFUME OF OLYMPUS

Alexander the Great's conquests in Asia and the discovery of the Spice Routes led to a 'perfume revolution' in Greece and the whole of the West. New aromas emerged with animal-based perfumes containing musk and ambergris. The Greek perfumers also played a part in the development of perfume ranges, inventing oils and fats scented with flowers, primarily iris, rose, lily and marjoram. Frankincense, myrrh, saffron and cinnamon were some of the most precious essences. Frankincense and myrrh came from southern Arabia, passing through Egypt, Syria and Phoenicia. The Greeks believed that ambrosia, the perfume of Olympus, gave the gods their immortality. For reasons of hygiene, and to guarantee them access to eternal life, the deceased were liberally doused in perfume and buried with their personal possessions, which included their perfume bottles. For the Greeks, perfume had very strong religious connotations.

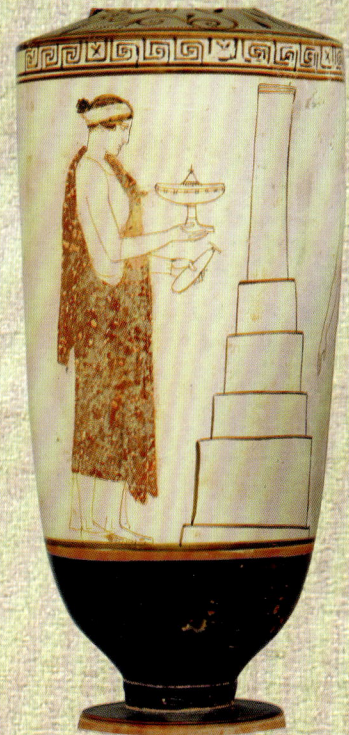

A woman in front of a tomb holding a cylindrical clay bowl (plemochoe) and a small pottery piece containing perfumed oil (alabastron), ancient vessel (lekythos), Greece, fifth century BCE.

SECULAR USE: PERFUME IN ROMAN TIMES

The Roman Empire placed the greatest importance of all on cosmetics and perfume. Although perfume was little used in ancient Rome, the Romans gained a better knowledge of the art of perfumery when they came into contact with the Etruscans and Phoenicians. It was one of the main substances they brought back from their conquests. Roman colonization and the resulting trade introduced spices, incense, perfume baths and the use of saffron for personal grooming to what is now the Italian peninsula. The Romans maintained the Egyptian, Greek and Oriental trade networks that brought scented products in their raw state from Arabia, Africa and India. Perfume production was commonplace in Rome and indeed the peninsula as a whole. We know that in Campania it reached almost industrial proportions, primarily due to the production of olive and almond oils and the vast range of flowers, roses in particular, that grew there. The Romans believed that many aromatic substances had medicinal qualities and their use of perfume for non-religious purposes, particularly at their many banquets and in their thermal baths, was almost excessive.

As far back as the first century BCE, each god had his or her own perfume: benzoin for Jupiter, aloe or agarwood (oudh) for Mars, saffron for Apollo, musk for Juno, cinnamon for Mercury and ambergris for Venus.

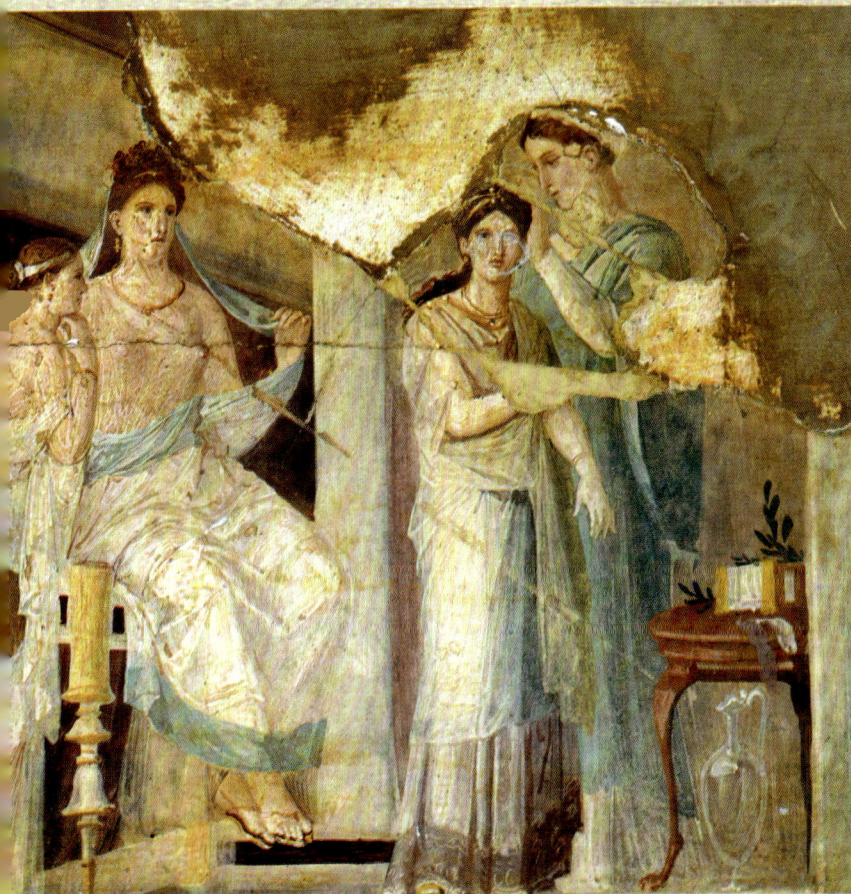

The washing and dressing of a young girl, fresco, Herculaneum, Italy, first century CE.

THE PERFUME ROUTE I: ANTIQUITY

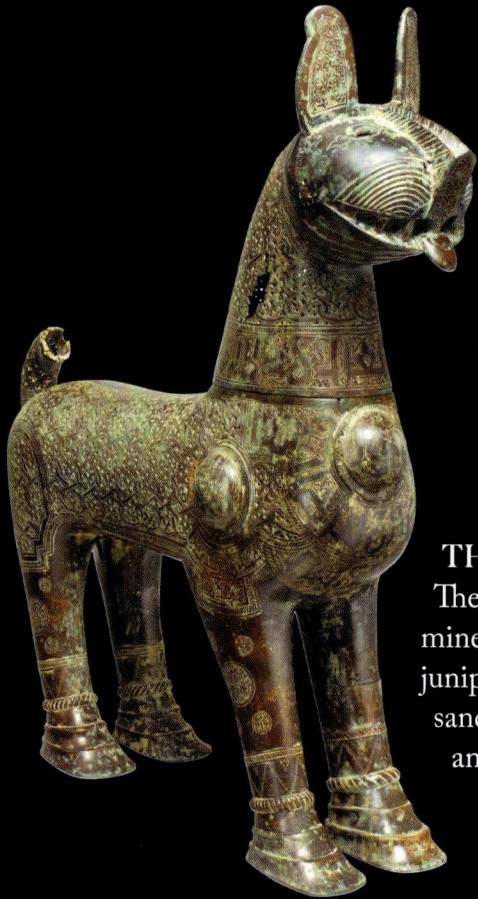

SINCE ANCIENT TIMES, PEOPLE HAVE BEEN DRIVEN TO TRAVEL IN SEARCH OF PRECIOUS PERFUMES. THIS QUEST TOOK THEM TO FARAWAY COUNTRIES, WHICH MEANT ROAMING FOR MANY MONTHS BEFORE THEY REACHED THE EAST OR THE MEDITERRANEAN. THEY WERE DRIVEN BY ONE GOAL – TO FIND AROMATIC PLANTS THAT WERE AS VALUABLE AS GOLD, AND VERY MUCH IN DEMAND.

THE NILE VALLEY

The Near East was an abundant source of fragrances, from rose to myrtle, iris, jasmine, crocus, violet, hyacinth, ginger, galbanum, styrax, opoponax, fenugreek, calamus, juniper, nard and cedar, to name but a few. Amber came mainly from the Arabian Sea, sandalwood and oudh from the Indies and the Indochinese peninsula. Frankincense and myrrh from Arabia and the Red Sea region passed through the Nile valley. Phoenicians and Cypriots excelled in the manufacture of perfumes and in the spice trade around the Mediterranean. They obtained their supplies from the Nile Delta, Arabia and the Red Sea region.

Transporting myrrh trees to be replanted in front of Queen Hatshepsut's temple in Deir el-Bahari.

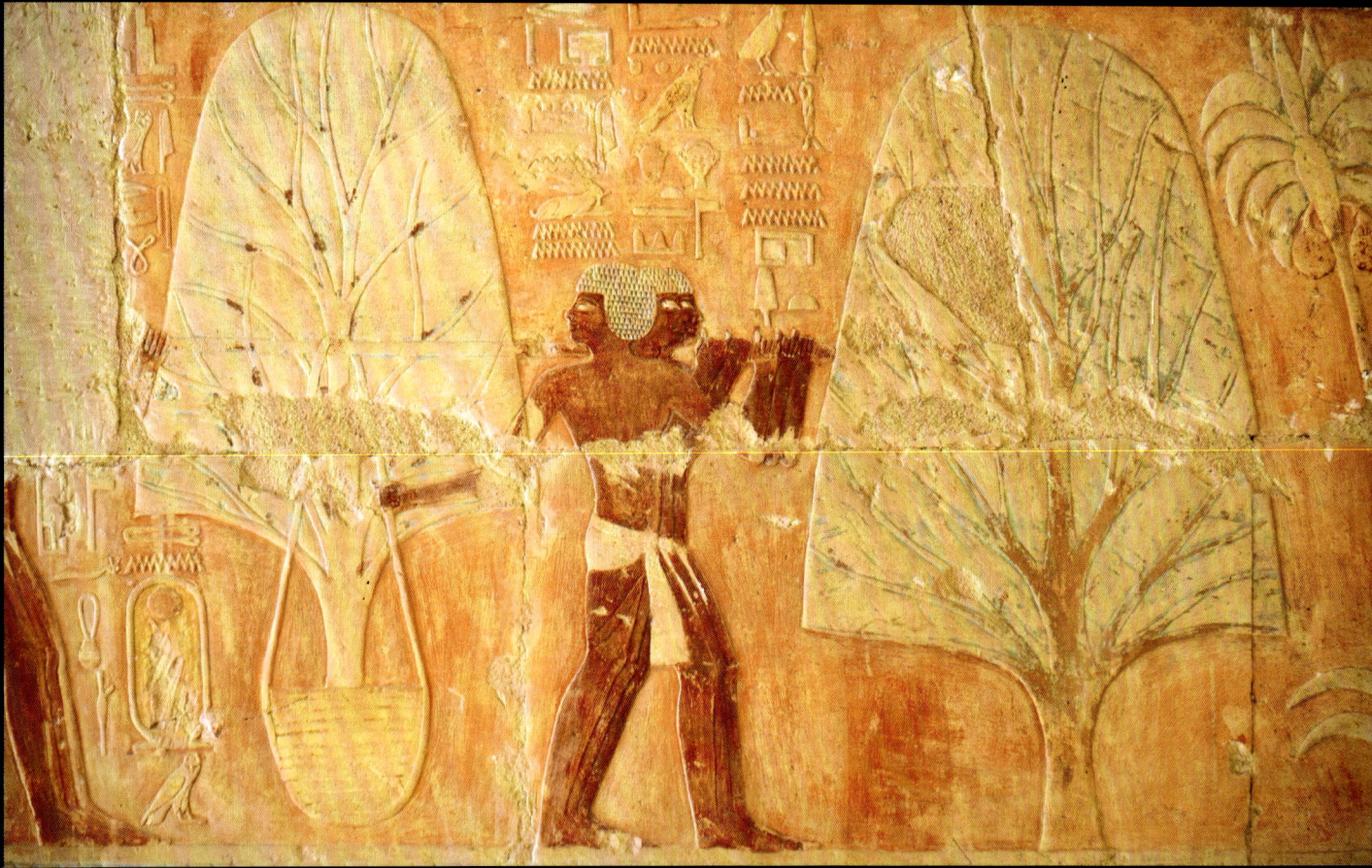

Queen Hatshepsut's expedition to the Land of Punt

The maritime expedition sent by Queen Hatshepsut in the first half of the fifteenth century BCE is a perfect example of the legendary quest for fragrances. At the queen's request, they were to bring back sufficient quantities of myrrh from trees native to the Near East, and the trees themselves, to satisfy the needs of the Egyptians. Five ships set off on a long and perilous journey from Thebes to the 'Land of the God', guarded by a giant snake, the perfume king. The exact route remains a mystery. Did the ships sail along the Red Sea coast, departing from ports such as Quseer or Ras Gharib? Or did they sail up the Nile? The Egyptians took 'Hathor, the Lady of Punt' gifts from the royal workshops. In exchange, they received gold, frankincense, ivory, wild animal skins and a cargo of aromatic plants and resins. They also uprooted 31 myrrh trees to be replanted in front of Queen Hatshepsut's temple in Deir el-Bahari. There were great festivities to celebrate the return of the expedition and the queen herself planted the myrrh trees in the gardens of Amun. However, the planting holes uncovered in the garden during archaeological digs indicate that the trees were unable to acclimatize to their new environment. Until the end of the Pharaoh civilization, the Egyptians would have to import their precious resins from Punt, that mystical land said to be located south of the Arabian Peninsula or in East Africa.

ALEXANDER THE GREAT'S EMPIRE

Alexander founded cities that would give rise to new and very profitable perfume routes on both land and sea. At that time, because of their religious, metaphysical and sociological value, perfumes were as expensive as precious metals. From his small kingdom of Macedonia, Alexander the Great conquered the Middle East and Central Asia, taking Greek civilization as far as India and bringing back the perfumes and the culture of the countries under his control. According to Plutarch, when Alexander saw the perfumed rooms and scented baths in Persia for the first time in October 331 BCE, after his incredible victory over Darius III (the 'king of kings'), he declared, 'So, that was what it was like to be a king, it seems.' The aromatic plants travelled from Petra's vast warehouses to Gaza, from where they were shipped to Greece and Italy.

THE SILK AND INCENSE ROUTE

The Romans, in turn, established five major routes to Asia for silk, rice, furs, precious stones and spices, which were transported by caravans across Chinese Turkestan and Persia then along the Euphrates valley. From the Middle Ages onwards, goods were shipped to Europe from Antioch or Alexandretta (in Turkey today) via Venice, Amalfi or Genoa. The convoys carrying incense, myrrh and cinnamon were duplicated by sea routes from China and Bengal, passing through Cochin, Bombay, Surat and Aden, then along the long Red Sea corridor to Alexandria from where the goods were shipped to Venice from the fifth century CE onwards.

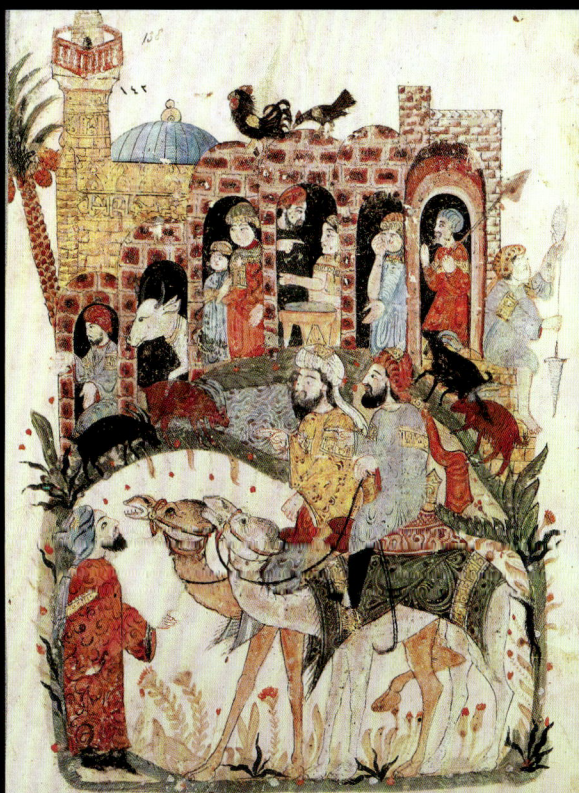

Merchants and caravans, miniature from Al-Hariri's *Maqamat* (Assemblies), Baghdad school, circa 1200–99

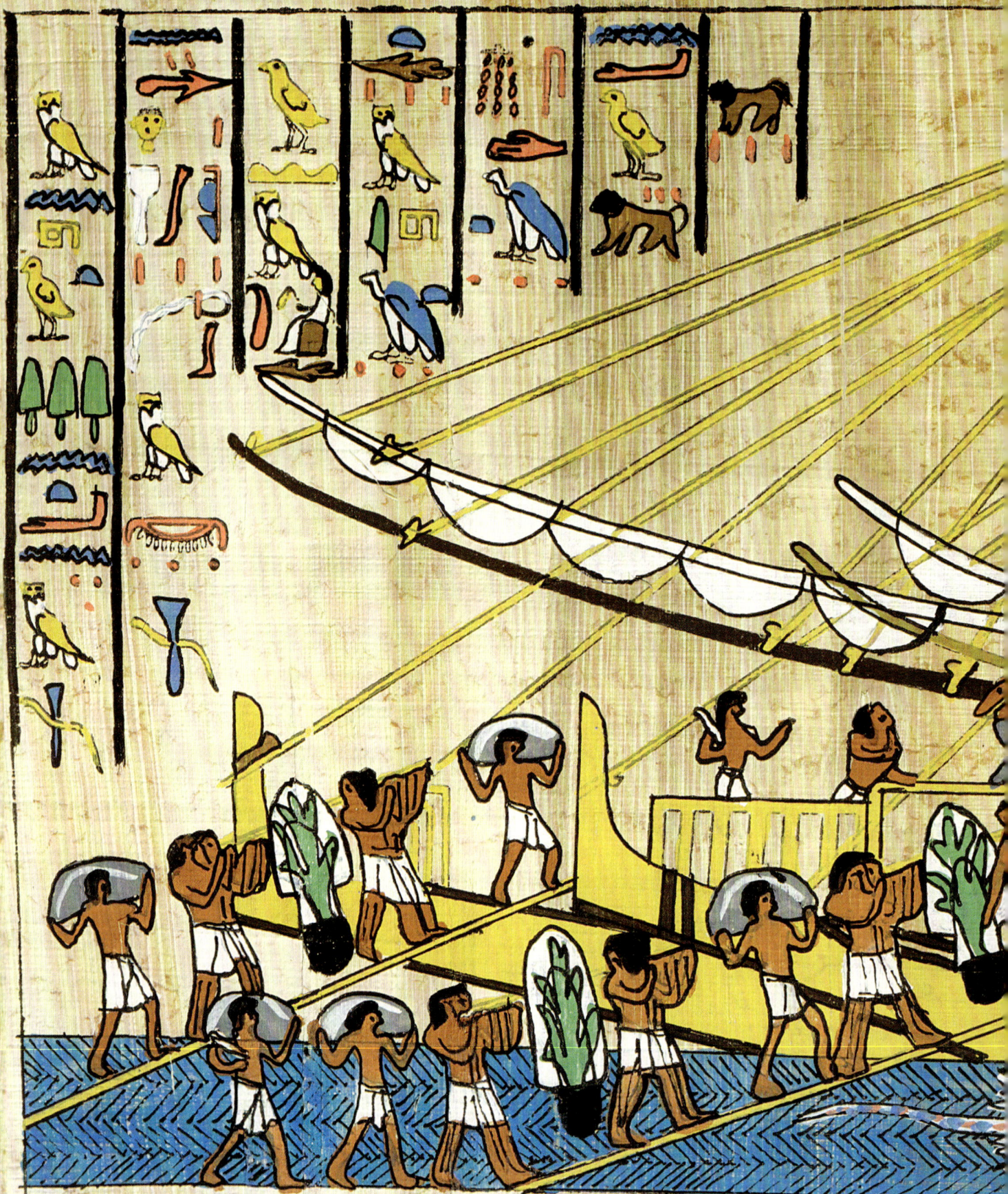

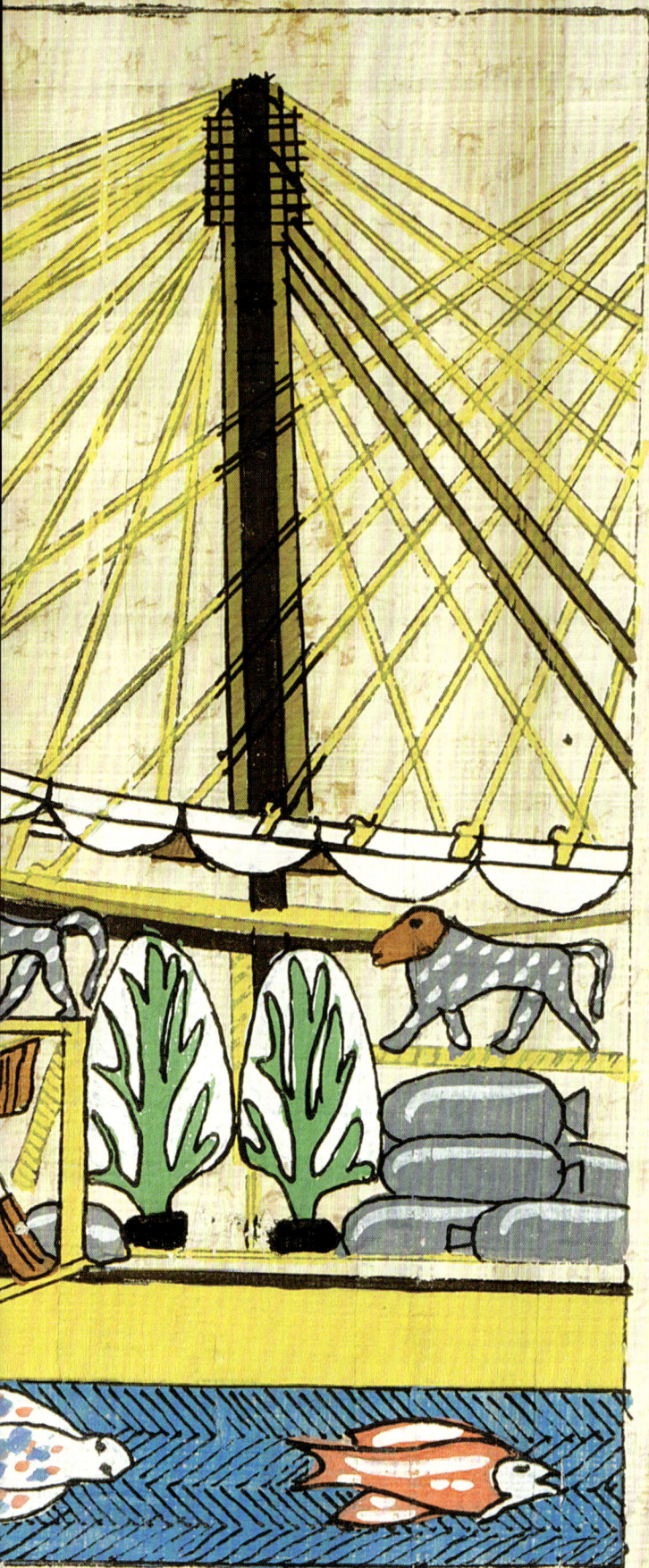

BYZANTIUM

Byzantium's position, standing guard over the entrance to the Bosphoran Kingdom, made it important to other Greek cities, particularly those in the Peloponnese region, for the trade in wheat, leather, wax and enslaved people. In the Hellenistic period, the Greeks established a cosmetics industry in the city. In the year 330, under the Eastern Roman Empire, the city was renamed Constantinople in honour of Emperor Constantine I, who had rebuilt and improved the city, naming it the imperial capital. As the terminus of the Silk Road, Constantinople saw its fortunes soar thanks to trade with Europe and the East, to such an extent that it became the most magnificent city of its time. Its people embraced an elegant lifestyle, with rosewater and soap used in the public baths.

CYPRUS

The island of Cyprus, birthplace of Venus, was also central to the trade in perfumes from the East as well as being famous for its oakmoss-scented gloves and vine-flower perfume compositions. It was close to Egypt and Asia, from where perfumed products arrived in Phoenician ships, adding to the many local resources such as rose, iris and thyme

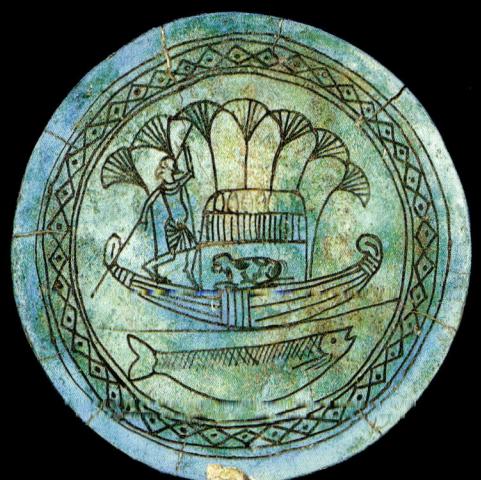

Above: Nile scene on an earthenware dish from a tomb in Enkomi, Cyprus, circa 1400–1200 BCE.

Left: Papyrus taken from the temple in Deir el-Bahari, Luxor, Egypt, recounting Queen Hatshepsut's expedition to the land of Punt.

RAW MATERIALS AND THE FIRST PERFUMES

PERFUME WAS OMNIPRESENT IN THE ANCIENT WORLD, USED FOR SPIRITUAL PURPOSES AND FOR BODY CARE. THE FIRST FRAGRANT SUBSTANCES WERE MAINLY RESINS AND PLANT-DERIVED RAW MATERIALS USED AS EARLY AS 4000 BCE IN FUMIGATION RITUALS. THEY WERE INTENDED FOR THE GODS AND WERE THE PRESERVE OF ROYAL FAMILIES. MYRRH AND FRANKINCENSE WERE PARTICULARLY PRIZED BY THE EGYPTIANS.

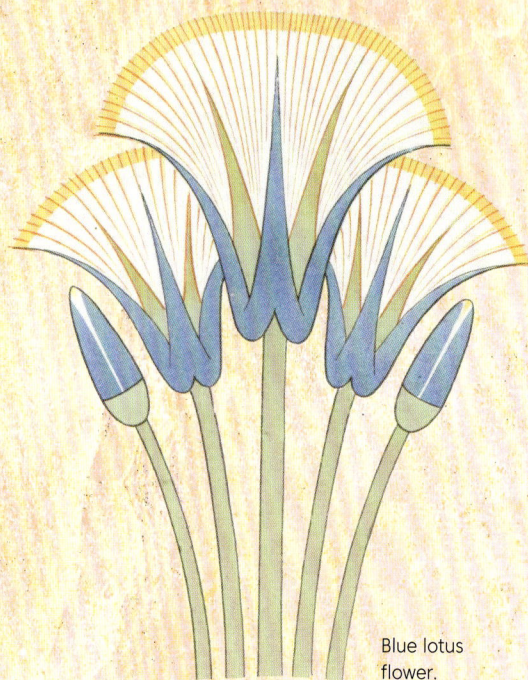

Blue lotus flower.

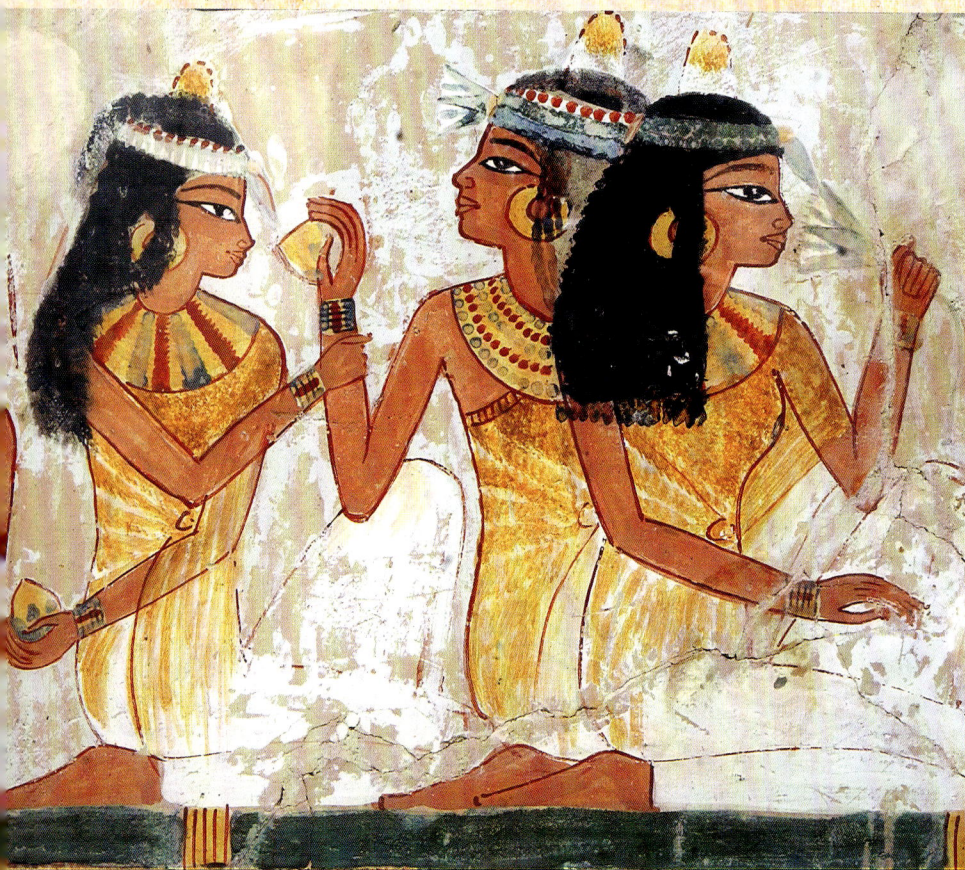

Scene of a funeral banquet, depicting two women each holding a mandrake fruit and a third smelling a lotus flower, fresco, circa 1390 BCE.

PLANT-DERIVED MATERIALS

Since ancient times, perfumes have been made from plant-derived raw materials such as blue lotus flowers, whose scents were deemed to come from the gods. Thought to carry creation god in their calyx, they are associated with the myth of creation and feature heavily in Egyptian iconography. Along with the papyrus flower, they symbolize the union of Upper and Lower Egypt, the two parts of the kingdom. Other Egyptian plants used included sweet galangal, narcissus, ben oil (from *Moringa*) and benzoin. The first floral notes can be traced back to the Mycenaean civilization, where sage and especially rose oils were used.

Some raw materials were very precious because they had to be imported. These included opoponax, and frankincense brought back from the mysterious Land of Punt, which Queen Hatshepsut tried to acclimatize to Egyptian soil (see page 13). In ancient times, the Nile valley became a transit area for *Boswellia* and *Commiphora*, gum resins from Arabia and the shores of the Red Sea (see box, facing page). Other imported aromatics of foreign origin were conifer resins and oils, terebinth resin and mastic from the Near East and eastern Mediterranean. Gradually, imports from the north diversified, but the southern trade routes were the most sought-after, becoming the object of Egyptian covetousness and supremacy.

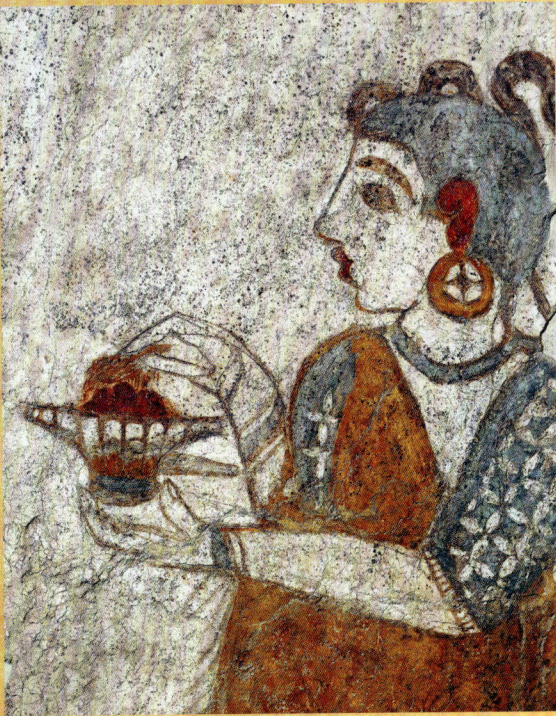

Incense and resins

White incense, or frankincense, is a resinous gum obtained by cutting the bark of the *Boswellia sacra* tree, which produces a natural sap on contact with air. According to Egyptian legend, incense was brought by a sacred Phoenix, as recounted by Ovid (43 BCE–17 CE) in Book 15 of his *Metamorphoses*. Considered to be a gift from the gods, it accompanied prayers and offerings in daily rituals. It was also a component of the embalming resins used in funeral rites.

The Egyptians also prized the precious resin extracted from *Commiphora myrrha*, or myrrh tree, which grew at an altitude of about 1000 metres (3281 feet) in Somalia, Ethiopia, Sudan and the Arabian Peninsula. Myrrh preserved the body during embalming and also revived the spirits of the faithful. It was a perfume for both life and death.

Fresco depicting a priestess burning incense, sixteenth century BCE.

THE FIRST PERFUMES

There is documentary evidence from ancient Mesopotamia that the first perfumes took the form of scented oils. The many variations available included primarily chufa, linseed, lettuce seed, sesame and ben oils scented with herbs, spices and flowers such as marjoram, white violet, blue lotus, narcissus, iris and rose.

In ancient Egypt, perfumes and aromatic plants played a key role in the daily rituals performed in temples. Many recipes for liturgical perfumes and burning gums and resins survive today. Among them, sonter (terebinth resin) was said to have the power to revive objects and places and so was used to extol the gods and awaken statues each morning. All these compositions were made by priests (the first perfumers), who were duty-bound to make three offerings each day: resin in the morning, myrrh at noon and kyphi, the great sacred scent, in the evening.

Egyptian relief of women gathering lilies, circa 664–525 BCE.

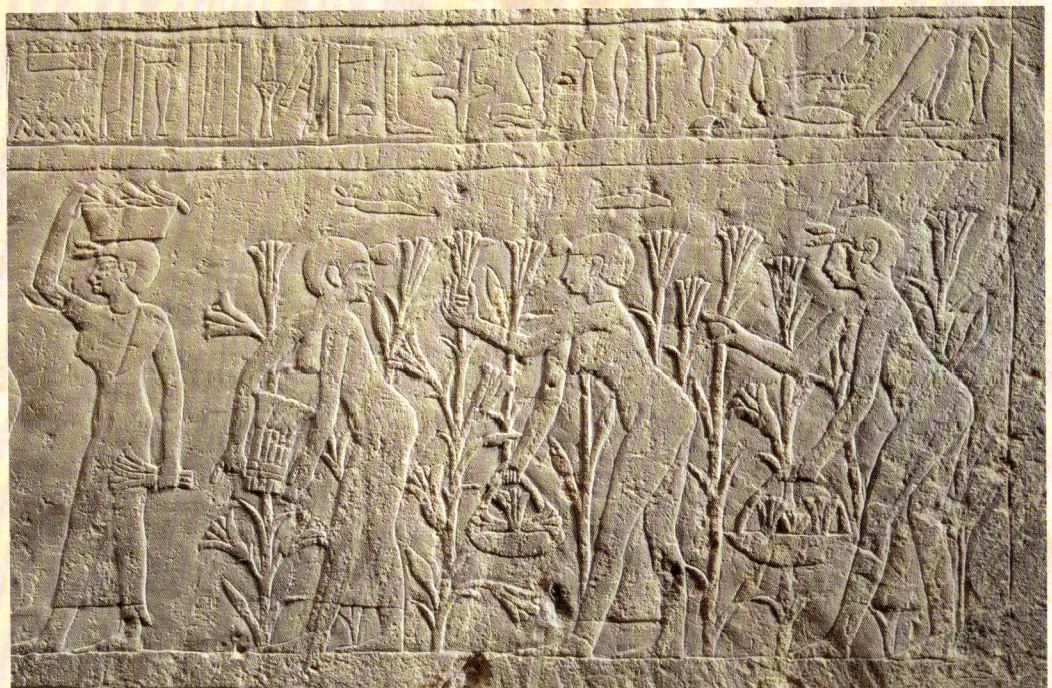

MENDES PERFUME

According to Pliny the Elder (*Natural History* Book XIII, 4, 5, 63), Mendes perfume, which took its name from Lower Egypt's administrative capital in the Nile Delta and was also known as heken oil, became very popular in ancient Egypt. It comprised ben oil scented with myrrh, cinnamon and resin.

KYPHI

From all the different specimens collected, kyphi was a perfume for burning containing over a quarter resin (myrrh, mastic and terebenthine) and almost the same proportion of fragrant woods and roots. It was a gentle scent with resinous and balsamic qualities, vanilla and oriental notes from styrax and a myrrh finish. Each of its ingredients, whether myrrh, frankincense or styrax, had its own special liturgical purpose. Its name translates as 'twice-good perfume' because it was burned by Egyptian priests in homage to the god Ra and was also known for its beneficial properties in humans.

It is thought that the kings and queens of predynastic Egypt (4000–3000 BCE) used this elegant composition to convert their life force to a spirit during funerals.

There are two recipes originating in the Edfu laboratory, which was typical of Ptolemaic and Roman temples, but the preparation could vary and ingredients were substituted according to what was available. This is why the Egyptian and Greek ingredient lists are not exactly the same. As a panacea, this sacred perfume reigned supreme in the ancient world.

METOPION

This is another famous scent that earned ancient Egypt its great reputation for perfumes. It was a complex composition of bitter almond oil extracted in Egypt, to which was added omphacion (green olive oil), cardamon, fragrant reed (*Acorus calamus*), honey, wine, myrrh, balsam seeds, galbanum and terebenthine.

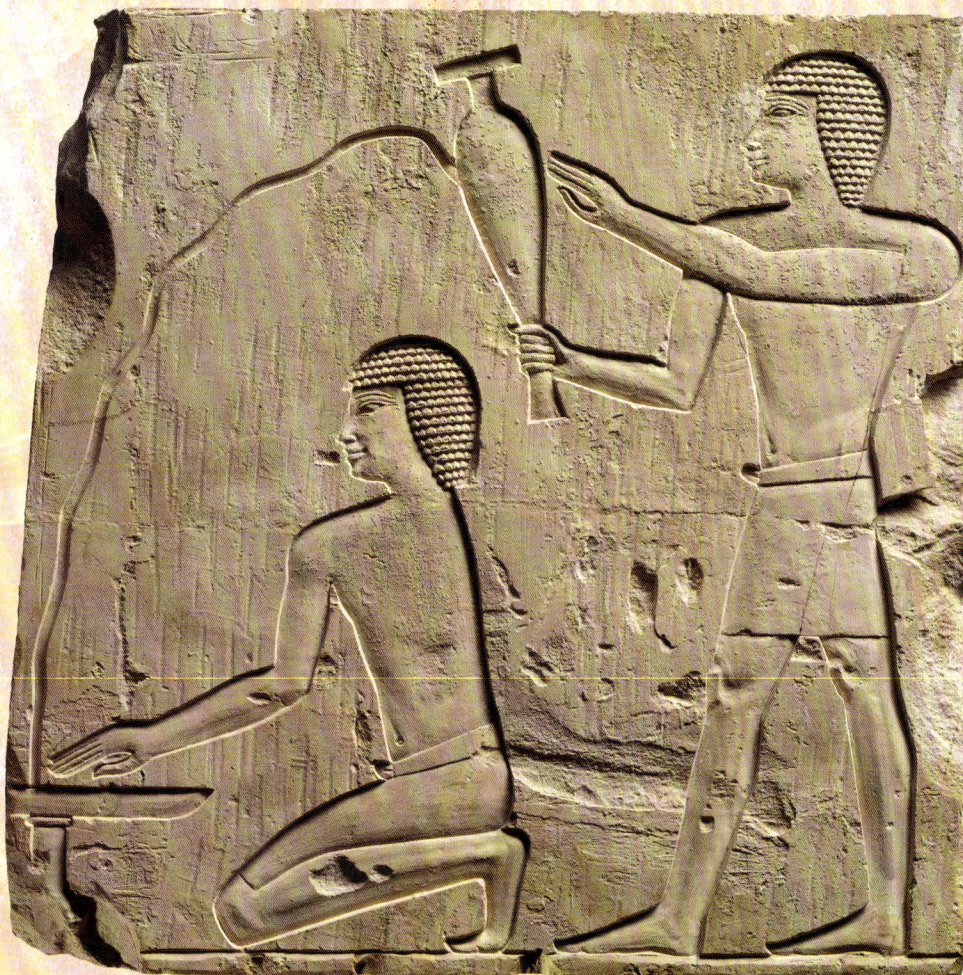

Priests during a funeral ritual, circa 667–647 BCE.

THE ROYAL PERFUME

The royal perfume is said to have been created for the Parthian king. Hereditary enemies of Rome, the Parthians were descendants of the multi-kingdom Arsacid dynasty, which was founded in 250 BCE and ruled the Persian Empire. At the time, because they dominated much of the world, the Persians were able to import many raw materials. The perfume caused a sensation in Rome and Pliny the Elder revealed its secret composition: 'Let us now talk about the ultimate in perfumes, the best of the best. I want to talk about the royal perfume, so named because it is prepared by the Parthian kings. It comprises ben oil (myrobalan or myrobolan), costus (from the Indus), black cardamon (from Nepal), cinnamon (from Sri Lanka), nut juice (Somali mokor), cardamom (Malabar ginger), nardostachys (Indian citronella), marum (*Teucrium marum*, a Libyan labiate), myrrh, cassia (Arabian cinnamon), styrax benzoin, labdanum (cistus), balm, *Acorus calamus* (a fragrant reed), fragrant rushes from Syria, oenanthe (or vine flower), malabathrum (Indian bay leaf), Cinnamomum tamala (Chinese cinnamon), henna, aspalathos (thorny broom), panax (Syrian opoponax), saffron, tiger nut, marjoram, lotus, honey and wine. None of these components of this scent is grown in Italy, despite the fact the country ruled the world.' *Natural History* (Book XIII, 17–18)

It is not known if this catalogue of ingredients was a figment of his imagination, but Pliny believed that its complexity marked it out as a perfume of quality. For the Romans, it was the symbol of the Pax Romana period. The emperors believed that smelling good made them feel like Alexander the Great, the king of kings, who had a god-like status in their eyes.

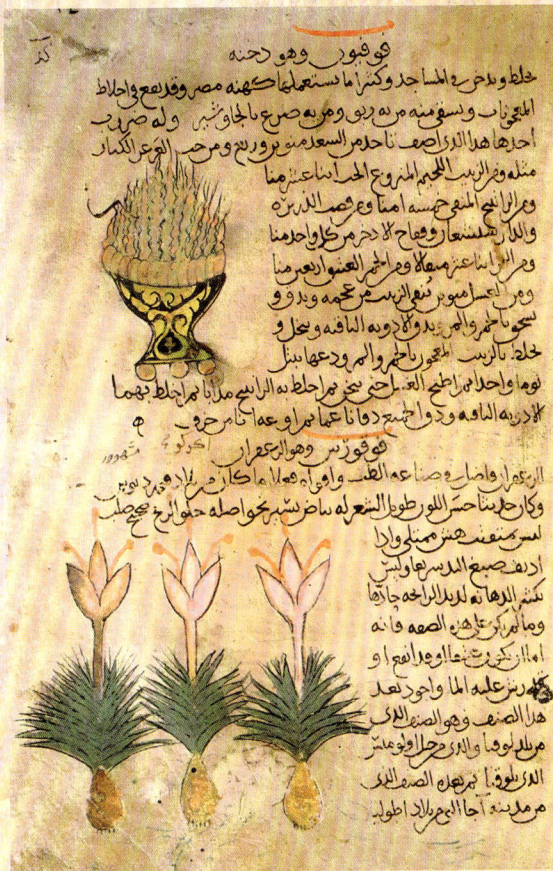

Ancient document depicting a bowl of burning kyphi, circa 987–990 CE.

Psyche and Cupid making perfume, Roman fresco, circa 50–79 CE.

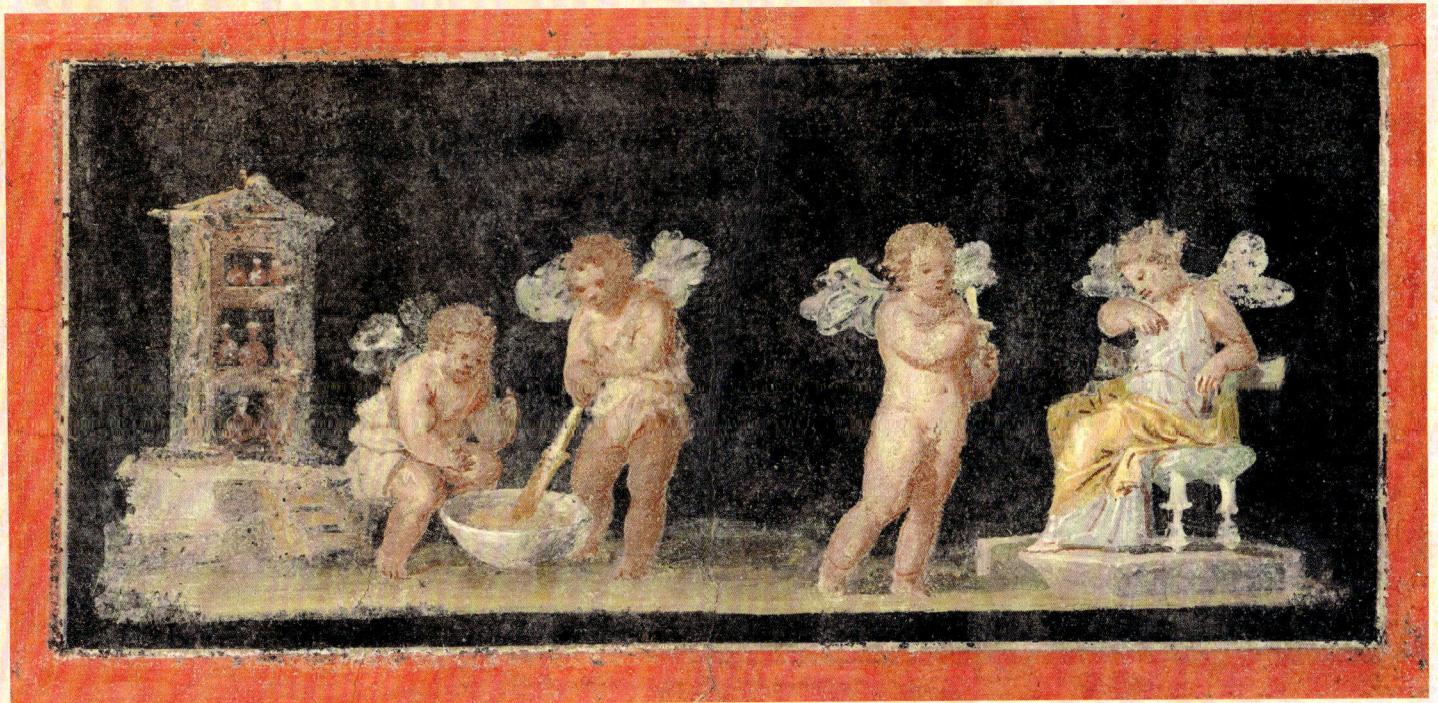

USAGE IN ANCIENT TIMES

PERFUME WAS OMNIPRESENT IN
THE ANCIENT WORLD, USED FOR
SPIRITUAL AND RELIGIOUS PURPOSES
AND FOR BODY CARE. IT REACHED
THE ENTIRE MEDITERRANEAN AREA
AND WAS ADOPTED BY THE GREEK
AND LATIN CIVILIZATIONS, WHO
USED IT IN THE SAME WAY AS THE
EGYPTIANS. THIS WAS THE GOLDEN
AGE OF ANCIENT PERFUME

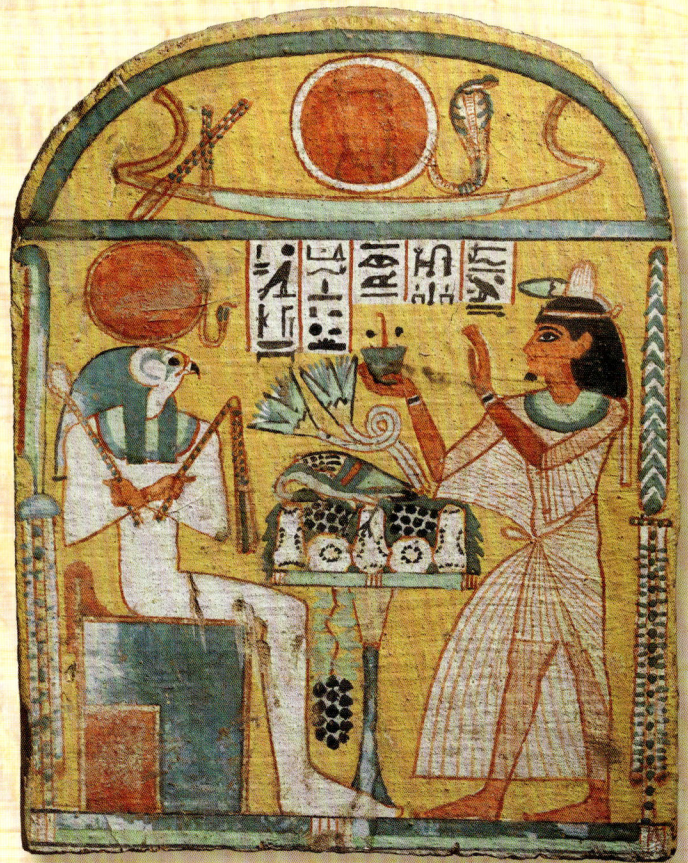

ANCIENT EGYPT: PRIMARILY SACRED USE

In the Pharaonic era perfume was used daily in secular spheres, but its main function was religious. Priests performed their daily rituals in temples filled with many different aromas. Perfume offerings were made to the gods. Incense and flowers were offered to the deities and to the king, represented by the priests, and there were at least three perfume fumigations each day.

Small wooden stela of Aafenmut showing the deceased, dressed in a robe draped round a tunic, offering incense to the seated sun god, Ra-Horakhty, circa 924–899 BCE.

Four young women, dressed in elaborate attire and wearing wigs adorned with lotus flowers and balm-filled cones, play music at a banquet held in honour of the deceased, mural, Nebamun's tomb, Egypt, 18thDynasty, 1350 BCE.

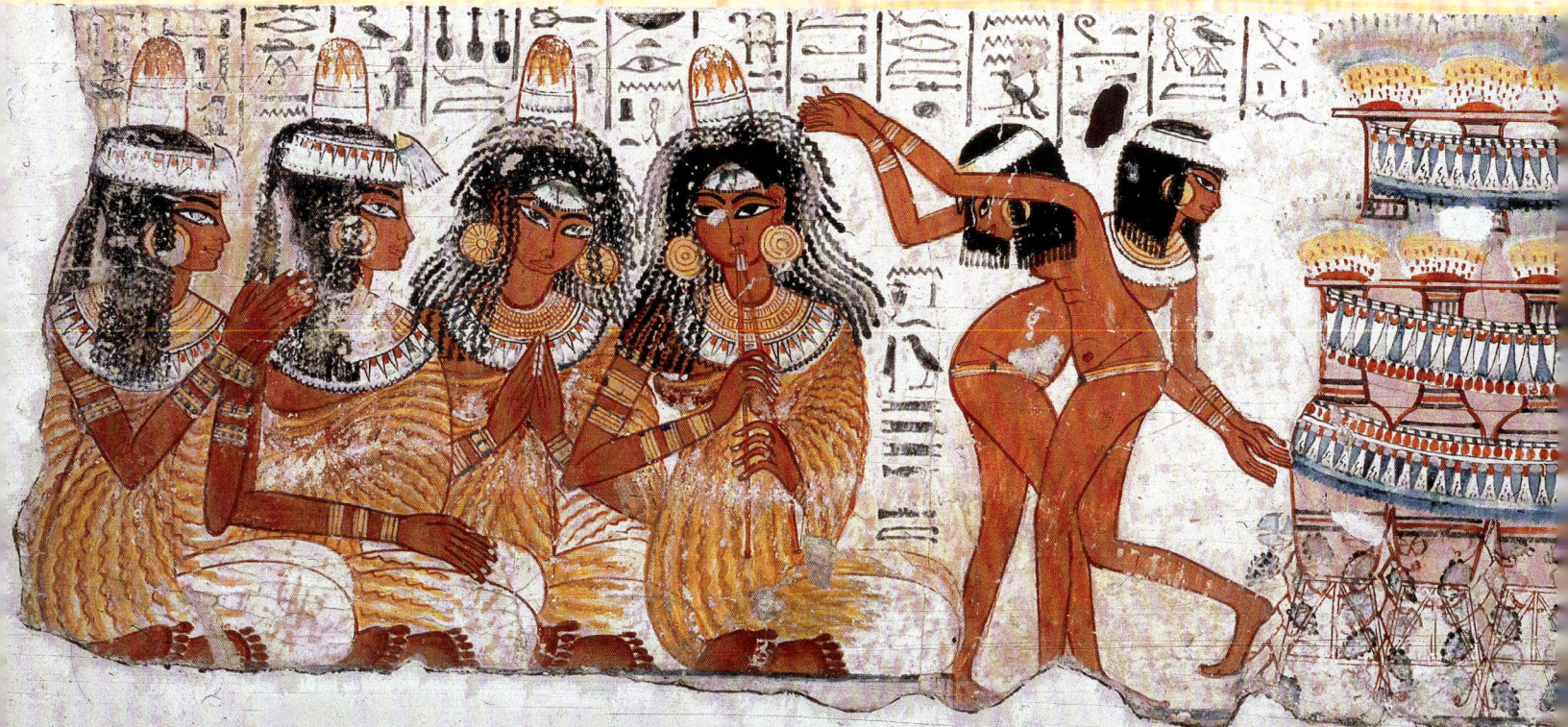

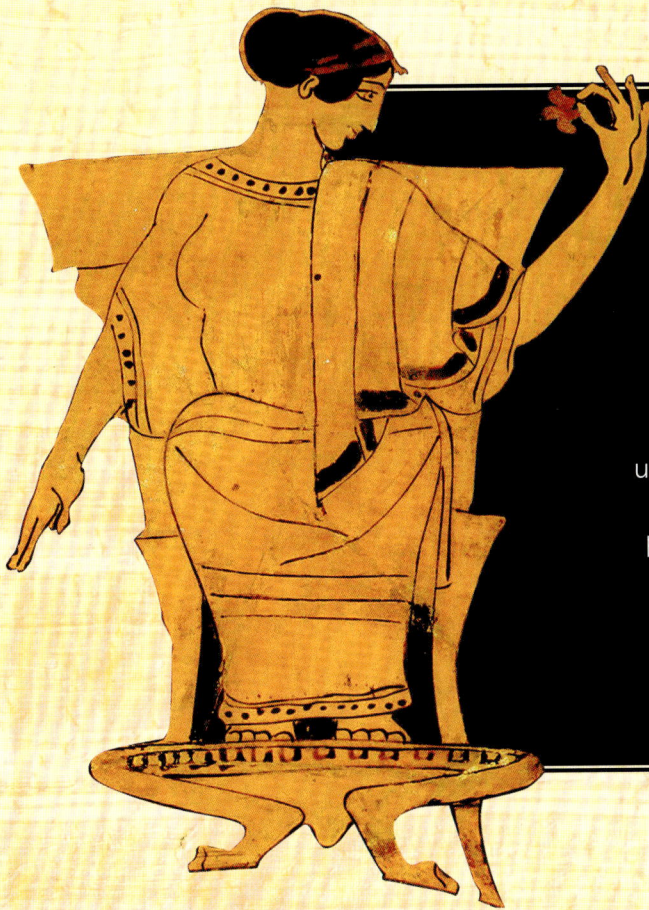

Woman with a rose, detail of a Greek
red-figure vase, fifth century BCE.

Perfume for seduction and festivities

Already in Egyptian times, perfume played a major role in seductive relations. Ptahhotep wrote: 'If you are a good and accomplished man, love your wife with sincerity and loyalty. Satisfy her and dress her in the knowledge that perfumes are the best way to care for the body.' Makeup, unguents, oils and balms were often used for pleasure and seduction but remained the preserve of the upper classes. Cleopatra was known for her particular use of perfume. She organized banquets where flowers were thrown on the floor, fragrant waters were sprayed, scented braids covered the walls and, on her orders, incense was burned both to impress and honour her guests.

SWEET SCENTS FOR THE GODS AND THE HEREAFTER

The Egyptians perfumed statues of their gods with incense and scented balms to bring them back to life. The families of pharaohs and priests themselves wore makeup and perfume and women's bodies were rubbed with scented balms as part of a purifying ritual. After death, the body had to be prepared for its journey to the hereafter. During the embalming ceremony, it was anointed from head to toe and then covered in bandages and scented holy oils to keep it sweet-smelling for eternity and also mask the smell of excrement, which symbolized mortal life, darkness and evil. The fragrance neutralized the odour, thereby guaranteeing the passage into the afterlife and immortality. The ceremony ended with fumigations to ensure the well-being and serenity of the deceased.

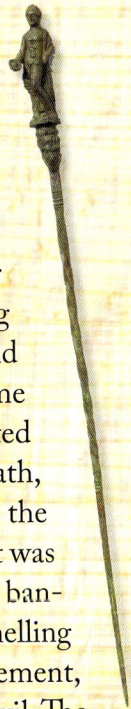

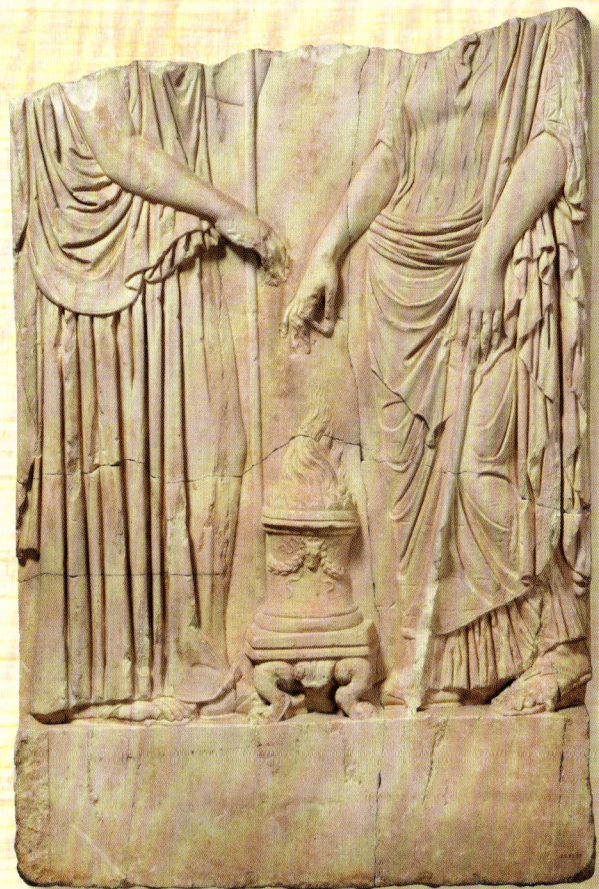

Above left: Stick from an ancient oil bottle, used to douse the body with perfumed oil.

Above: Roman copy of a Greek relief, probably depicting Demeter and Persephone beside an incense burner, fifth century BCE.

21

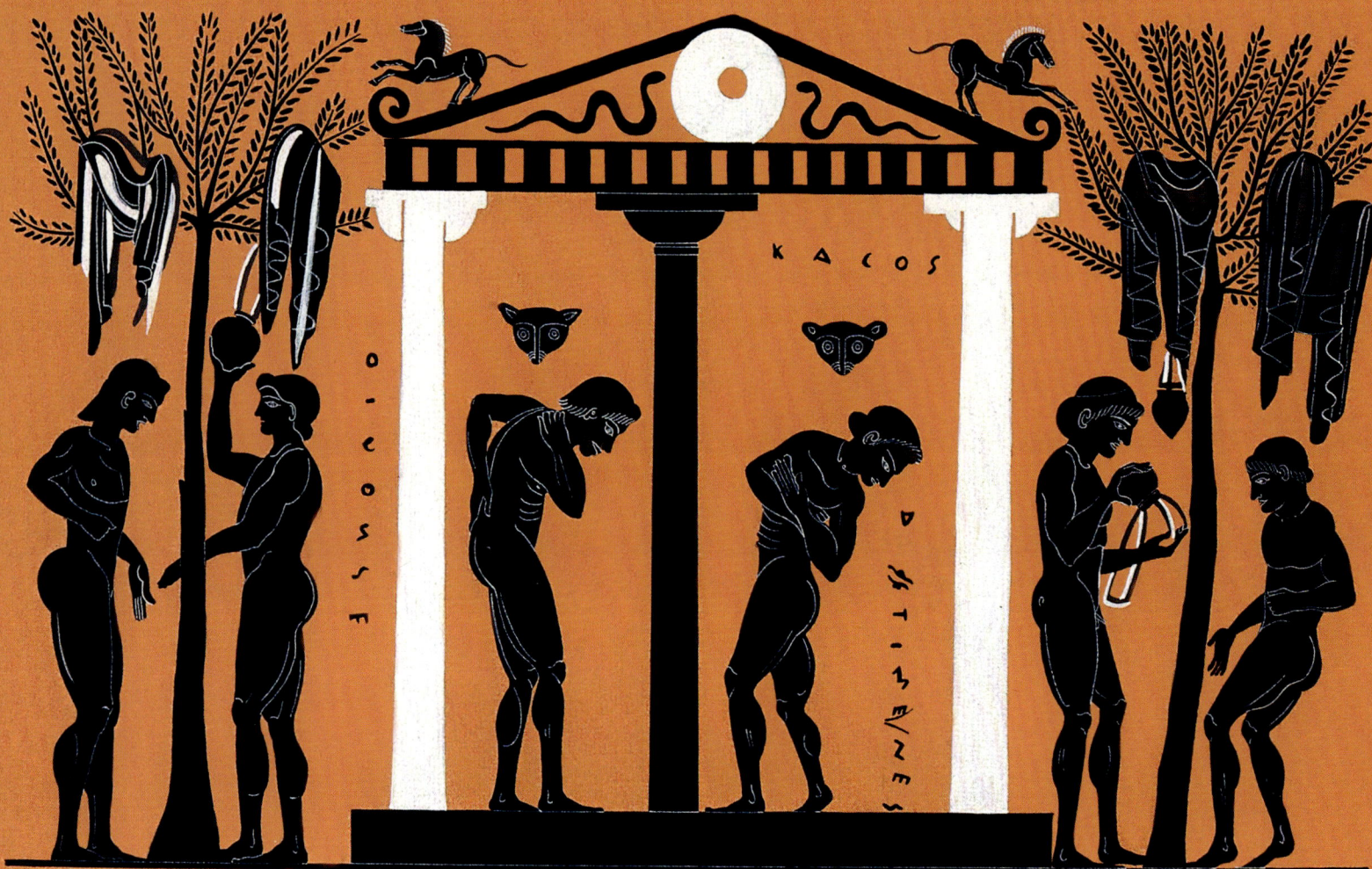

Men washing in public baths in Greece, after an Attic black-figure hydria attributed to the Antimenes Painter, sixth century BCE.

ANCIENT GREECE: AMBIVALENCE AND THREE FUNCTIONS

The use of perfume became commonplace among the Greeks from the end of the seventh century BCE. It had three functions: as a condiment for food and for religious and erotic purposes. As in other cultures, the desire for immortality went hand in hand with sweet smells. In temples, perfumes were offered to the gods and each had their preference – rose for Aphrodite, for example.

Perfume symbolized the strength and exuberant lifestyle attributed to the inhabitants of Olympus. Daubing oneself with perfume brought one closer to divinity. Not only did it smell divine but it gave a glow associated with the radiant beauty of the deities who lived on Olympus. This is why statues of the gods and funerary steles were doused in perfumed oil.

In day-to-day life, perfume was also used for the rites of passage which marked the beginning of life and the journey to the hereafter, such as birth, marriage and funerals. Very little use was made of perfume for body care, however. Plato, in *The Republic*, suggested that perfume corrupted the mind; when fragrances were used for seduction, they had an almost negative connotation.

ANCIENT ROME: MAINLY SECULAR USE

In ancient Rome, as in the Eastern world and ancient Greece, perfume offerings were part of religious and funeral rituals, and perfumes were also widely employed for their therapeutic properties. However, it was non-religious use that prevailed during this period. Upper-class men and women bathed frequently in baths fragranced with lavender, rose, jasmine and other perfumes. A lady of the ruling classes would begin her toilet by removing her makeup and applying a beauty balm. She would then gargle with saffron or rose and chew flavoured gum as she slid into a jasmine, lavender or rose bath. A slave would then give her an aromatic massage and spray her body with the same perfumed water she had first used as a mouthwash.

At banquets, diners ate under mists of extremely rare essences as they ate asparagus dipped in perfumed oils, served in fragrant wooden dishes, and drank rose- or myrrh-flavoured wines. Between courses, they were sprayed with floral water.

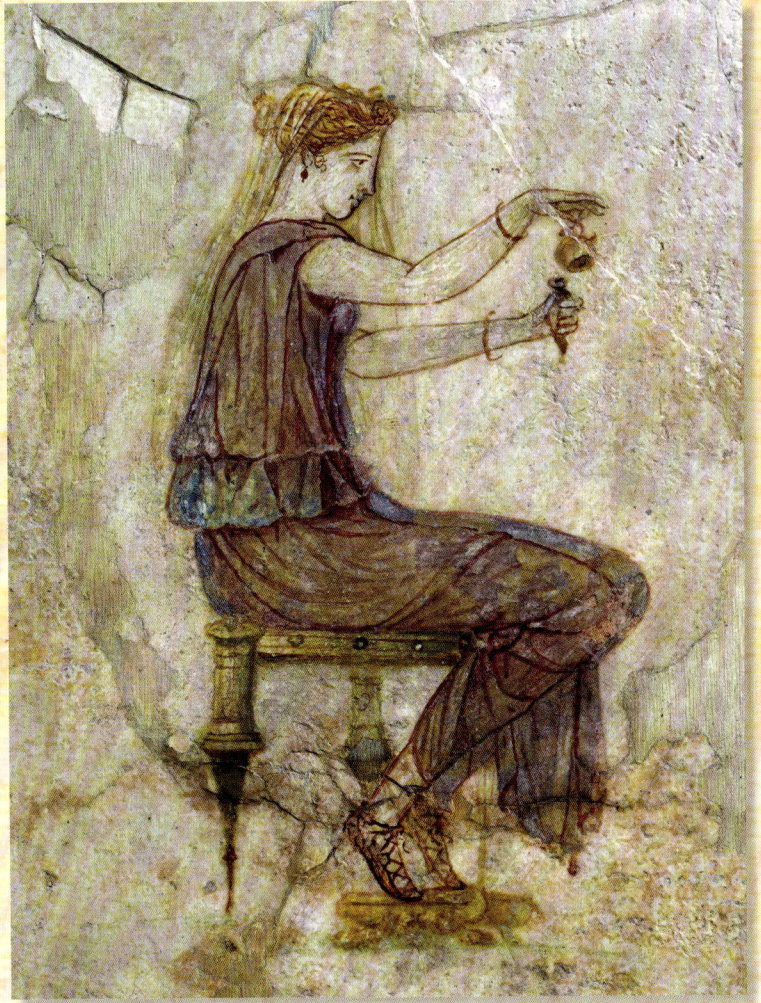

Roman fresco depicting a seated woman decanting perfume.

Painted wooden spoons and perfume utensils from Ancient Egypt. Illustrations from 1878 by Émile Prisse d'Avennes (1807–79)

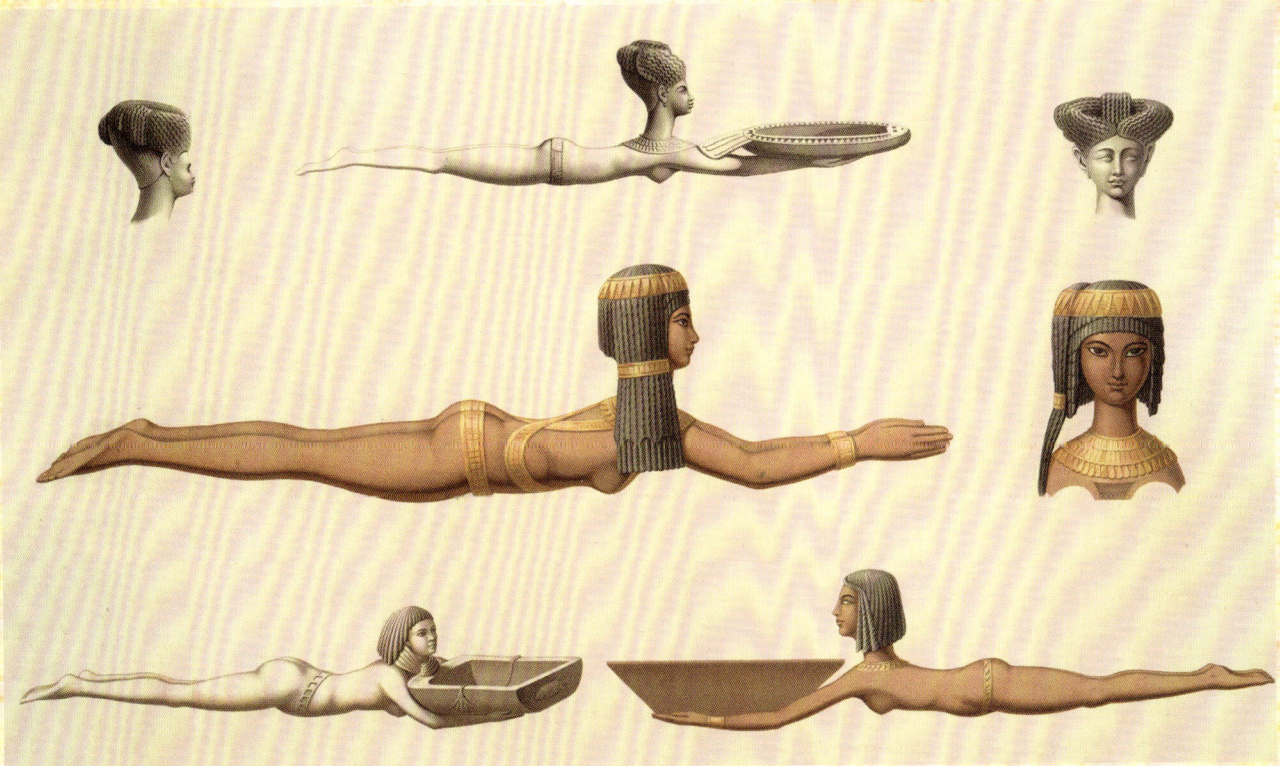

THE GOSPELS: DIVINE OFFERINGS

Although the Christian Church paid little attention to bodily cleanliness and rejected non-religious use of perfume for fear that it would incite lust, it did continue to use sacred incense, a tradition inherited from Greece and the East. There are several mentions in the Gospels of divine offerings to Christ in the form of perfume, including gold, frankincense and myrrh, brought to Jesus on his birth by the Three Wise Men. The gold symbolized Christ's royal status, and frankincense his divine origin. Myrrh was offered because it linked body, mind and soul and, as it signified death and mourning, served as a reminder that Christ, sent by God, was truly human and mortal. Another example is Mary of Bethany anointing Christ's body with prized perfumes (myrrh, aloe and nard) after his death. In the words of Jesus, 'When she poured this perfume on my body, she did it to prepare me for burial' (Matthew 26:6–12; Mark 14:3–8; John 12:1–7). Here, he is emphasizing the burial ritual, a portent of his future resurrection and transfiguration. Indeed, the name Messiah given to Christ alludes to the perfumed oil, just as Christos means 'anointed' and refers to the chrism, or holy anointing oil, used since the sixth century CE.

The Three Wise Men, detail of a mosaic from the Basilica of Sant'Apollinare Nuovo in Ravenna, sixth century.

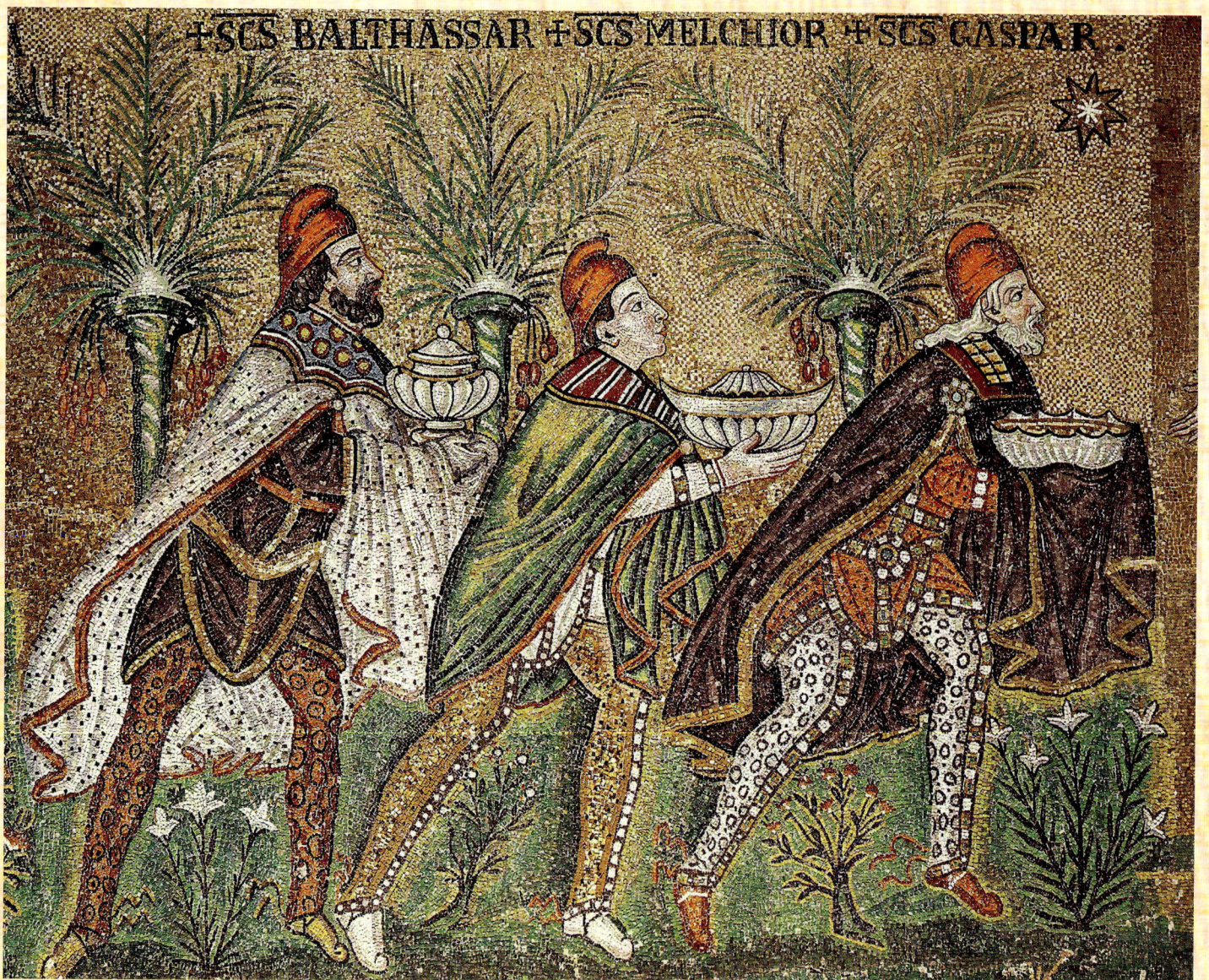

+SCS BALTHASSAR +SCS MELCHIOR +SCS GASPAR

ARABIA AND RELIGIOUS PURIFICATION PRACTICES

In the seventh century, Islam established itself in the Arabian Peninsula, the birthplace of the kingdom of Sheba, which produced and exported perfumes in large quantities. It is to these perfumes that Arabia owes the immense power of attraction it has enjoyed since ancient times. Islam did not hinder or put a stop to the production and use of fragranced essences – quite the opposite. The Prophet Mohammed liked perfumes, used them regularly and advised his people never to refuse a fragrance: 'Perfume your homes with frankincense and savory [...] Take a bath on Fridays, apply perfume and change your clothes.' We also know that he used musk before he set off on a pilgrimage and on his return. According to tradition, he taught a number of religious purification techniques because foul smells were a sign of evil emanating, whereas nobility of character exuded sweet aromas. Perfume stood for all things pleasant and was the opposite of animality. It was also an excellent way to prepare for entering the sacred space of the mosque. Praying and presenting yourself to God demanded purity, expressed through absolute cleanliness and a pleasing aroma.

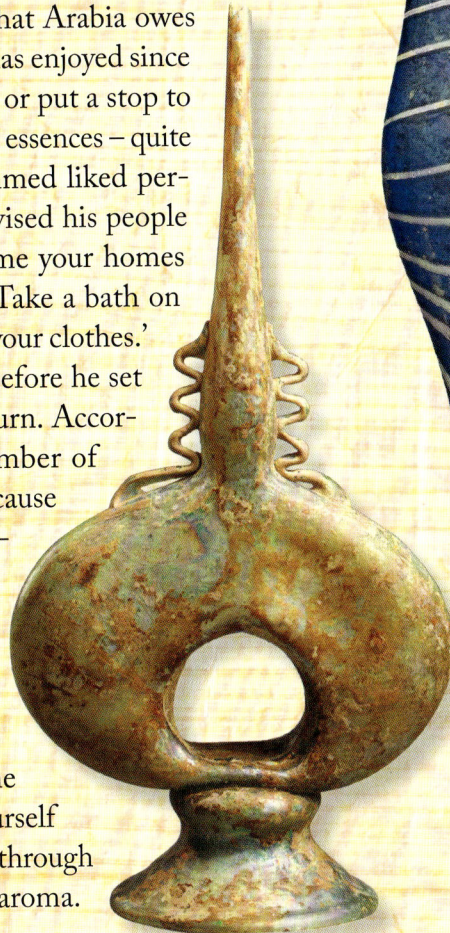

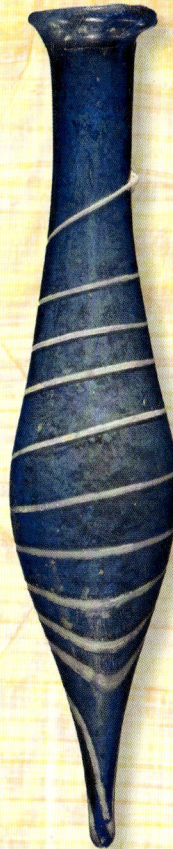

The first glass bottles appeared in the Roman Empire in the first century. These were made in Aleppo, Syria

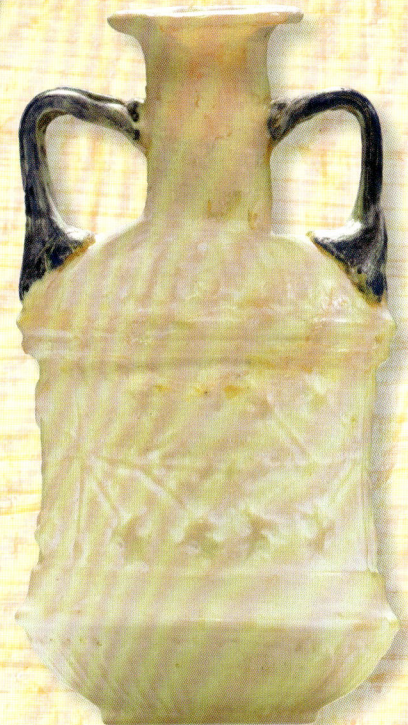

THE PERFUME ROUTE II: THE MIDDLE AGES AND THE RENAISSANCE

LONG BEFORE VENICE BECAME PERFUME CAPITAL IN THE MIDDLE AGES, CHRISTIAN KNIGHTS WERE BRINGING BACK INCENSE, AMBER, ALOE AND ROSEWATER FROM THE EASTERN MEDITERRANEAN. THE PORTUGUESE AND SPANISH OPENED UP NEW MARITIME ROUTES TO THE FAR EAST AND COUNTLESS INDIA COMPANIES WERE FORMED.

VENICE: PERFUME CAPITAL OF THE MIDDLE AGES

The trade that began in the Mediterranean after the Crusades (1095–1291) continued in the Middle Ages. Most ships set sail from the Italian ports of Venice and Genoa and the two city states achieved great power as a result. Between the tenth and sixteenth centuries, Venice was the perfume capital because it had a monopoly on the spice trade. Raw materials from India and Sri Lanka passed through Venice, the City of the Doges, in the holds of Arabian ships en route for Europe. One of the Venetian merchants, Marco Polo (1254–1324), famously travelled to China and recounted his story in his book *The Travels of Marco Polo*. While held captive in Genoa (a rival city to Venice), and after an absence of 26 years, he dictated an accurate description of the Kublai states and the East. He also talked of the many spices traded there, such as Tibetan musk, ambergris ('the gold of the seas'), cinnamon, cloves, saffron and ginger. Perfumes from the East were brought to Europe via Venice from Alexandria, Damascus, Gaza and the Black Sea ports of Sinope and Trebizond, transported by land caravan or by Arab sailors across the Red Sea and the Persian Gulf.

Caravan transporting the Polo brothers, with their son and nephew Marco, miniature from a map in Abraham Cresques' *Catalan Atlas*, 1375.

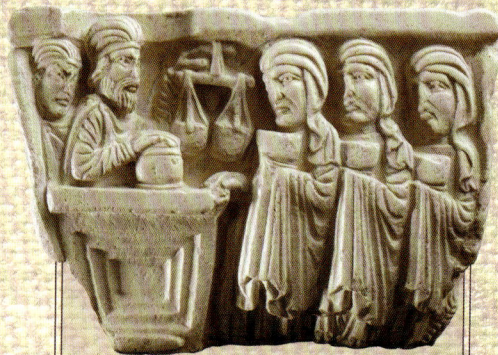

Venice: city of pleasure

In the sixteenth century, Venice was still a city of pleasure, with perfume very much present thanks to the abundance of aromatics. It was used everywhere, including in food and on tables and plates at banquets; sauces were thinned with rosewater and packed with spices. Carnival costumes, fans and masks were fragranced with musk and ginger. Therefore it was only natural that the first European treatise on perfume should be written in Venice around 1555 by alchemist Girolamo Ruscelli and translated into English as *The Secrets of Alexis*. It was also at this time that Venice established glassworks in Murano, which would flood the whole of Europe with their creations.

Perfume and balm merchants, marble relief, Italy, thirteenth century.

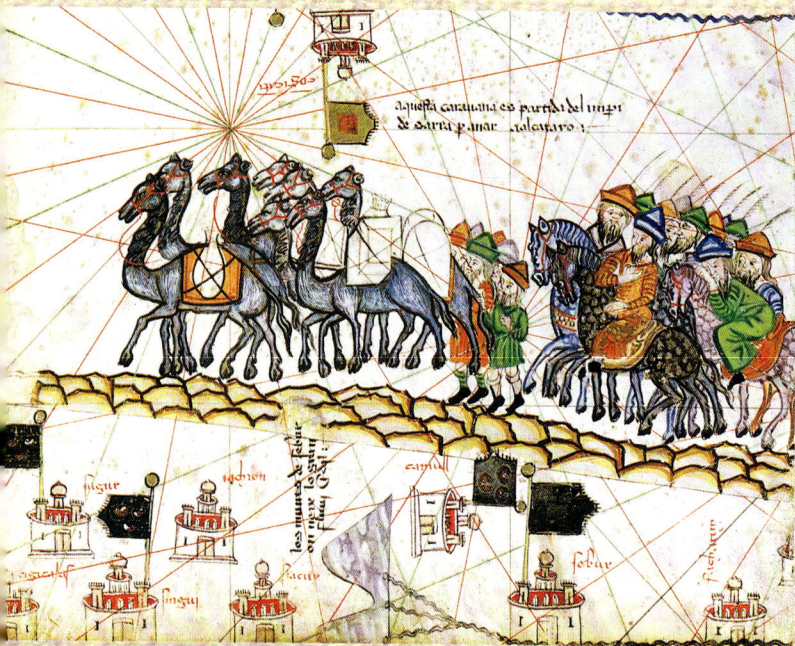

THE ERA OF THE EXPLORERS

In the fifteenth century, when the Ottoman conquest had blocked traditional routes to the eastern Mediterranean, Europe had to look towards the ocean. Portugal led the way in the search for an alternative route. In 1488, Bartolomeu Dias rounded the Cape of Good Hope, the southernmost tip of Africa, and a maritime route to India opened up to the East, securing the Portuguese a monopoly on spices throughout the sixteenth century. In 1498, Vasco de Gama reached the spice-rich city of Calicut in India and brought back coriander, pepper, ginger, saffron, paprika and more. The Portuguese were also the first to drop anchor at the Moluccas for nutmeg, in Japan and Ethiopia for rice and tea, and on the African coast for coffee and peanuts, adding to the pineapples, bell peppers, tomatoes and potatoes they had already brought back from the New World. On behalf of Spain, Christopher Columbus sailed to the Greater Antilles in 1492, and then made four return trips, thereby opening up a new route westwards. In 1519, Hernán Cortés arrived on the Mexican coast at Veracruz and took cocoa beans and vanilla pods back to Charles V of Spain. Between 1519 and 1522, Ferdinand Magellan, on behalf of the Spanish crown, was the first to circumnavigate the globe to reach the spice-rich islands from the west.

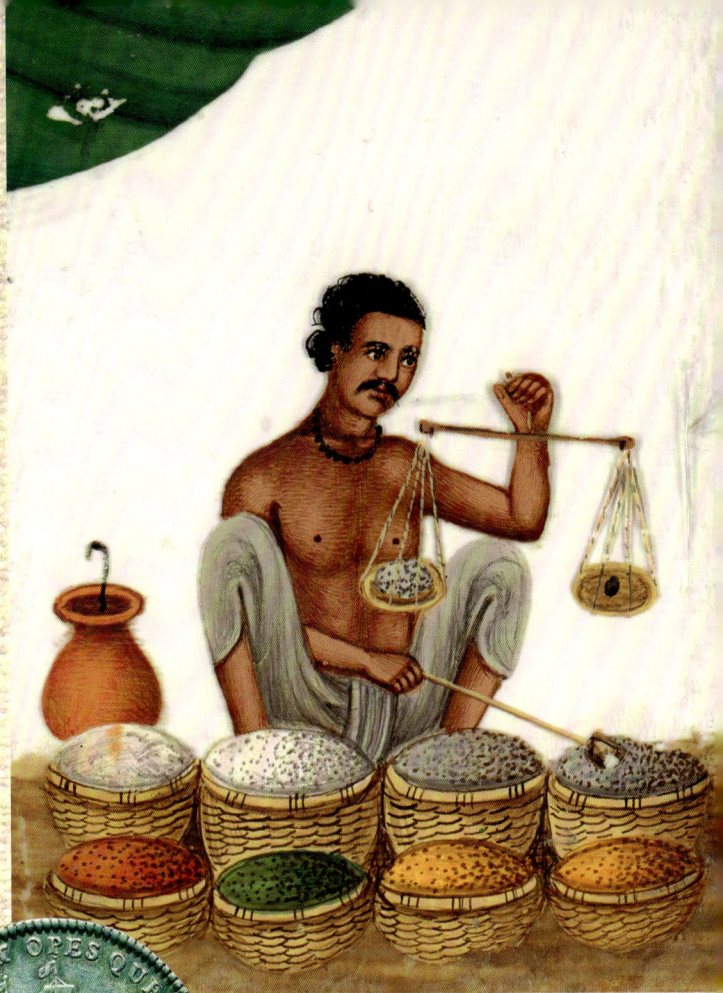
Spice seller with his scales.

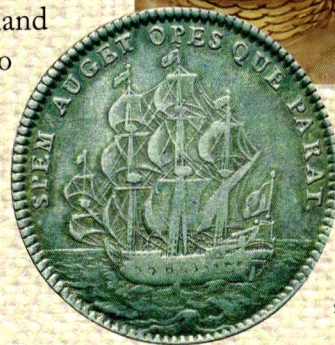
East India Company token depicting a sailing ship, circa 1723.

Mauritius: a vast botanical garden

In 1664, Jean-Baptiste Colbert set up the French East India Company and many ships sailed from Lorient port to new trading posts in India. In 1715, the French established a colony known as Isle de France - now Mauritius - and created a botanical garden there to grow spices. They got their supplies of pepper from the Malabar coast and cinnamon from Sri Lanka. They also loaded their ships with star anise and galangal from southern China, but the venture turned out to be less successful than expected. Pierre Poivre persuaded the French East India Company that it would be a good idea to introduce spices to Mauritius by smuggling in nutmeg (*Myristica fragrans*) seedlings and later, in 1767, Dutch clove and pepper plants.

THE INDIA COMPANIES

In the mid-17th century, competition was fierce among European powers to build colonial empires that could provide capital and commercial riches. This was the impetus for the establishment of the India companies, which enabled Europeans to conquer and exploit land and turn trading posts into colonies. With the Dutch East India Company, which was becoming one of the cornerstones of Dutch capitalist power and imperialism, began a new era driven by greed and a quest for the monopoly of the trading routes, including the spice trade. The Dutch took over the entire production of cloves, nutmeg, mace, cinnamon and pepper, and controlled the selling price of these commodities in Europe.

RUDIMENTARY PROCESS UNTIL THE END OF THE MIDDLE AGES. THE MATERIALS WERE GROUND, BOILED AND MIXED WITH ANIMAL FATS OR INFUSED. HOWEVER, ONE INVENTION, DISTILLATION, WAS REVOLUTIONARY IN CHANGING THE PROCESS. THE GREEKS WERE ALREADY FAMILIAR WITH THE ANCIENT FORM OF THE TECHNIQUE, WHICH WAS THEN DEVELOPED IN THE TENTH AND EVOLVED CONSTANTLY UNTIL THE FIFTEENTH CENTURY.

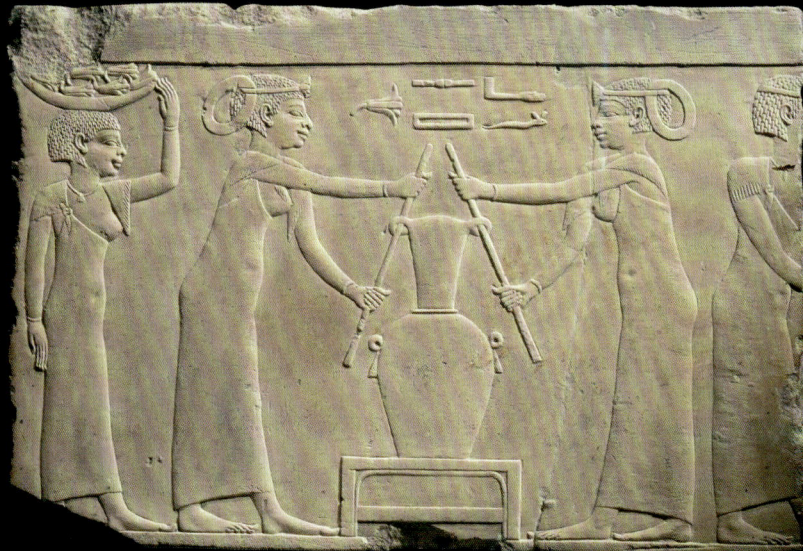

Women pressing lilies to make perfume, Egyptian relief, circa 664–525 BCE.

THE ART OF PERFUME

Little is known about the techniques and processes used to make perfume in ancient times. We do know that the ingredients were boiled in water and then in oil in a long process that could last between 10 days and 3 months. They were then wrung out and filtered through wool or linen cloths and the resulting product was stored in jars. The Mycenaeans probably used alcoholic maceration with honey and fruit in wine. Olive oil was still a popular base but safflower, almond and poppyseed oil was also used, as were animal fats. In Cyprus and Crete, archaeologists have discovered perfumers' workshops, in which they found apparatus such as magnifying glasses, sieves, mortars, pestles and pitchers. The Egyptians developed three techniques: enfleurage, which involved sprinkling flowers onto fatty substances; maceration in hot or cold oil; and pressing. Most of the perfumes were solid and burned in temples during rituals, such as the sacrificial burning of bull-shaped perfume animals by the Greeks.

Avicenna: pioneer of distillation

The ancient Egyptians did not know about distillation. Most of their aromatic preparations were aqueous or slightly alcoholic decoctions obtained primarily by cooking resinous or oily substances. We know that the Greeks had alembics (stills), because Aristotle was familiar with distillation, but the Arabic name (al'inbiq) was popularized in Europe by the Persian philosopher and physician Avicenna (987–1037), who formalized the process. In the early eleventh century, he used distillation to isolate rose scents to produce a mix of rosewater and essential oil. In Arab medicine, red roses were used to combat infection and Avicenna cooked roses as a specific cure for consumption.

ALCOHOL DISTILLATION

A century after Avicenna, further progress was made when doctors at the Salerno school in Italy developed alcohol distillation, the cornerstone of modern perfumery. It was their translations of the Arabic treatises (which were translated again a little later, in the thirteenth century, by the Andalusians) that introduced the process to the Western world. With the advent of the alembic (still) and alchemy in the West in the twelfth century, the production of rose attar (rose essential oil) became commonplace. In the Muslim world, the Damascus oasis in Syria in particular, rosewater was widespread because it was made by distilling rose petals with water without the need for alcohol. In India, attar was a non-alcoholic scented oil obtained by distilling sandalwood oil with flowers, primarily roses. When Muslims arrived in India, the use of distilled essences began to spread and as a result the Arabic word *attar* (derived from *itr* meaning 'perfume') became part of the word for perfumer, pharmacist and herbalist.

Under Moorish rule, Arab perfumers set up shop in Granada, Spain, selling perfumes and also potions made from ambergris and musk. At the time, the word 'amber' was used for vanilla- and labdanum-based oriental preparations with delicate, powdery notes, which were often described as delicious and sensual. Ambergris had been an iconic perfume ingredient since ancient times, alongside frankincense, myrrh and musk.

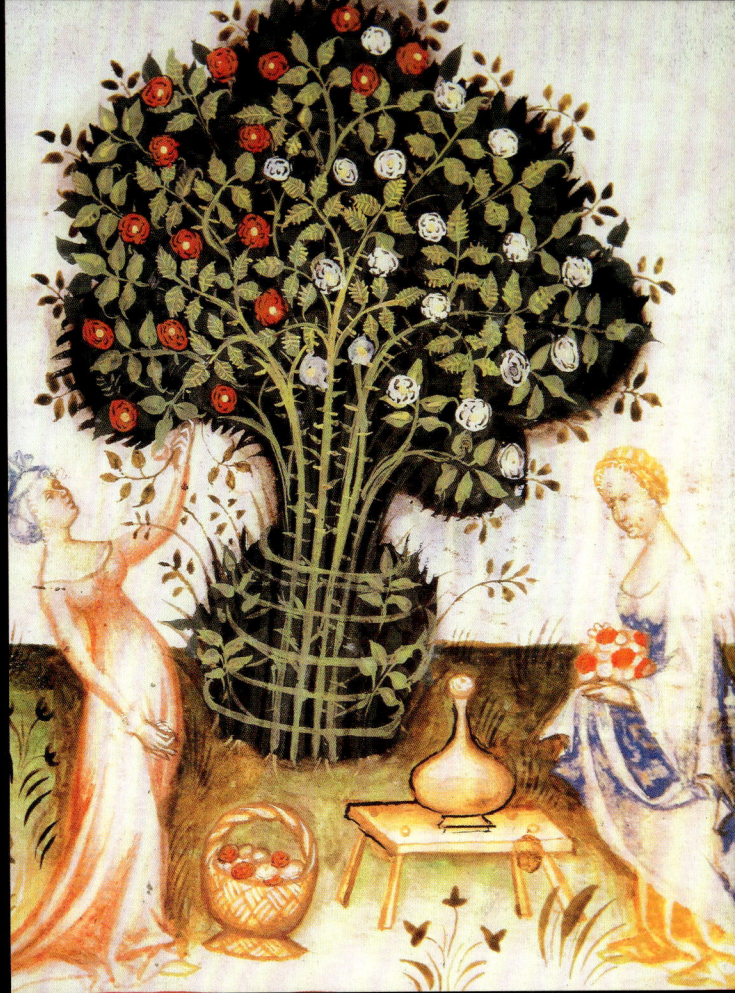

Women picking roses to use the petals to make rosewater. Illumination from a fourteenth-century health manual.

ARNALDUS DE VILLA NOVA AND ALCOHOL IN PERFUMES

In the fourteenth century, the doctor, chemist, astrologer and theologian Arnaldus de Villa Nova practised medicine in Montpellier in the south of France. He also taught at the university there. He developed the first essential oils and also discovered sulphuric, hydrochloric and nitric acids. Having learned the principle of distillation in Cordoba, he applied it to wine to make stronger 'spirit of wine' and was the first scholar to use alcohol in perfume. The alcohol helped to make *eau de feu* ('fire water'), a spirit precipitated by heat. All these discoveries contributed greatly to perfume making because the traditional medium, oil, could be replaced with a volatile, neutral product. The process was used to produce an elixir (meaning 'most precious medicine'), which was drunk to procure radiance from within. In the West, the first scented water was Eau de la Reine de Hongrie (1370), followed by Eau de Cologne (1695).

Miniature on parchment depicting alembics (stills) and the first distillation processes, fourteenth century.

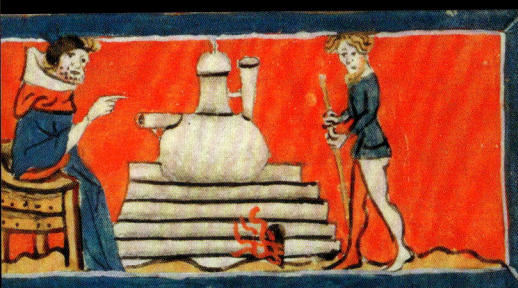

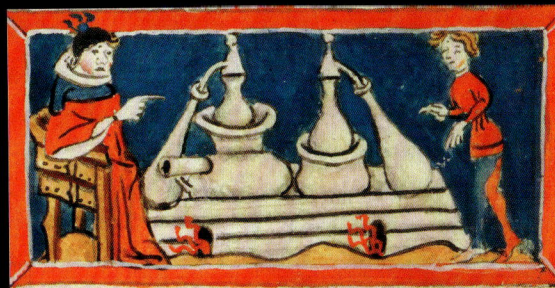

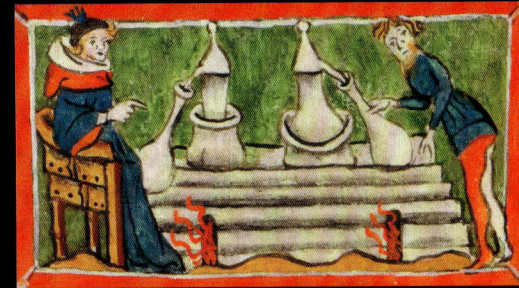

PERFUME AS A REMEDY

PERFUME HAS ALWAYS BEEN USED FOR ITS
THERAPEUTIC QUALITIES, AS SOME OF THE RAW
MATERIALS SUCH AS MYRRH, LAVENDER AND
ROSEMARY ARE NATURALLY ANTISEPTIC. IT BEGAN
TO BE EMPLOYED AS A REMEDY IN ANCIENT TIMES
WITH THE BIRTH OF AROMATHERAPY. IN THE
EARLY MIDDLE AGES, PERFUME WAS POPULAR
FOR ITS HEALING AND PROTECTIVE
PROPERTIES DURING EPIDEMICS.

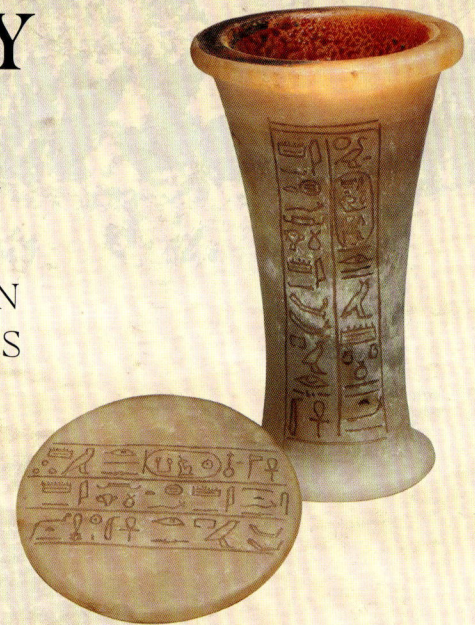

THE BIRTH OF AROMATHERAPY

In the ancient world, in Egypt, Greece, Rome and throughout the East, the use of aromatics extended beyond religion to healthcare and hygiene. With so many purification practices, a vast pharmacopeia of aromas was established. Whether used for religion or personal hygiene, the aim was always to dispel the abhorrent, as pleasant aromas were purifying. Fragrant essences were burned to combat some contagious diseases, making aromatherapy the oldest form of medicine.

Egyptian priests, who were also doctors, believed that illnesses were caused by supernatural forces (the gods). They administered perfumes to the sick, supposedly to appease the gods. Some of these fragrances were included in the pharmacopeia: kyphi for instance, which was known for its calming and sleep-inducing properties. Medicinal recipes and their methods of absorption are included in the Ebers Papyrus, produced in 1555 BCE.

Balms had purifying properties and were thought to repel harmful elements. They were also combined with natron, a naturally occurring mixture of sodium carbonate, sodium bicarbonate, sodium sulphate and sodium chloride, to make soap. And because they were thought to cleanse the soul and purify the mouth before divine worship, they were swallowed or used as mouthwash.

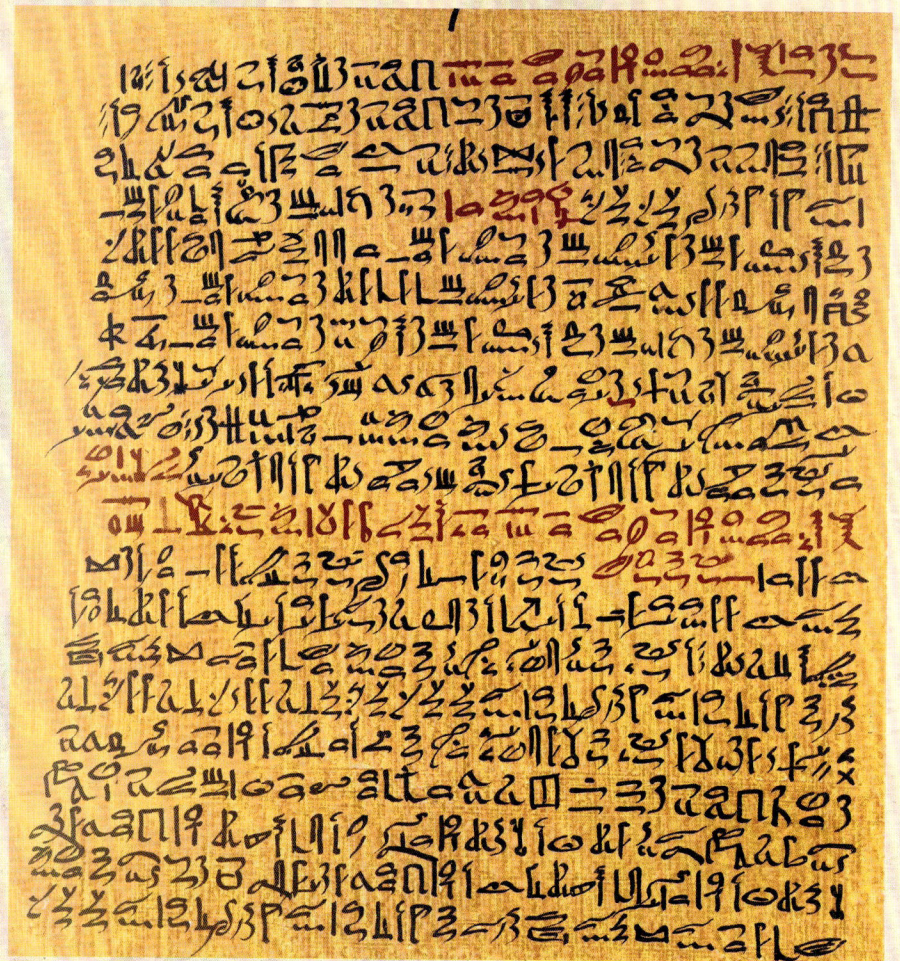

Above: The Ebers Papyrus, one of the oldest medicinal treatises of Pharaonic Egypt, circa 1555 BCE.

Top of page: Vessel for body-care balm, dating from the 18th Dynasty, circa 1479–1458 BCE, from Hatshepsut's temple in Deir el-Bahari.

Health-giving aromatics

Frankincense was used as incense and for culinary and medicinal purposes. Because it has antiseptic properties, it could be mixed with food or oil to treat tooth decay and bronchitis. Myrrh was used in mummification to preserve the flesh, and it also helped to combat gastric pain and asthenia (chronic weakness). Women concocted remedies from anise, cedarwood, garlic, cumin, coriander, quince, fennel, thyme and juniper berries. Fumigation preparations contained dried frankincense, terebinth resin, chufa, melon or Phoenician reed.

Perfumed oils, balsamic essences and balms protected the skin from dehydration and were also excellent for sunburn. A rose- and iris-scented oil named bakkari was very popular with women. 'Egyptian perfume' was an expensive cinnamon and myrrh composition that was said to be effective against a wide range of ailments.

Medicinal plants used in Mesopotamia in the second millennium.

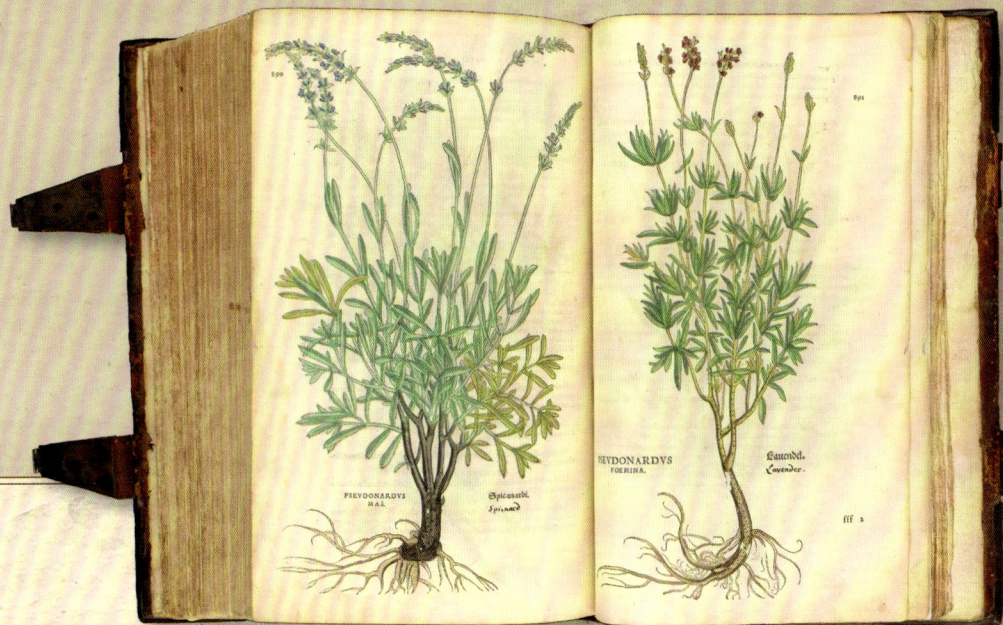

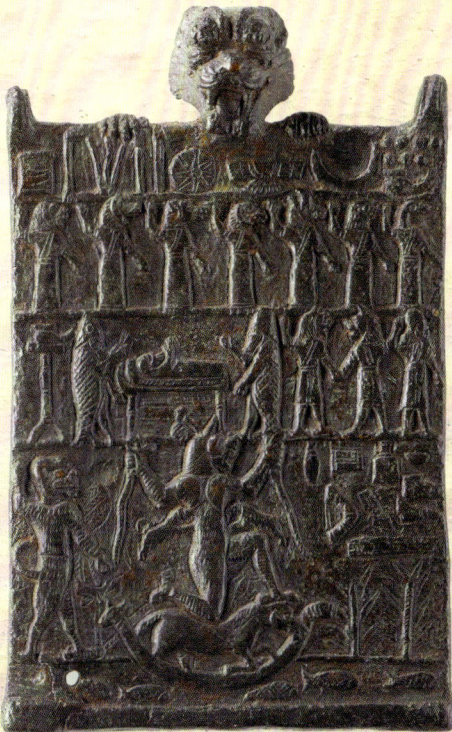

MESOPOTAMIA IN THE SECOND MILLENNIUM

The Sumerian and Babylonian perfume pharmacopeia listed plants such as myrrh, asafoetida, thyme, fig, pyrethrum, saffron and oleander. We also know from tablet inscriptions the names of resins in common use, including styrax, galbanum, terebenthine, myrrh and opoponax. As in Egypt, salves and balms were employed in medicine and beauty.

The Babylonians, too, believed that illness was caused by the supernatural so, to banish the demons responsible, patients were given bitter, foul-smelling products, while pleasing aromas were reserved for worshipping the gods of salvation. Practices combining medicine and magic, which involved burning figurines made of wood or fat in the fire of healing and purification, came about to combat the fear of these demons and to avoid upsetting the gods. Some 250 medicinal plants and 120 animal substances were used!

Greek protection plaque against the demoness Lamashtu, also known as a Hell Plaque, circa 750 BCE.

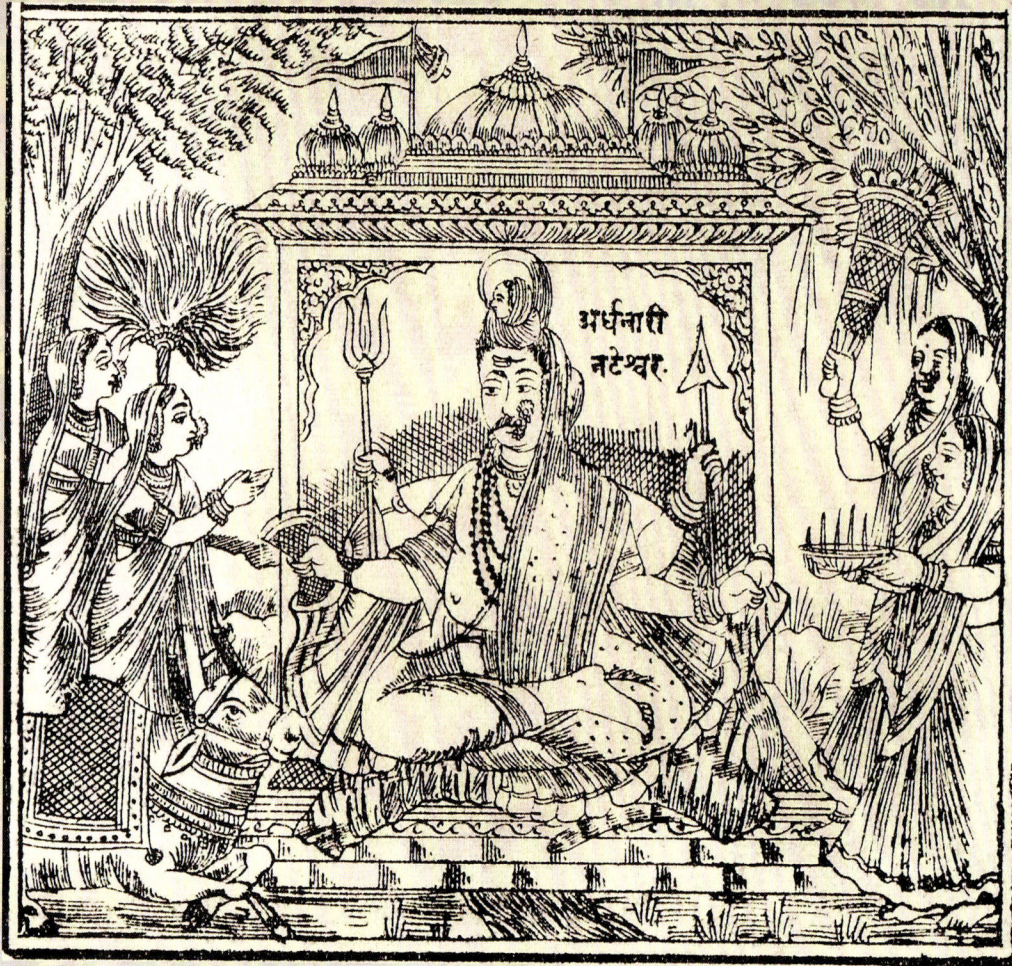

In India, Lord Dhanvantari is known as the physician of the gods and the god of Ayurvedic medicine. As a god specializing in healthcare, he is said to have invented and made the first medicinal plant-based treatments and other natural remedies.

INDIA AND PERFUME AS THE CELESTIAL COMPONENT

Traditional Indian medicine is centred around the wind, the cosmic force considered to be the soul of the world. This force is represented in yoga by the breath. Breathing practices are linked to perfumes, which provide the celestial component. Therapeutics are therefore based on incantations and magical practices that combine countless aromas of plants and flowers chosen for their colours, shapes and fragrance. The healing qualities of these plants and flowers were gradually discovered and brought together in a coherent system known as Ayurveda, or Ayurvedic medicine.

HIPPOCRATES' PERFUME PRESCRIPTIONS

Little by little, perfumes used in religion began to be prescribed for medicinal purposes. Greece was at the confluence of knowledge and experience spanning several millennia, from Egypt in the south, Mesopotamia in the north, and the peoples of the East and of the Danube and Central Europe in the west. Naturally, as medicine developed so did ideas, which to some extent were influenced by myths and magic. In Athens, Hippocrates famously healed the sick of malaria and the plague by carrying out fumigations and burning fragrant wood. He believed that nature was the medicine of the sick and that success could only be achieved by promoting its effects. He prescribed perfumed balms, massages and oil and other aromatic substances, and recommended burning sage to treat some conditions. He also believed that the scent of saffron induced restorative sleep and pleasant dreams. In addition, it was Hippocrates who developed a perfume test, prescribing a range of aromas to women who were having difficulty conceiving. 'If a woman fails to conceive, and you want to know if she can, cover her in wraps and burn perfume underneath her: if the odour passes through the body and out at the mouth and nostrils, she may be deemed capable of conception.'

Greek warriors and perfumed oil

Throughout Greece, physical exercise was performed naked. Bodies were rubbed with scented oil to relax the muscles and moisturize the skin. Before combat, the Greeks doused their houses and pets with perfume, and warriors also covered their bodies with perfumed oils or creams to protect themselves from the Mediterranean sun and mask body odour. After battle, scented oil was used to treat wounds. Homer described the ailments and injuries the Greeks suffered and the first tentative treatments. In the *Iliad*, we learn that Hecamede prepared an aromatic potion with magical properties (Book XI).

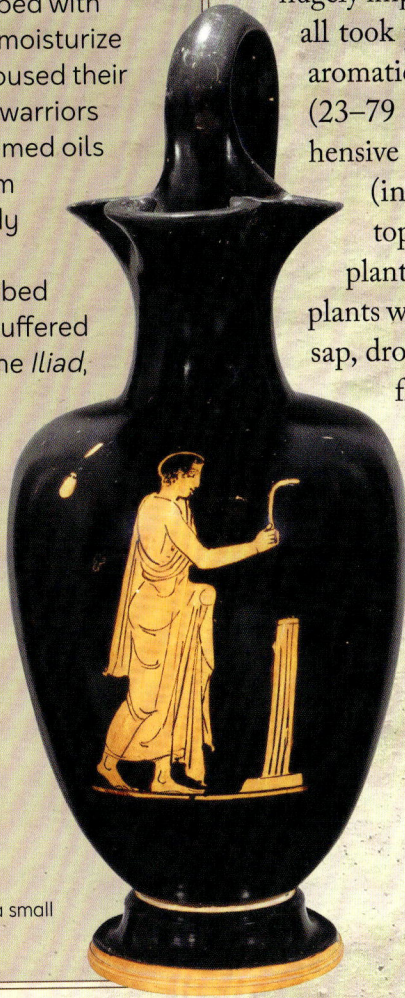

Greek vase depicting a young man holding a strigil, a small tool used to scrape and clean the skin.

PLINY THE ELDER, ROMAN HERBALIST

Baths, massages and physical exercise were also hugely important in ancient Rome. These activities all took place in an atmosphere perfumed with aromatic oils. It was a Roman, Pliny the Elder (23–79 CE), who produced the most comprehensive work on the matter. His *Natural History* (in particular Books XII to XIX) covers topics including botany and describes exotic plants and trees. In it, we learn that aromatic plants were harvested for their roots, stems, bark, sap, droplets, wood, shoots, flowers, leaves and fruit. In Books XXII to XXXII, the author also describes the remedies derived from these plants. His history provides encyclopaedic knowledge that was passed down through the generations from the Middle Ages to the nineteenth century.

The Roman public baths, lithograph.

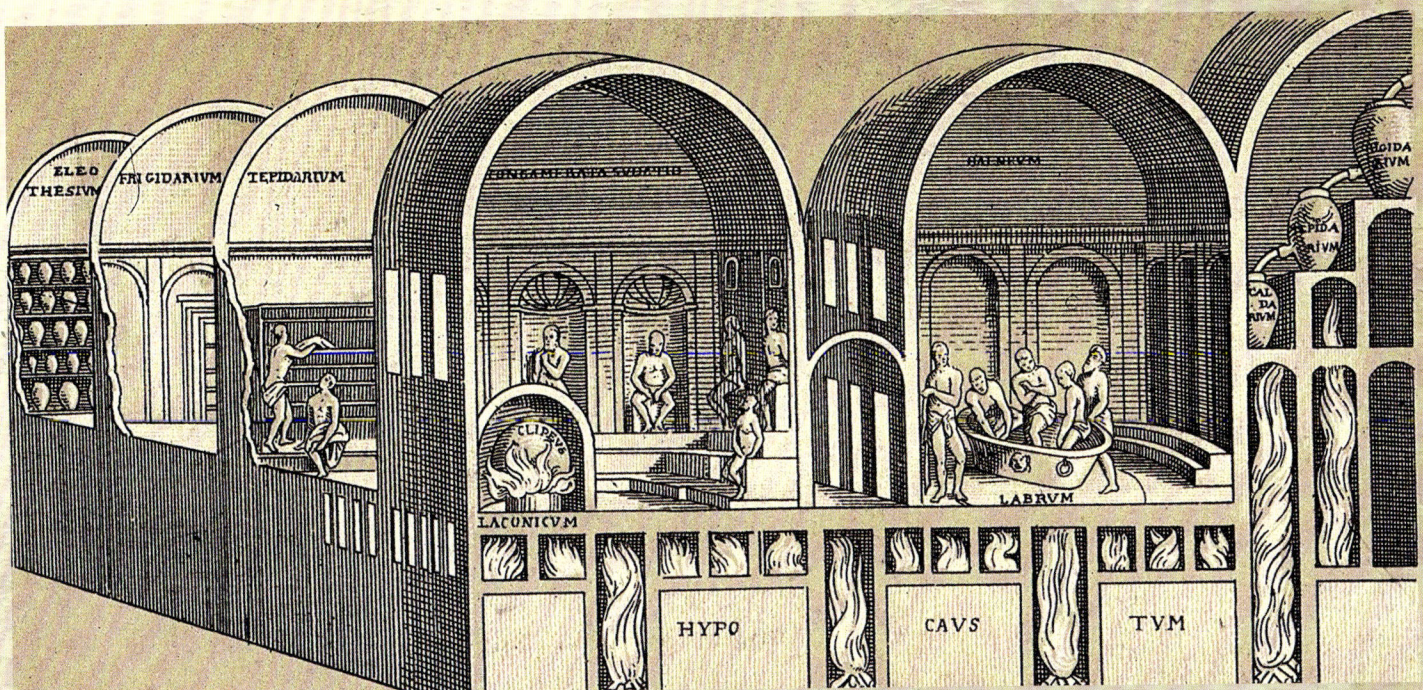

THE IMPORTANCE OF THE EAST

At the height of the Roman Empire (second century CE), the Near East was filled with the most intoxicating aromas. Five centuries later, Islam would take root in all the civilizations of the Mediterranean Basin, including Persia, which provided a gateway to Asia and India, the source of herbs, drugs and perfumes. From Samarkand to the Atlantic Ocean, the Islamic wave expanded to become a vast empire, and perfumes played their part in the conquest. Perfume, women and children were all components of the Prophet Mohammed's vision of paradise. Scholars and doctors were honoured in Baghdad, the land of roses and then capital of the Islamic world. The great Persian scientist and physician Abu Bakr al-Razi (865–925) built a hospital there, where he produced a compilation of analyses of 113 works under the Latin name Continens. This classification provided the basis for a vast observation-based pharmacopeia, demonstrating the importance of the trade in medicinal and aromatic plants between East and West.

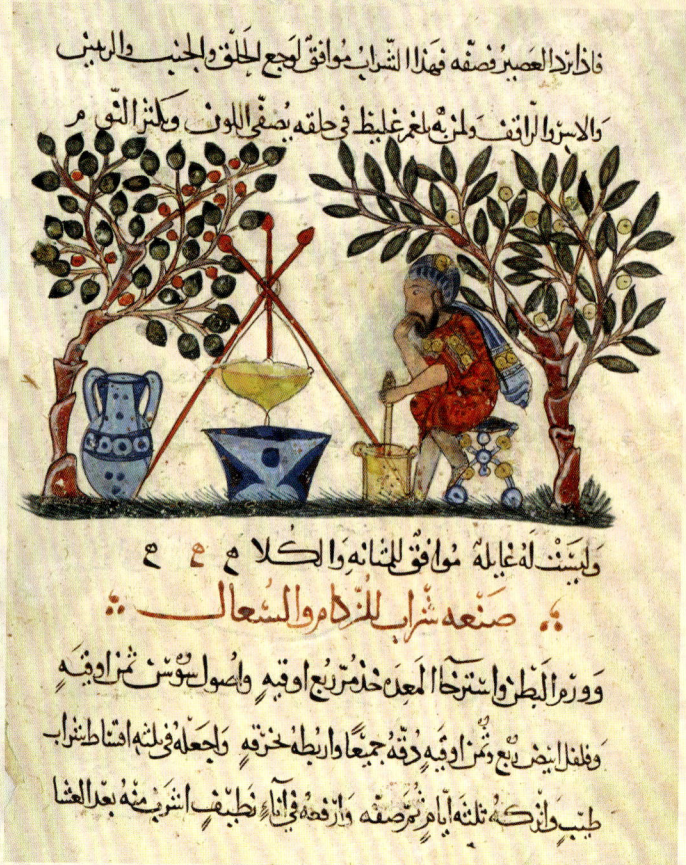

Right: Recipe for a cold-and-cough remedy, discovered circa 1913, probably originating in the Baghdad region.

Below: Persian miniature depicting the bedroom of Ghiyath al-Din Muhammad, in which a servant is spraying perfume, 1495–1505.

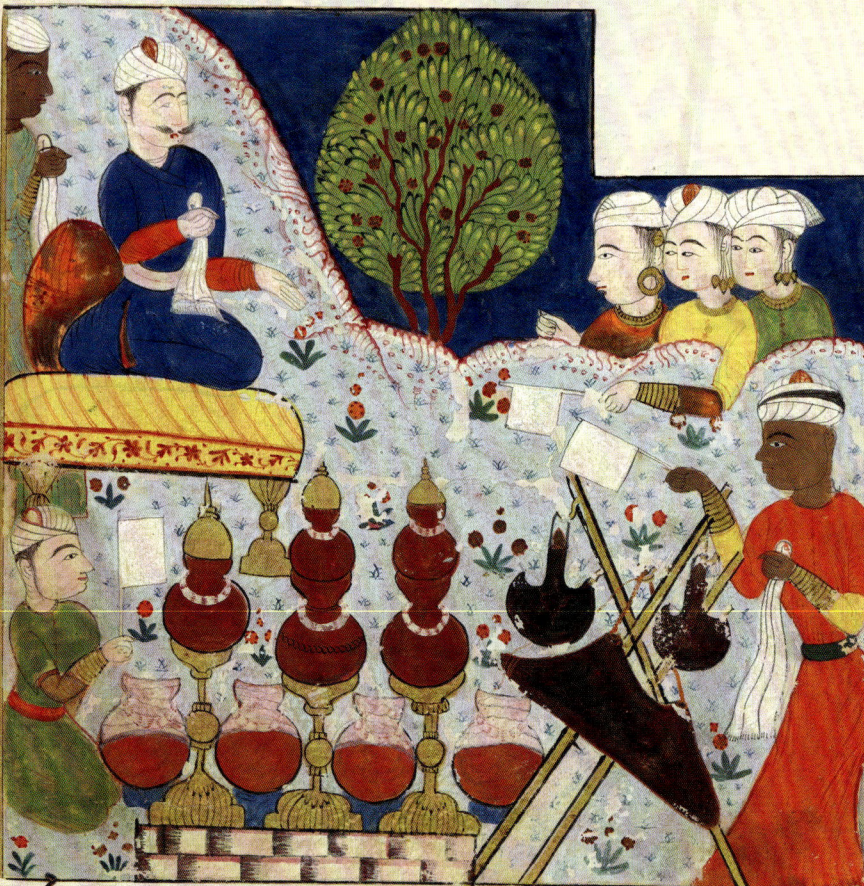

THE EARLY MIDDLE AGES

Perfume use declined in Europe, partly because the Church saw fragrance as frivolous due to its links with the pagan world. However, when Christian knights returned from the Crusades (1096–1291), they brought back aromatics, incense burners and perfume burners, and also frankincense, amber and aloe. In France, damask rose was imported by Robert de Brie (1254–1270) and *Rosa gallica*, the apothecary's rose, is said to have been brought back from the Holy Land. In the thirteenth century, the Venetians capitalized on the Crusades to secure a monopoly on the trade in luxury products and perfume ingredients supplied by the trading posts on the Black Sea and Cyprus. Many written works documented the medicinal properties of perfume recipes, with scent considered to be the 'soul of the medicine'.

THE CHURCH AND MEDICINAL PLANTS

In the Middle Ages, use of medicinal plants was widespread in religious communities. 'Simples' were medicinal remedies made from plants, and the herb garden or garden of simples was home to all the plants associated with God or the devil. The clergy made scented waters and other elixirs. The work of Hildegard of Bingen, a twelfth-century German Benedictine abbess and mystic, is one example. She recorded her visions and expanded her body of work with one collection on divine aromas and another on the causes of illnesses and their cures. In her *Scivias* (1152), we find recipes and observations on her favourite health-giving plants and their therapeutic properties. Healthcare and knowledge were still linked to religion. Monks had an extremely accurate, and empirical, knowledge of the medicinal properties of plants. At an abbey, the herbalist had an important role as apothecary and doctor. Some of the plants, such as soothing thyme and camomile, were used in first aid. Absinthe, mint and thistles were grown to treat stomach ache. German camomile and verbena were used for fevers, and artemisia, lemon balm and rue brought relief for women's menstrual pains. The characteristics of every plant, such as its shape, colour and fragrance, often obvious from its common name, hinted at what it might be used to treat. This was referred to as the 'doctrine of signatures'.

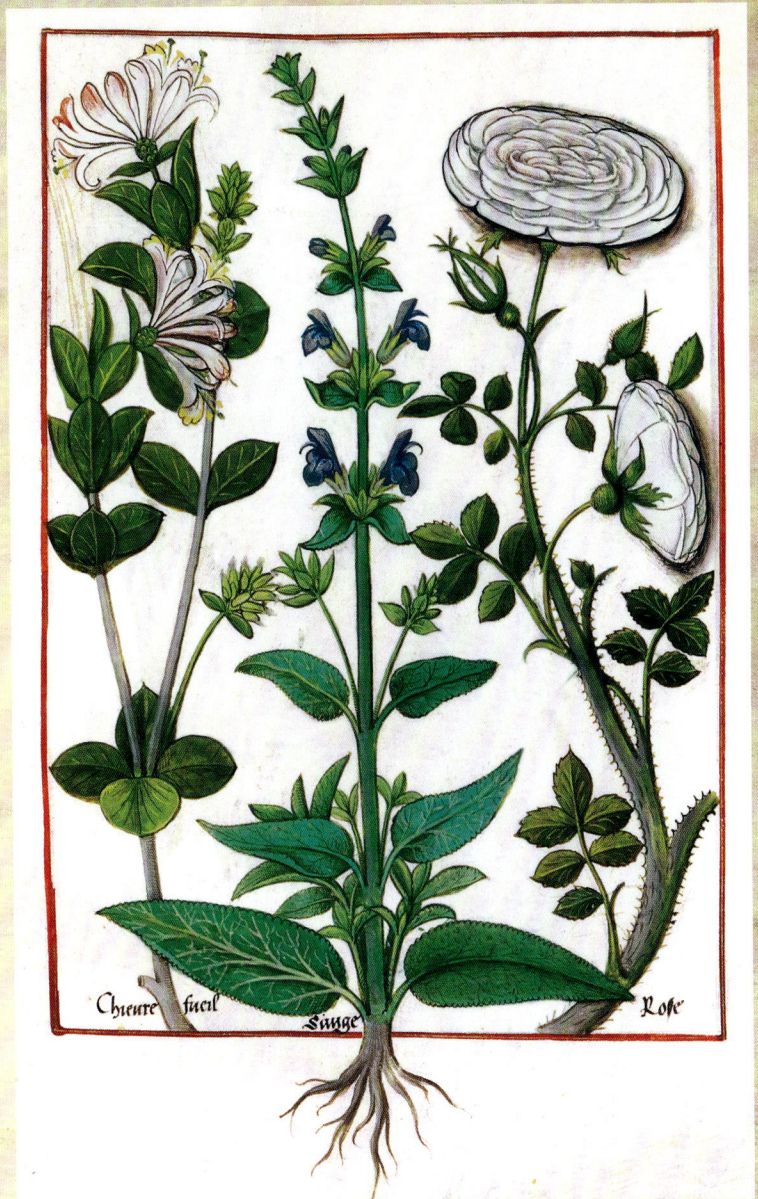

Honeysuckle, sage and rose. Illustration from Matthaeus Platearius' *Book of Simple Medicines*, fifteenth century.

For or against bathing?

The idea that water could be healing was common in the Middle Ages. In the thirteenth century, public baths were used widely in cities such as Paris, where there were dozens of bathhouses. Gradually, however, because there was the potential for excitement and arousal in the steam rooms, they became places of perdition and were strongly condemned by the Church. From the fourteenth century onwards, the baths were thought to be a source of contamination in times of plague: the steam was said to increase the porosity of the skin and let in unhealthy vapours. Thus, bathhouses were criticized no longer for religious reasons but on hygiene grounds. As a result, their number decreased, although royal residences in France such as Fontainebleau, and later Versailles, still had bathing apartments. Ambroise Paré, the first surgeon to King Henry II in 1551, ordered all public baths to be closed for good.

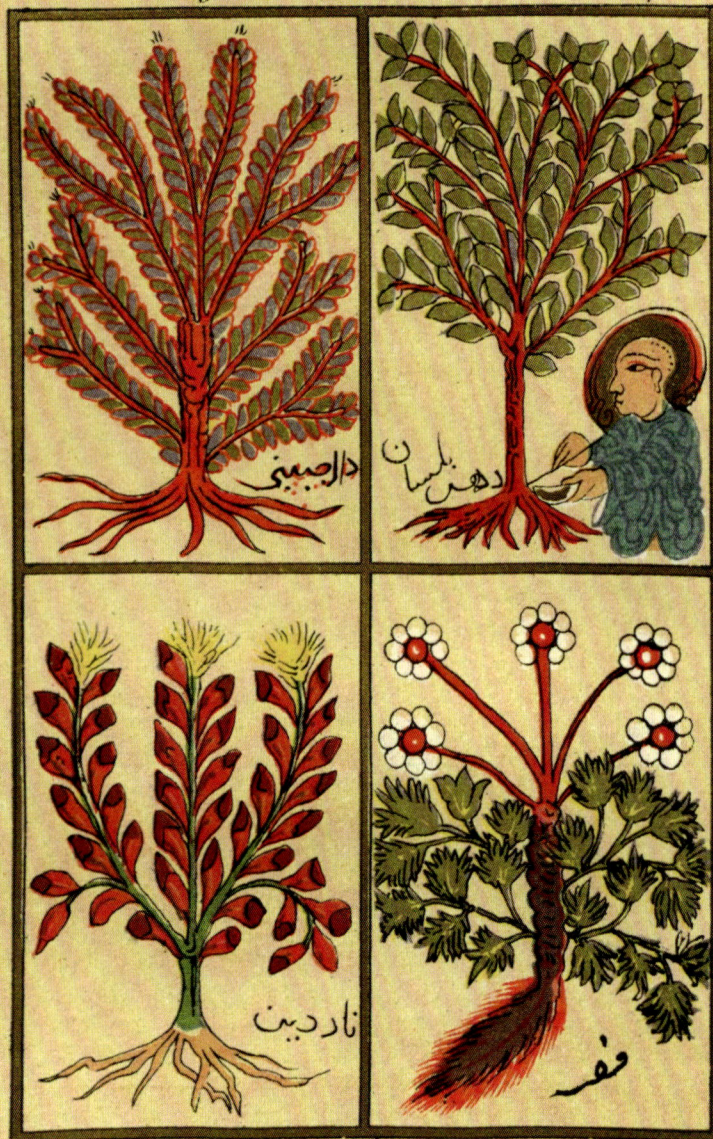

Above: Extract from the *Livre des Parfums* (Book of Perfumes) after a Persian manuscript from the seventeeth century: 'the principle perfumes of the Hebrews' from cinnamon to Balm of Gilead (used by physicians and perfumers in Ancient Greece and the Roman Empire), to nard and valerian.

Opposite: *Personification of Medicine, Pharmacy and Surgery*
Nicolas de Larmessin II, seventeenth century.

In the centre, on a raised platform, is the physician. He is wearing academic dress and his robe is composed of ancient and medieval books in which traditional Western medicine is transmitted. Among these volumes there are ones by Greek authors including Hippocrates and Galen, ones by medieval authors from the East, including Avicenna and Abu Bakr al-Razi, ones by medieval authors from the West including Bernard de Gordon and Arnaud de Villeneuve, as well as by the custodian of all medieval knowledge, Laurent Joubert. The physician gives six instructions to the two subordinates with more specialist qualifications: the surgeon and the pharmacist. On a table to the left there are glass vessels and a prescription with a long list of plants (senna, cassia, tamarind, rhubarb, manna) used for healing. Below, to the left, there is the apothecary figure with his pharmaceutical paraphernalia. His hat is a distillation flask. Bags filled with lily and laurel oils cover his chest. Various ointments, creams and syrups make up different parts of his body. To the right, there is the surgeon, whose body is bedecked with surgical instruments.

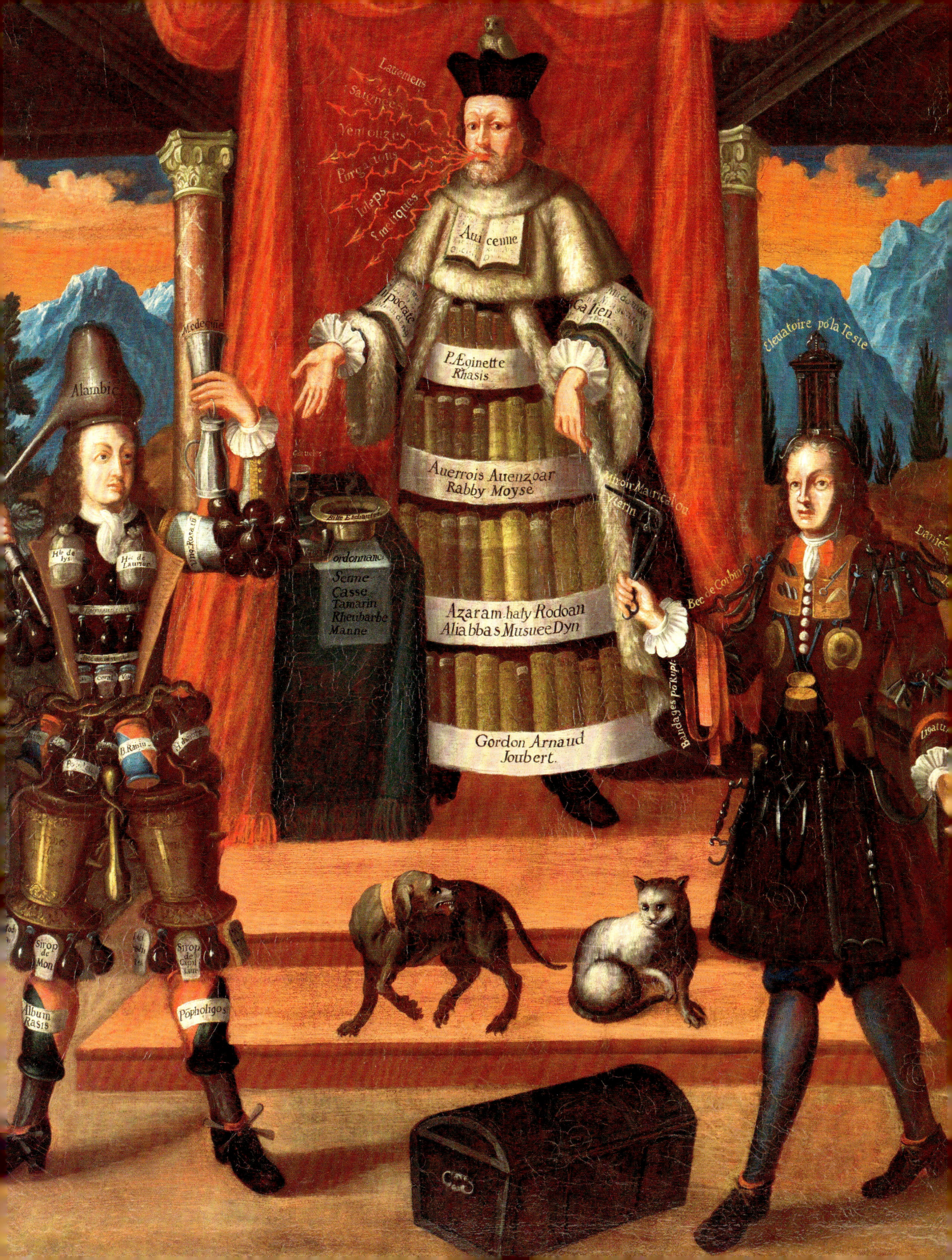

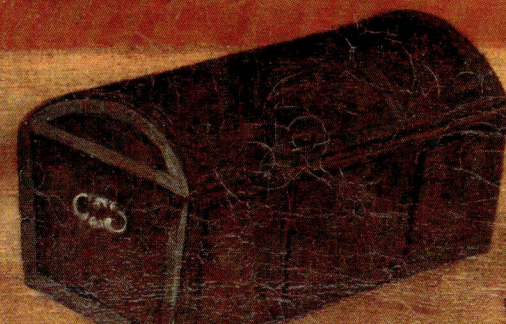

FROM REMEDY TO HYGIENE: BANISHING HARMFUL ODOURS

FROM THE END OF THE MIDDLE AGES,
PEOPLE ESCHEWED DAILY BATHING,
SO PERFUME WAS USED TO MASK BODY
ODOURS. FEARING THAT WATER TRANSMITTED
ILLNESS, CITY DWELLERS BATHED IN SCENTED
WATERS. ROYAL COURTS HELPED TO INCREASE
SALES OF PERFUME AS, NOW MORE THAN EVER,
IT WAS A SYMBOL OF DISTINCTION.

Above: Portrait of a woman holding a pomander, seventeenth century.

Below: A gold pomander beautifully decorated with precious stones, comprising six compartments for fragrances, circa 1600–25.

PERFUME: SYMBOL OF SOCIAL DISTINCTION

During the Renaissance, physiologists believed that epidemics could be spread in the air and by water. The air was purified with potpourri or by burning perfumes. Grooming was performed without water, by applying rose water, lotions and vinegars on the body. Lavender water was added to baths, although very few people now took them.

During this period, scent took on an element of theatricality and became associated with desire and social distinction. The sixteenth century saw the advent of the pomander, a receptacle to hold musk, amber, resins and other perfumed essences. It was an extremely sophisticated accessory, of Eastern origin, comprising a gold or silver ball, often encrusted with precious stones and pearls. Suspended on a ring from the belt, neck or finger, the pomander was recommended to ward off epidemics and treat digestive disorders.

Violet, lavender and orange blossom perfumes became increasingly popular among elegant noble ladies, who concealed sachets of fragrant flower petals or scented wood bark under their garments. The Royal Courts of England, France and Italy enlisted the services of well-known perfumers, who turned perfume into a status symbol. Members of the Court of Versailles often wrapped themselves in an aura of perfumes and other fragrant objects in the belief that they extended and magnified the self. Perfume was also considered highly effective in banishing harmful odours in palaces, where latrines were often neglected.

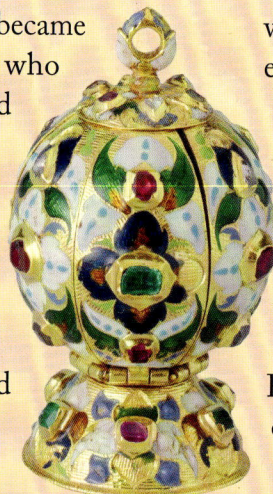

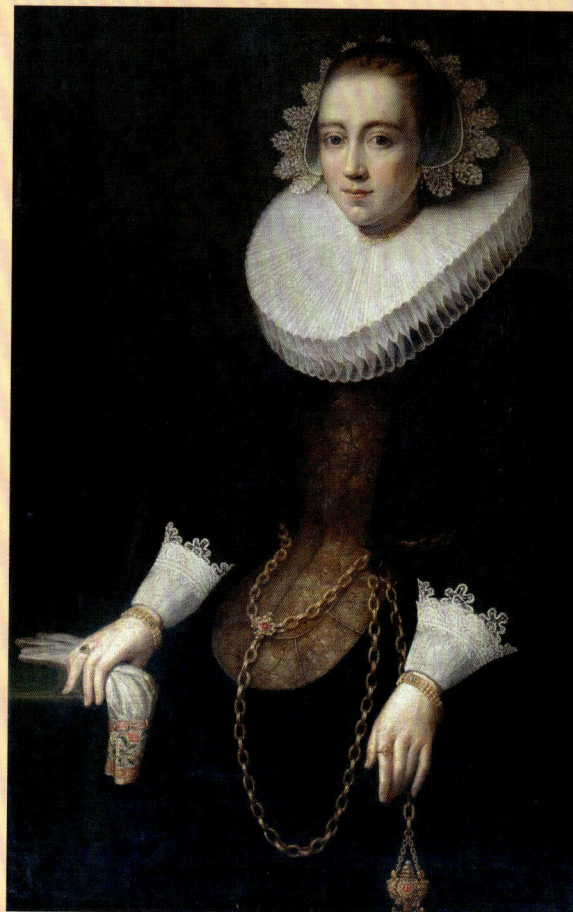

From the late sixteenth century onwards, people, fearing the transmission of illness in the air, changed their clothes regularly to keep clean. Hygiene, however, largely remained reserved for those at court. It would only become widespread in the eighteenth century, particularly in England where, compared to the rest of Europe, many enjoyed a simpler life, closer to nature.

England had its own long tradition of perfume. In fact it was during this period, in 1730, that a certain Juan Famenias Floris set up shop in London's elegant quarter of Saint James, at the back of a barbershop. Located at 89 Jermyn Street, where Floris is still based. It counted the likes of Elizabeth Pierrepont, Duchess of Kingston, among its clientele.

WARDING OFF EPIDEMICS

In France, the plague recurred in the seventeenth and eighteenth centuries, most markedly between 1720 and 1750 in Marseille, Aix, Arles and Toulon, where it wiped out half the population. Doctors told people to self-isolate and burn fragrant resins in their homes (incense, amber, musk, camphor, quince, juniper berries, sulphur, orpiment, antimony and even gunpowder). To approach someone with the plague, you had to wear a plague suit: a long, enveloping robe, as airtight as possible, a wide-brimmed hat and a mask with a beak filled with aromatic plants and perfumes to purify the air you breathed. Perfumers were responsible for disinfecting places, people and even animals.

Right: Doctor wearing a seventeenth-century plague suit. The long 'beak' held spices to mask the smell of corpses, and the eye sockets were covered by glass. The robe was made of leather.

Below: Stick with fumigator used by doctors to mask the odour of dead bodies when visiting plague victims.

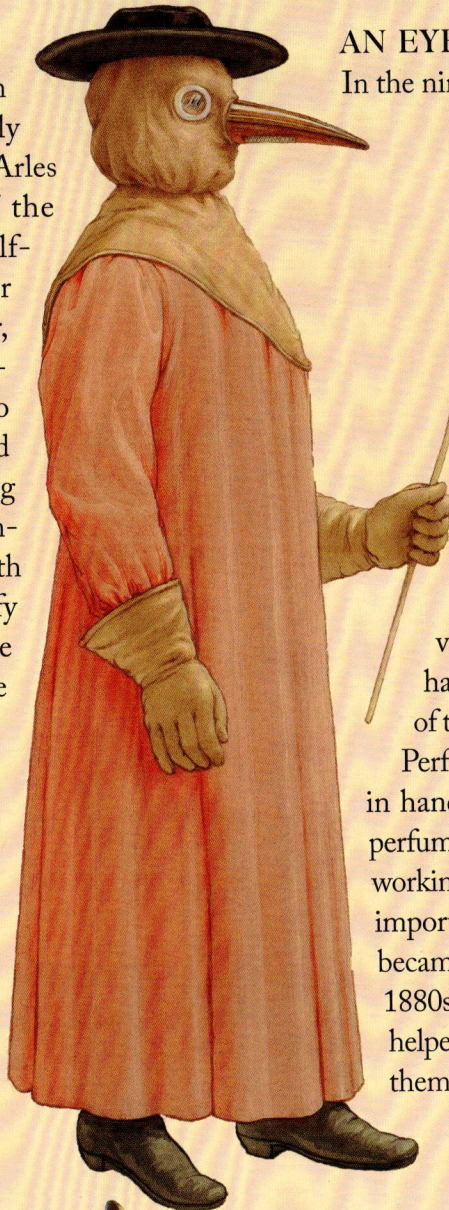

AN EYE ON HYGIENE

In the nineteenth century, people became more aware of hygiene and no longer dismissed cleanliness as unnecessary. Bathing, which had previously been recommended in moderation, was now seen to improve both skin and health. The perfume industry capitalized on the quest for cleanliness and made products to meet the needs of a hygiene-conscious and moralistic nineteenth-century society. Perfumed toilet soap replaced Castile Soap or Marseille Soap (a hard vegetable-oil soap), and in the second half of the century it accounted for half of the total output of the perfume industry. Perfume and hygiene continued to go hand in hand, contributing to the success of the perfume industry. From the 1830s, architects working to improve public health placed more importance on convenience, and bathrooms became an integral part of the home from the 1880s. Aside from luxury and well-being, it helped keep people clean which, in turn, kept them healthy.

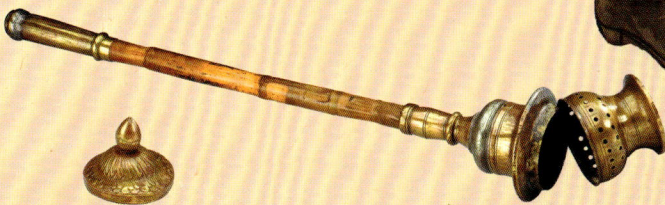

The invention of the water closet

From the mid eighteenth century, there was a personal cleanliness revolution that started in England. The English recommended washing regularly – hands and face daily and the whole body two to three times a week – to eliminate toxins. They invented the modern lavatory, called a water closet, where people could relieve themselves discreetly and hygienically. This fashion swept over to France and the Countess du Barry, last mistress of Louis XV, had one installed in her apartments at Versailles.

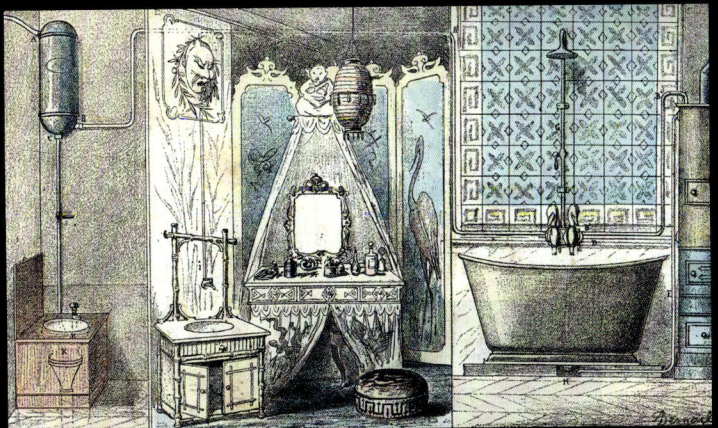

Water closet or bathroom in a Parisian appartment, circa 1887.

THE FIRST ICONIC PERFUMES

FROM THE FOURTEENTH CENTURY ONWARDS, ALCOHOL-BASED PERFUME GRADUALLY BEGAN TO INFILTRATE THE WEST (SEE PAGE 29). ALCOHOL DISTILLATION, AND THE CONDENSATION COIL, PAVED THE WAY FOR MODERN-DAY PERFUMERY AND THE FIRST ICONIC PERFUMES AND FAMOUS WATERS SUCH AS EAU DE COLOGNE.

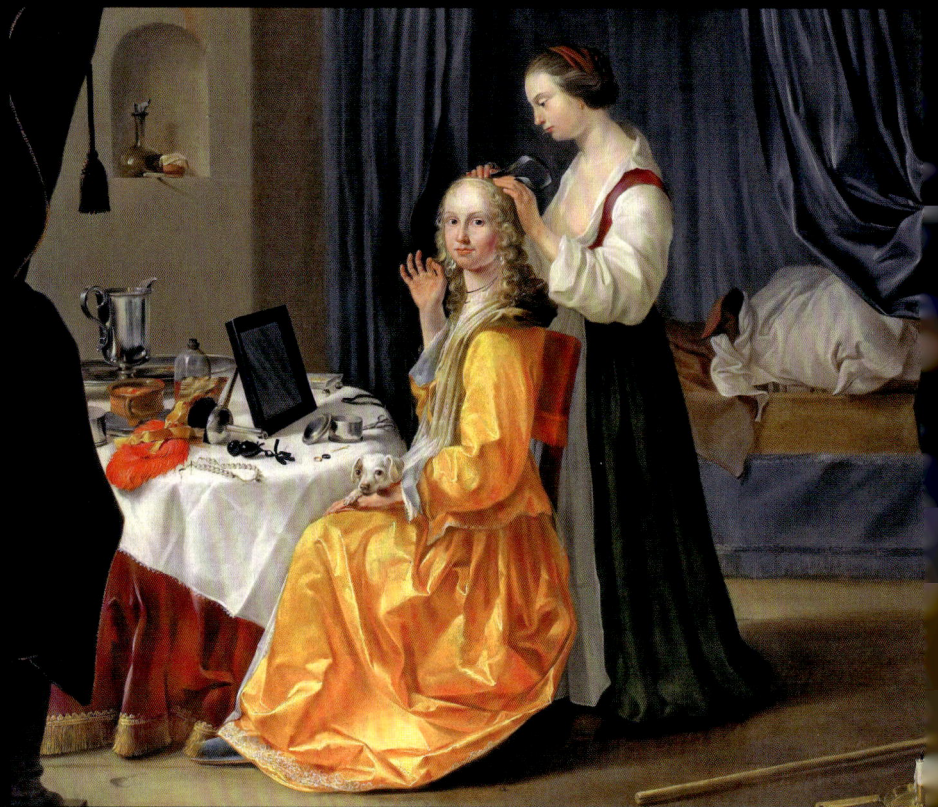

Painting of a young woman at her toilet, circa 1650–60.

QUEEN OF HUNGARY'S WATER

The story of the first Western perfume (1370), a sage, rosemary and marjoram distillate or alcoholate combined with cedar and lemon balm, is so far-fetched as to beggar belief. Isabella, Queen of Hungary, both elderly and infirm, was said to have been given this preparation by a hermit whom she had never met before. Having used the concoction for a year, she was so transformed that the King of Poland wanted to marry her. She declined, for love of Jesus Christ, believing the hermit to have been

his angel (see pages 42–3). But who was this mysterious Queen of Hungary? Was this story simply invented by a chemist in a quest to attract an aristocratic clientele, or indeed, by the perfumers of Montpellier, who had made it their speciality? Arnaldus de Villa Nova (circa 1235–1313) mentioned a similar thirteenth-century recipe for a rosemary tincture which he likened to 'drinkable gold'. The first reference to Queen of Hungary's Water (Eau de la Reine de Hongrie) appeared in 1660 in scholarly works, such as that by French chemist Marie Meurdrac, which were popular at the Court of Versailles.

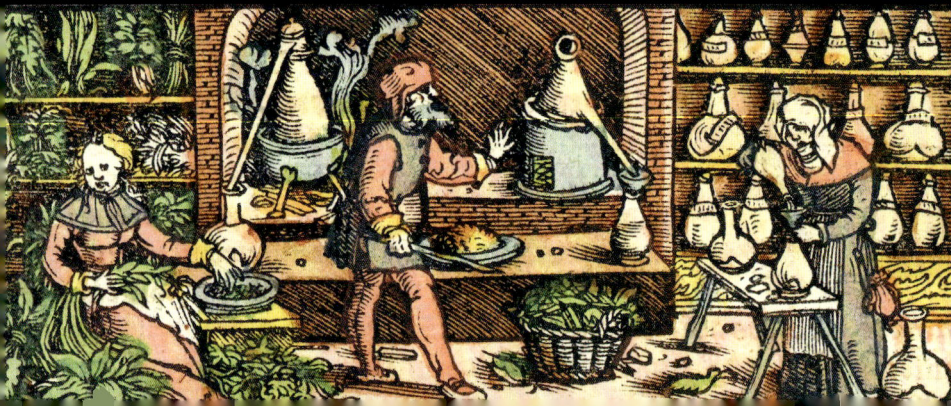

An old distillery.

A SCENT TO CURE GUNSHOT WOUNDS

A few famous products were developed in monasteries to combat a whole range of ailments. One example was arquebusade, an elixir distilled by monks in the sixteenth century from a range of aromatic plants, on the orders of the French king Francis I, to treat arquebus (gunshot) wounds. The product was found to be extremely effective for anxiety, headaches, toothache, sleeping problems, stomach ache and digestive disorders. Gradually, its use expanded beyond the king's riflemen to the general public. In the eighteenth and nineteenth centuries, it was so popular that Eau d'Arquebusade became a generic name. Pierre François Pascal Guerlain built his success partly on the back of this product when he opened his first boutique in 1828.

Right: *Melissa officinalis* or lemon balm.
Left: A bottle of Carmelite water.

CARMELITE WATER

Carmelite water (Eau des Carmes) or melissa water was another famous and very effective plant-based revitalizing remedy of the time. Also known as Carmes water, it combined the therapeutic properties of 14 plants and nine spices, among them *Melissa officinalis* (lemon balm), which gave its name to the mixture. Lemon balm had been grown for centuries as a medicinal plant and used by doctors in Spain. It was introduced to France from Spain in the tenth century by Benedictine monks. The invigorating blend of Carmelite water was developed by a sixteenth-century French herbalist, who disclosed his secret formula to Father Damien, a member of the Confrérie des Carmes Déchaux, a religious order based in rue de Vaugirard in Paris. The monks firmly believed in the effectiveness of this water and decided to make it themselves. It became one of the favourite remedies of Cardinal Richelieu, who used it to obtain relief from his persistent migraines and digestive problems.

Right: A monk at work. Could it be Father Damien preparing his secret Carmelite water recipe?

Far right: Four thieves' vinegar, late eighteenth century.

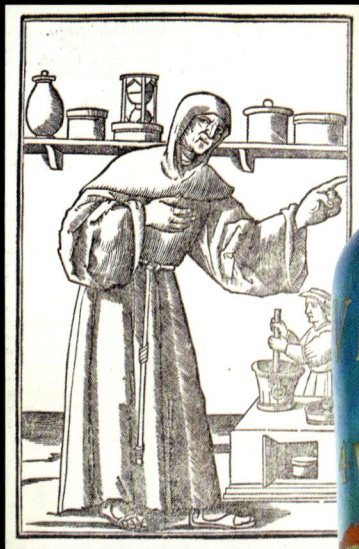

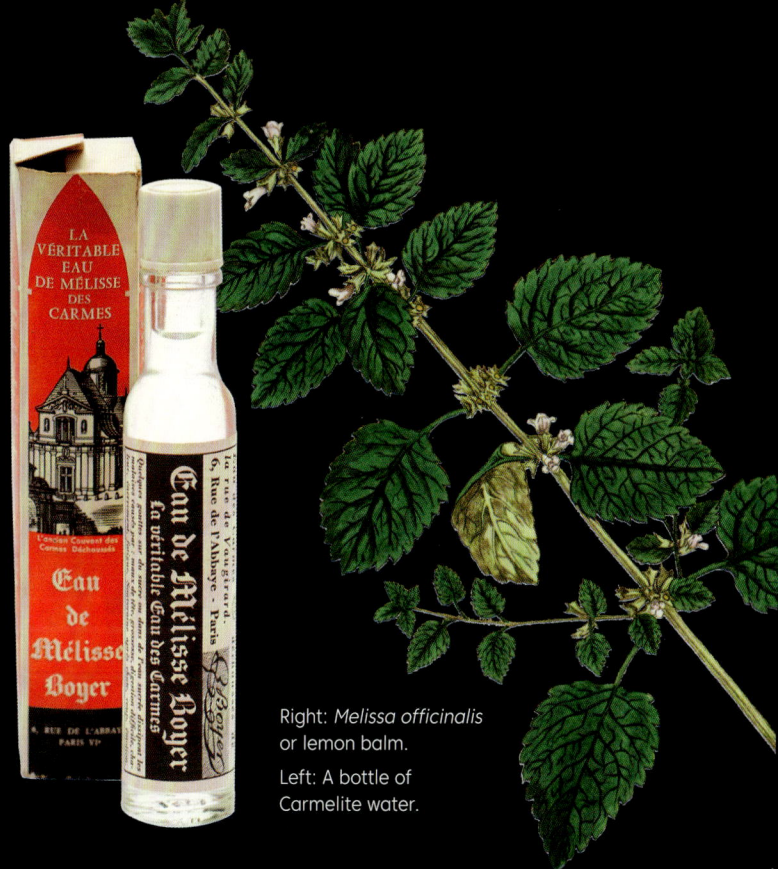

FOUR THIEVES' VINEGAR

Many legends tell the story of this famous product, which is linked to the plague. The story goes that in the early eighteenth century, when the government of the city of Marseille (or Toulouse, according to other sources) could find no way to stop the devastation caused by the plague, four unscrupulous robbers were pillaging the city. They appeared to be immune to the disease, so could easily enter houses and steal from the sick. Brought before the courts, they offered to disclose the secret of their immunity in exchange for a lenient sentence. If the legend is to be believed, they were rubbing their bodies, particularly their hands and faces, with a maceration of garlic vinegar and lots of aromatic herbs such as sage, rosemary, mint, cinnamon and nutmeg, mixed with camphor. The recipe, subsequently published and recommended to the public, proved to be very effective. Because of its dermatological and antiseptic qualities, *vinaigre des quatre voleurs* (four thieves' vinegar) was recognized as a useful remedy against contagious diseases and listed in medical treatises as early as 1748. It was sold in pharmacies as an antiseptic for external use until 1937.

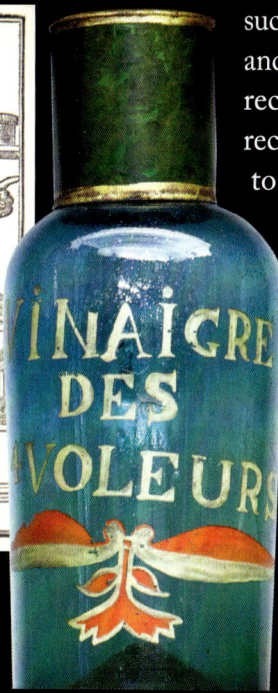

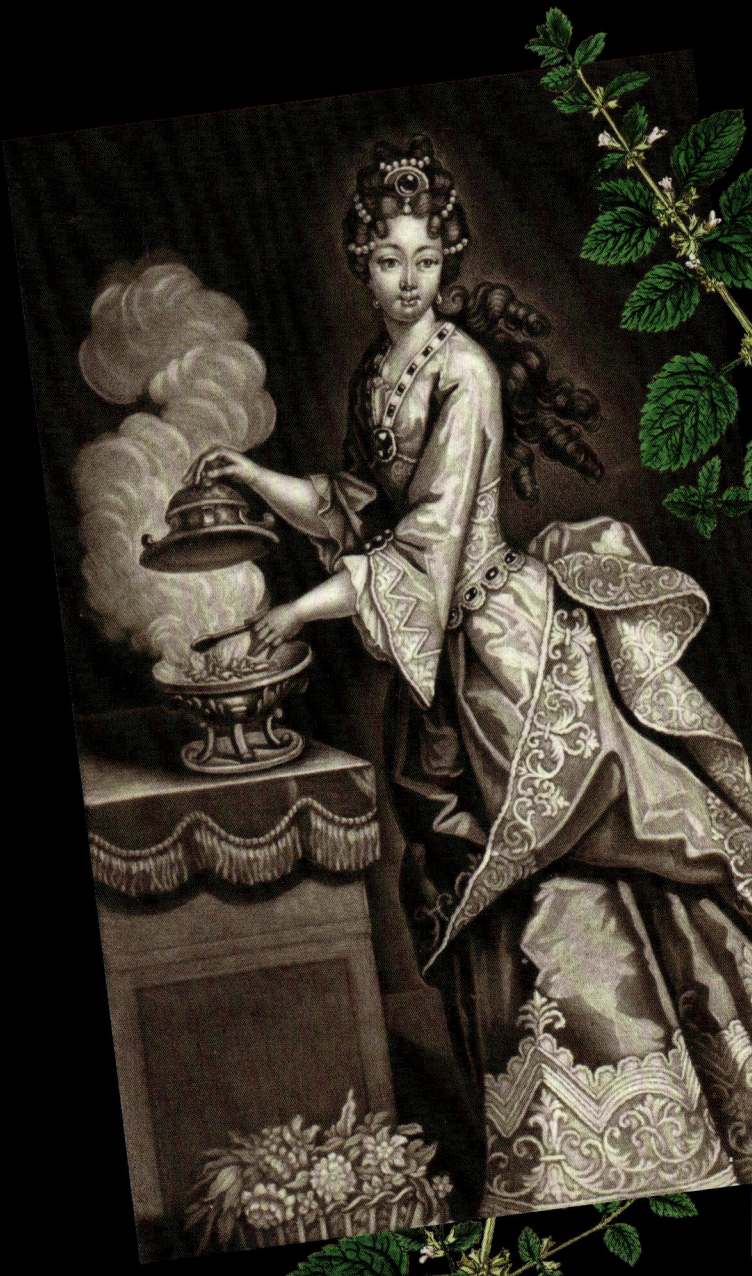

LA BEAUTÉ ET LA SANTÉ.

SECRETS
CONCERNANT
LA BEAUTÉ ET LA SANTÉ.

DIX-HUITIÈME PARTIE,

Contenant la description de divers Parfums qui ont des proprietez Medecinales.

CHAPITRE PREMIER.

Des Liqueurs distilées.

Eau de la Reine de Hongrie.

EN la Cité de Bude Capita'e d'Hongrie fut trouvée écrite la suivante Recepte dans les Heures de la Serenissime Princesse DONNA ISABELLA, Reine de ce Royaume.

Translation:
SECRETS
CONCERNING
BEAUTY AND HEALTH
EIGHTEENTH PART
Concerning the description of various perfumes with medicinal properties

PART ONE
On distilled liquors
Queen of Hungary Water
In the city of Buda, capital of Hungary
the following recipe was found
in the Hours of the Serenissima Donna Isabella
Queen of this Kingdom

I, DONNA ISABELLA, Queen of Hungary, aged seventy-two years, who is sick in the limbs and suffering from gout, used for a whole year this recipe given to me by a hermit, who I had never seen; it had such an effect on me that while I am healed, I have also regained strength, to the point of looking so beautiful the King of Poland wanted me to marry; but I refused for the love of Jesus Christ, and believing that the recipe was given to me by an angel:

Take the distilled water, four times thirty ounces, twenty ounces of rosemary flowers, put them all in a vessel to infuse them, then distil them in an alembic in a bain-marie, and keep the water for the next usage. While the Queen of Hungary Water is not a gentle perfume, many people like its strong scent and breathe it in frequently; so much so, it is fitting that is be included as it is here in the book.

SECRETS CONCERNANT

Moy DONNA ISABELLA Reine d'Hongrie, âgée de 72. ans, infirme de membres & gouteuse, ay ufé un An entier de la préfente Recepte, laquelle me donna un Hermite que je n'avois jamais vû & n'ay fceu voir depuis, qui fit tant d'effet fur moy, qu'en mefme temps je gueris & recouvray les forces, en forte que paroiffant belle à chacun, le Roy de Pologne me voulut époufer, ce que je refufay pour l'amour de N. S. JESUS-CHRIST, croyant qu'il me l'avoit envoyée par un Ange.

PRENEZ Eau de Vie diftilée quatre fois trente onces, fleurs de Romarin vingt-onces, puis mettez ces chofes dans une Cucurbite, pour les faire infufer pendant cinquante heures, enfuite dequoy vous le diftilerez au Bain-Marie, & vous conferverez l'eau qui en diftilera pour l'ufage fuivant.

Quoy que l'Eau de la Reine d'Hongrie ne foit pas un parfum fuave; néanmoins bien des gens en aiment l'odeur forte & la flairent inceffamment, fi bien qu'elle ne pouvoit avoir dans ce Livre une place plus convenable que celle-cy; Mais comme elle a d'ailleurs des vertus admirables, tant prife interieurement qu'appliquée exterieurement, j'ay crû qu'on ne feroit pas fâché de les voir icy décrites auffi bien que fon ufage.

LA BEAUTÉ ET LA SANTÉ.

1. Appliquée à la Nuque du Col, aux Tempes & aux Poignets, elle repare les efprits diffipez, débouche les Nerfs obftruez, & par ces deux effets augmente la memoire, affûre le jugement, donne de la force & de la gayeté, & par une fuite neceffaire foûtient la force de tous les fens exterieurs.

2. Tirée par le nez elle foulage beaucoup la Migraine & abbaiffe mefme les vapeurs par fa feule odeur.

3. Mife dans les oreilles avec un peu de coton elle diffipe affez ordinairement la pituite & les vents qui caufent le tintement & bourdonnement qui diminuënt la faculté d'ouir.

4. Appliquée fur les coftes & fur les Hypocondres elle fert à la Pleurefie, elle foulage les douleurs de cofté, elle débouche le Foye & la Ratte, & par ce moyen elle furvient à la Jauniffe, aux Coliques bilieufes & aux autres Maladies qui dépendent de l'obftruction des vifceres.

5. Imbibée dans des Rofties de pain & appliquée fur le Nombril elle appaife prefque toutes les douleurs du ventre.

6. Un petit linge imbibé de cette Eau & appliqué fur les Paupieres fortifie la vûë affoiblie par une chutte habituelle de larmes ou de ferofitez.

7. Appliquée fur tout le Corps, elle fert merveilleufement à l'Apoplexie, à la paralyfie, à la Goutte, aux Rhumatifmes, & generalement aux Maladies qui dépendent d'un dépoft de pituite & de Serofitez irritantes.

8. Si on fomente fouvent avec cette Eau les Tumeurs, les Contufions & les Echymofes qui viennent de chuttes ou de coups, elle les refout tres-puiffamment.

9. Meflée avec l'eau d'Argentine elle amortit les brûlures, les puftules & les enleveures du Vifage.

Pour l'Eau rouge de la Reine de Hongrie, voyez au Chapitre quatriéme de la dix-feptiéme Partie.

Extract from *Secrets Concerning Beauty and Health* by Nicolas de Blégny, describing the usage and benefits of Queen of Hungary's Water, seventeenth century,

It has such admirable virtues both inside and outside, I thought there could be no objection to seeing them set out here, along with its usage.

1. Applied to the nape, temples, wrist, it repairs dissipated spirits, unblocks obstructed nerves, and by these two effects increases memory, improves judgement and gives strength and gaiety.
2. Inhaled through the nose, it eases migraines, even its vapours just through their smell.
3. Placed in the ears on a cotton, it dissolves the mucus and the wind that can cause tinnitus and whirring that can reduce one's hearing.
4. Applied to the ribs and hypochrondrium, it eases pleurisy, side pains, it unblocks the liver and the spleen; and in this way, prevents jaundice, bile and other illnesses related to visceral obstruction.
5. Imbibed in slices of bread and applied to the navel, it soothes almost all stomach pains.
6. A small cloth soaked with this water and applied to the eyelids, fortifies one's failing sight after a torrent of tears […]
7. Applied all over the body, it serves wonderfully to treat apoplexy, paralysis, gout, rheumatism, and generally all illnesses related to mucus and secretions that cause irritation.
8. If one has frequent use of this water, tumours, contusions and bruises that come from falls and knocks, will be powerfully countered.
9. Mixed with Argentine water, it alleviates burns, boils and removes them from one's face.

For the Queen of Humgary's red water, see the fourth chapter of the seventeeth part.

PERFUMES FROM THE EAST

THE PERFUMER'S SKILL AND EXPERTISE WOULD BE
NOTHING WITHOUT THE FRAGRANT RAW MATERIALS FIRST
DISCOVERED IN ARABIA, EGYPT, INDIA AND TURKEY.
THE SOFT, POWDERY, VANILLA AND ANIMAL NOTES OF
THE ORIENTAL INGREDIENTS ARE THE EPITOME OF LOVE
AND SENSUALITY, OPULENCE AND DISTANT LANDS.

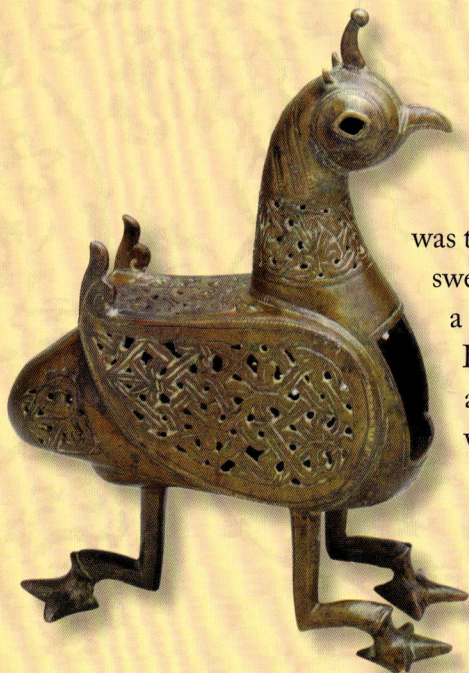

THE EAST, LAND OF EVOCATIVE SCENTS

For three thousand years, the world has been luxuriating in the intoxicating fragrances from the East and South Arabia (known as Arabia Felix in ancient times), the lands of the most opulent sacred scents. The Greek historian Herodotus was the first to describe the perfumes of Arabia: 'The whole of Arabia exudes a divinely sweet scent.' Here, perfume was synonymous with beauty and seduction and also had a certain romantic nostalgia. A lover's name was forever associated with a fragrance. Back in the year 1000, the Arabs perfected the art of distillation to extract essences and produce rosewater, which they used to purify mosques and other places of worship and also, because of its voluptuous scent, for beauty and hygiene purposes.

Bird-shaped oriental bronze censer, dating from the twelfth or thirteenth century.

AN INVALUABLE ART

Since ancient times, bottles of the most exclusive perfume have been encased in metal, hard stone, glass or ceramic. The caliphs surrounded themselves with precious gold or silver incense burners and Arabs were famous for their expert use of fire to produce metalwork, deemed to be the most exquisite art of all. Because of this and the fact that aromatics cost as much as gold, the citizens of Arabia were reputed to be rich and living a life of opulence. Ever since the Queen of Sheba had visited King Solomon with a caravan laden with aromatic substances, fragrances had pervaded the whole of the East. These rare commodities were so sought after that their trade extended to the Mediterranean Basin, including Greece and Rome, Europe, Egypt, Persia and as far as China.

Arab sailors held the monopoly on perfume ingredients for many years and made their fortune from frankincense, which was more precious than gold. Its location made the island of Cyprus a trading hub, and it became very famous for perfumes from the East. Under Moorish control, Arabian perfumers set up shop in Granada, Spain. Due to the Barbarian invasions and the fall of the Western Roman Empire in 476, perfume making declined in the West, to recover in the twelfth and thirteenth centuries thanks to merchants trading with the East, the Venetians and Arabs in particular.

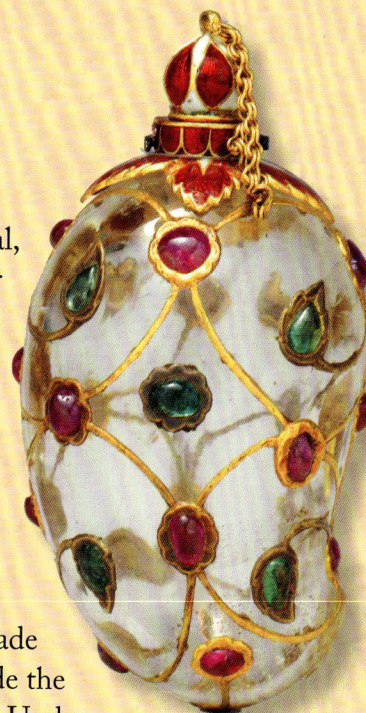

Mango-shaped Mughal Empire bottle decorated with gold and precious stones, mid seventeenth century.

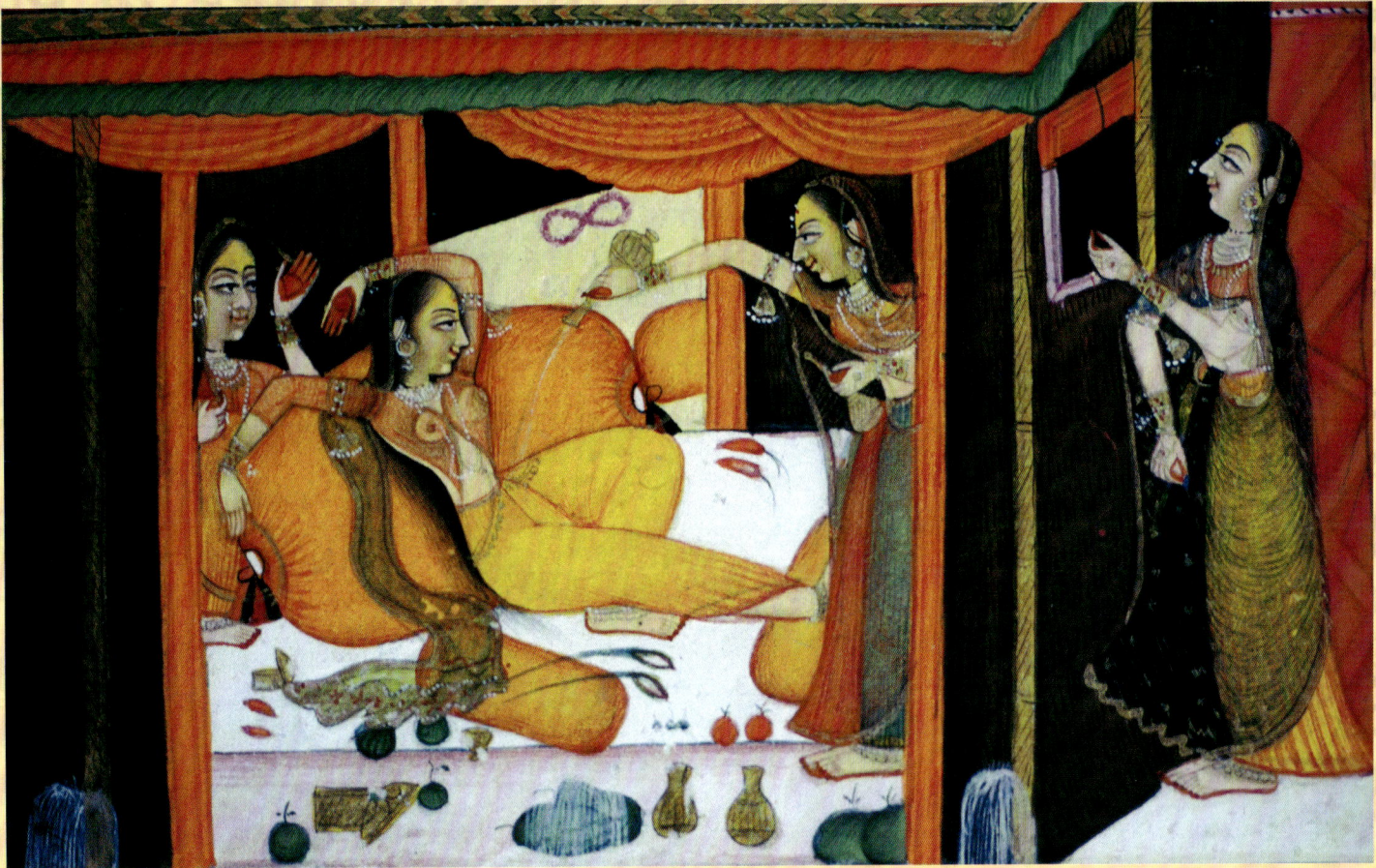

Miniature depicting a woman in a tent being doused with rosewater, Bundi school, Mughal empire, eighteenth century.

MYSTICAL INDIA

Since the dawn of time, perfume has occupied a prominent place in both religious and secular circles in India. It is closely associated with a number of gods, who are worshipped with flowers, incense sticks and aromatic essences. There are many different names for perfume in India as a result of the country's many influences and evolving culture. From the early Vedic period until the present day, different parts of plants (the resin, leaves, roots, flowers and wood) have been used in rituals, pharmaceutics and cosmetics. At marriage ceremonies during the time of the Maharajas, a 'perfume man' would use a stick to spread essences onto parts of the groom's body.

IMPERIAL CHINA, A HAVEN OF INSPIRATION

In Chinese, the words 'perfume' and 'perfumed' are both represented by the character *xiang*, which is also found in culinary preparations and place names and is used to describe the Buddha. The word has existed in the Chinese language for well over 2,000 years. In the second half of the first millennium, the notion of fragrance was expanded to incorporate moral values such as, for instance, virtue for the Confucians and supreme wisdom for the Buddhists. Buddha statues are sometimes carved from sandalwood and so are 'sweet smelling', both physically and metaphorically.

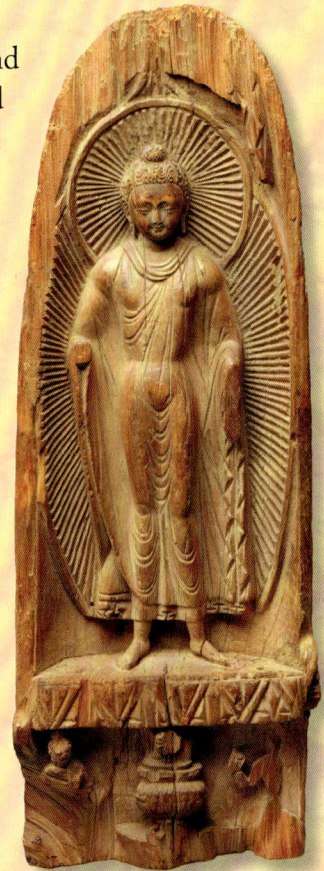

Centrepiece of a three-part travelling shrine depicting Buddha with a radiating halo in a mandorla, China, fifth to sixth century.

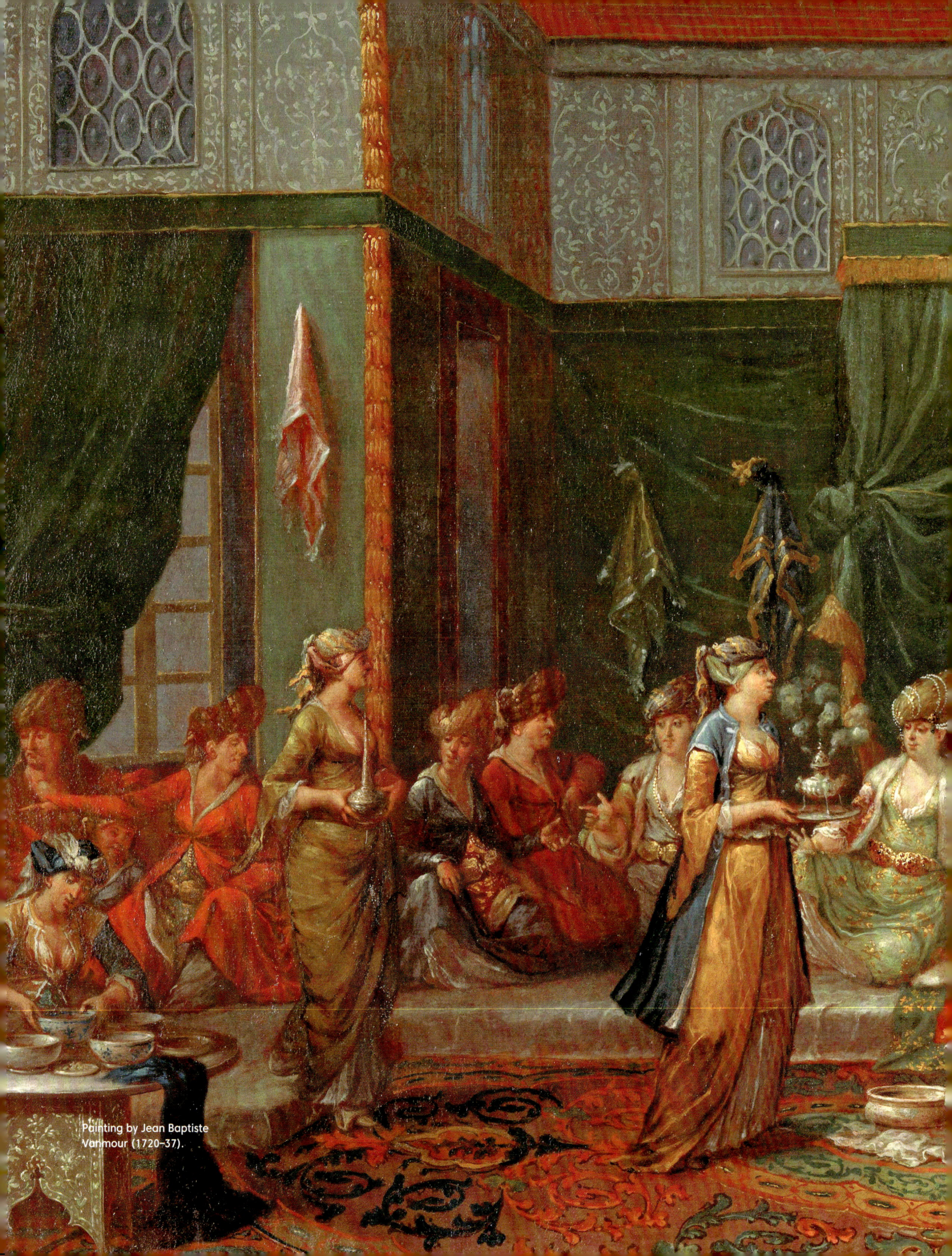

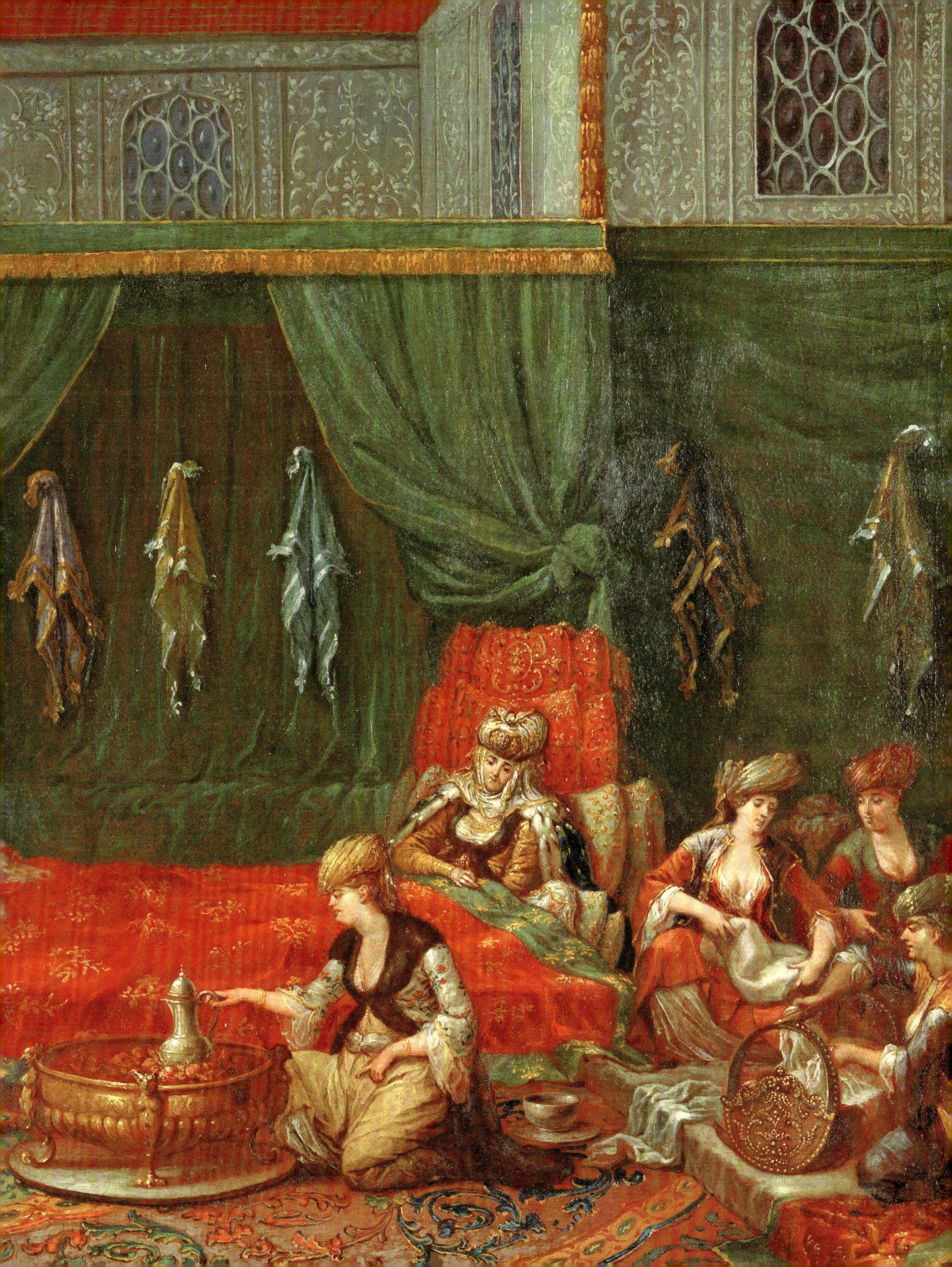

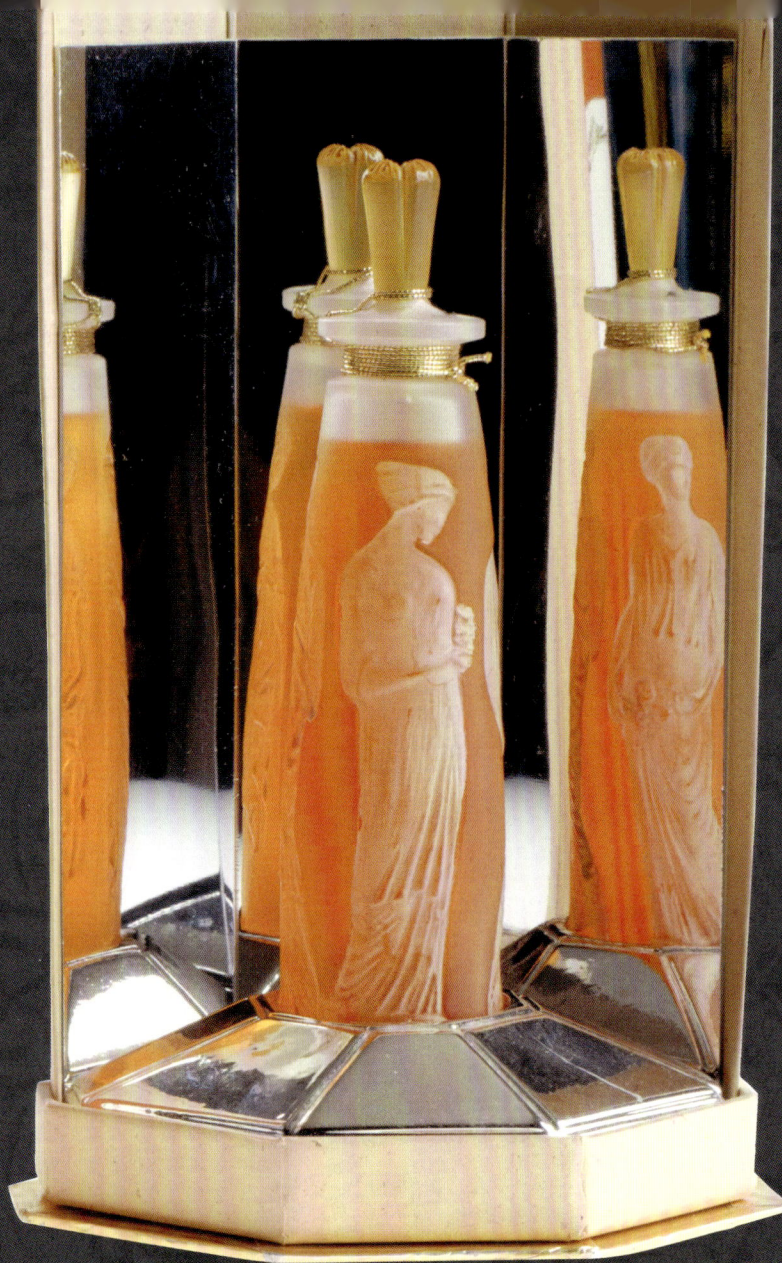

FRANÇOIS COTY AND THE AMBER REVIVAL

The nineteenth century, often referred to as the period of modern-day perfumery, saw the appearance of many scents called Eau des Sultanes, Eau de Shéhérazade, Parfum de Harem and Amber Eau de Cologne, a nod to the traditional Eastern note. In 1905, the soon-to-be-famous perfumer and polymath François Coty's creative genius seemed to know no bounds (see also page 80). His flagship scent Ambre Antique (Old Amber) paved the way for a new perfume family, the ambers. These combined exotic flowers and essences with the traditional amber scent, a

fusion of vanilla and the sweet opiate notes of balsams, precious woods and musk. He brought the fragrance up to date by using a synthetic base, Ambreine Samuelson, for the first time. It was created for him by the chemist Samuelson, and it became the basis of all his formulas. The same theme was later revived in Coty's Styx (1911) and Émeraude (1921).

Ambre Antique by Coty, 1995 revival of the bottle designed by René Lalique. The bottle is decorated with a series of women and comes in a pretty box. Limited edition.

REFINEMENT IN THE LAND OF THE RISING SUN

In Japan, where frankincense was known as *ko*, perfumes for burning had long garnered favour with the educated elite and nobles of good taste. At the Heian Imperial court in the eleventh century, the aristocracy indulged in highly competitive 'perfume tournaments' called *ko-awase*, which required competitors to identify subtle, yet complex, wood and aromatic compositions for incense. The preparations, which could last for weeks, were described by a lady of the court, Murasaki Shikibu, in *The Tale of Genji*, one of the oldest stories from the Imperial period.

Under the influence of Zen Buddhism in the sixteenth century, incense moved away from secular society and the aristocratic elite of the Imperial Court to be used as an aid to concentration and religious meditation. During *ko-do* (the way of fragrance) ceremonies, celebrants were required to 'listen to the incense'. Known as *ko-o-kiku*, the art was as loaded with meaning and codes as *ikebana* (flower arranging) and the tea ceremony.

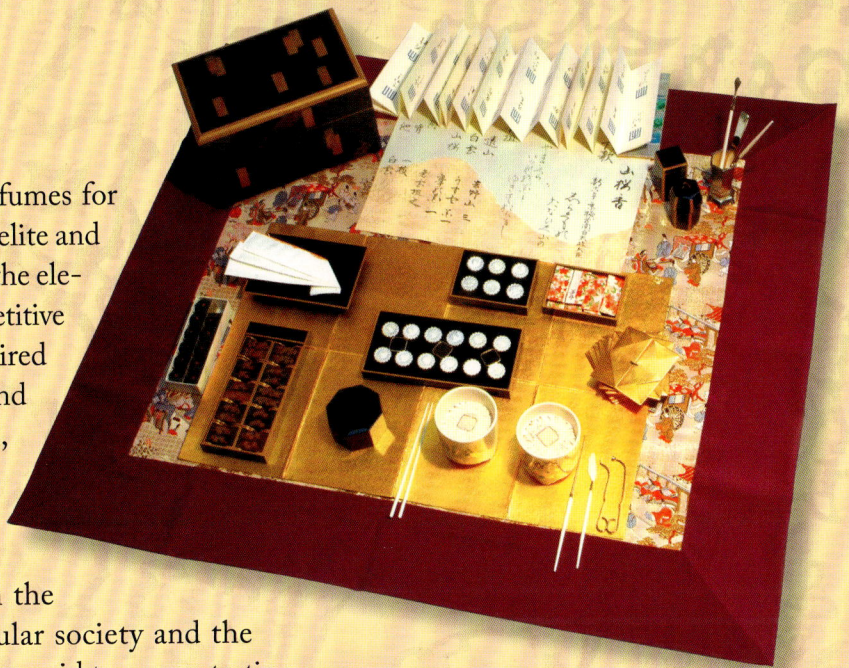

Takasago kodo: a game that involves identifying wood mixes by their smell and then matching them with symbols, Japan, twentieth century. International Perfume Museum, Grasse, France.

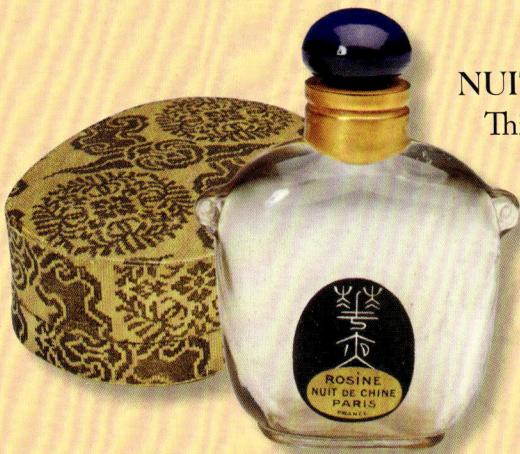

NUIT DE CHINE BY PAUL POIRET

This perfume, from 1913, embodies Paul Poiret's love of Oriental art, which was also reflected in his fashion. It comes in an imitation jade glass bottle not unlike a classical Chinese opium snuff box. The name is also written in Chinese characters. It is a warm heady blend of patchouli, jasmine, rose, cinnamon, clove, vetiver, labdanum, amber and musk. To accompany his perfume, he created the slogan 'Je ne prêche pas l'économie, je ne vous parle que d'élégance, achetez Nuit de Chine,' which translates as something like, 'Forget economy, elegance is what matters. Buy Nuit de Chine.'

MITSOUKO BY GUERLAIN

Jacques Guerlain's creation (1919) was one of the first perfumes to seamlessly combine natural and synthetic ingredients. It is a sensuous chypre (a heady sandalwood-based perfume) with mossy, earthy notes enhanced by the addition of peach-scented aldehydes. At a time when Europe was infatuated with the culture of the Far East, the fragrance took the name of the heroine of Claude Farrère's 1909 novel *La Bataille* (The Battle), which tells the tale of the impossible love affair between a Japanese admiral's wife, called Mitsouko, meaning 'mysterious', and a British naval officer during the 1905 Russian–Japanese war.

No scent without sun

Never in its history has perfume come from cold regions. For this reason, the perfume industry could not exist without the floral and aromatic resins and precious woods that have always come from sunny Eastern climates. For the West, the East is a land of fantasy and dreams. Orientalism, a Western literary and art movement of the nineteenth century, is the embodiment of this concept. It highlights the West's interest at the time in Arab cultures, particularly those of Turkey and the Maghreb. Perfumers were truly fascinated by the opulence and exoticism of the East, and each expressed their vision in their own unique way.

SHALIMAR BY GUERLAIN

At once fresh and light and rich and sensual, Shalimar (1925) is a perfume of paradoxes. It comes in a beautiful stupa-inspired bottle designed by Raymond Guerlain for the 1925 Paris Exhibition. Jacques Guerlain's masterpiece takes its name from the gardens of Shalimar, which is Sanskrit for 'temple of love'. Located in Lahore, they provided a backdrop for the seventeenth-century love affair between the Mughal emperor Shah Jahan and his beloved wife Mumtaz Mahal. After her death, Sha Jahan had the Taj Mahal built near Agra as her mausoleum.

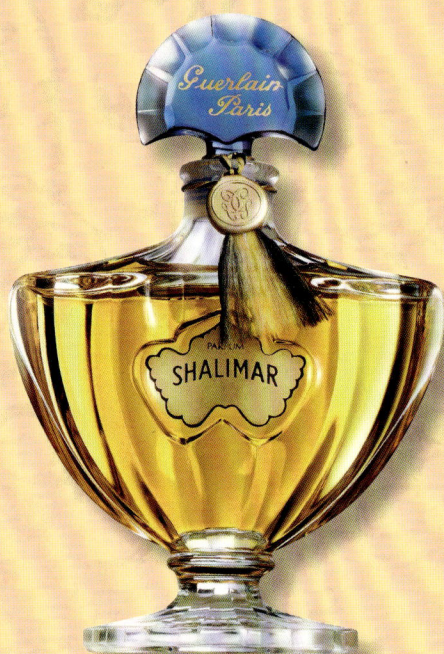

AMBRE SULTAN BY SERGE LUTENS

This heady, generous perfume from 1993 commemorates Serge Lutens' first trip to Morocco in 1968. An artist of many passions – photography, drawing, film, fashion and, of course, perfume creation – he was one of the very first perfumers to make a feminine fragrance with dominant Atlas cedar notes, his 1992 Féminité du Bois. That same year he opened his Palais-Royal boutique in Paris for the Shiseido brand to showcase luxury perfumes and long-forgotten ingredients. Greatly inspired by Middle Eastern culture, Serge Lutens experienced a shock to the senses when he first visited the Marrakesh souk, where cedar notes blended with synthetically scented amber resin. His Ambre Sultan was created to celebrate this delightful mix of fragrances and pay homage to the rulers of Morocco.

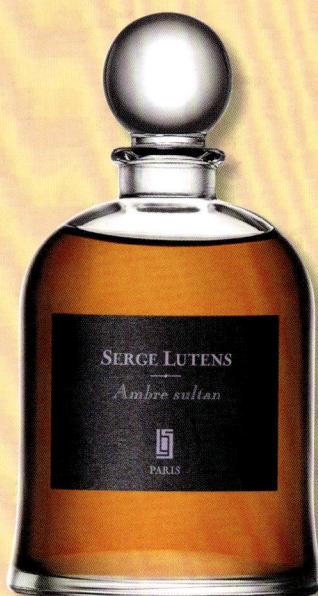

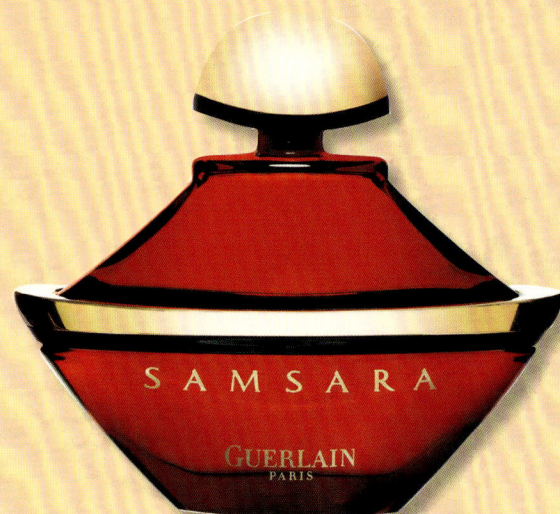

BYZANCE BY ROCHAS

In the city of Byzantium, the most magnificent of its time, the sixth-century Empress Theodora's gown had glittered with precious stones, according to a contemporaneous mosaic in Ravenna, Italy. The Ottoman Empire destroyed Byzantium, taking control and renaming it Constantinople, in 1453. But the grandeur and opulence of the former Byzantium inspired many perfumers, including Parfums Rochas, who in 1987 created a light, delicately floral oriental perfume for which they used the city's French name, Byzance. An abundance of rose and jasmine, cedar, sandalwood and musk add a sense of opulence. The blue bottle with its gold medallion is also very much in keeping with the Byzantine style.

SAMSARA BY GUERLAIN

The name Samsara has roots in southeast Asia, coming as it does from a Sanskrit word which means 'cycle of birth and rebirth', the wheel of life. The red of the bottle is a sacred colour in Buddhism and the perfume itself, from 1989, is a beautiful expression of sandalwood, an Indian wood and one of Jean-Paul Guerlain's favourite raw materials. It is combined with jasmine sambac, a sacred flower collected at dawn by women singing love songs and offered up in Hindu temples. The warmth of the accord is prolonged by vanilla and tonka bean and the bottle, by Robert Granai, was inspired by a statue of a Cambodian dancer. This highly concentrated perfume also revived the fashion for Eastern fragrances, but in a

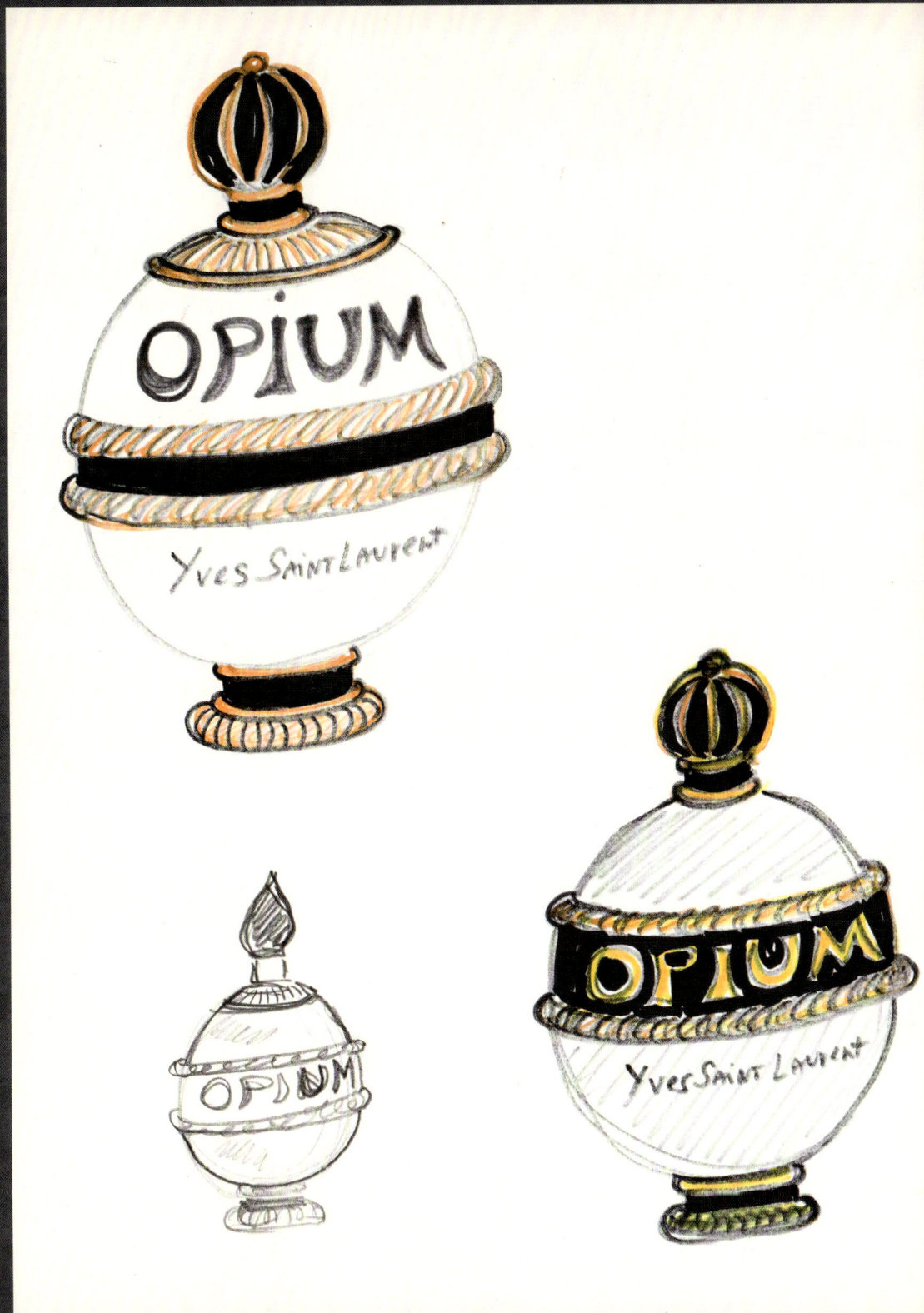

Research sketch for Opium perfume bottle, circa 1977.
Musée Yves Saint Laurent Paris.

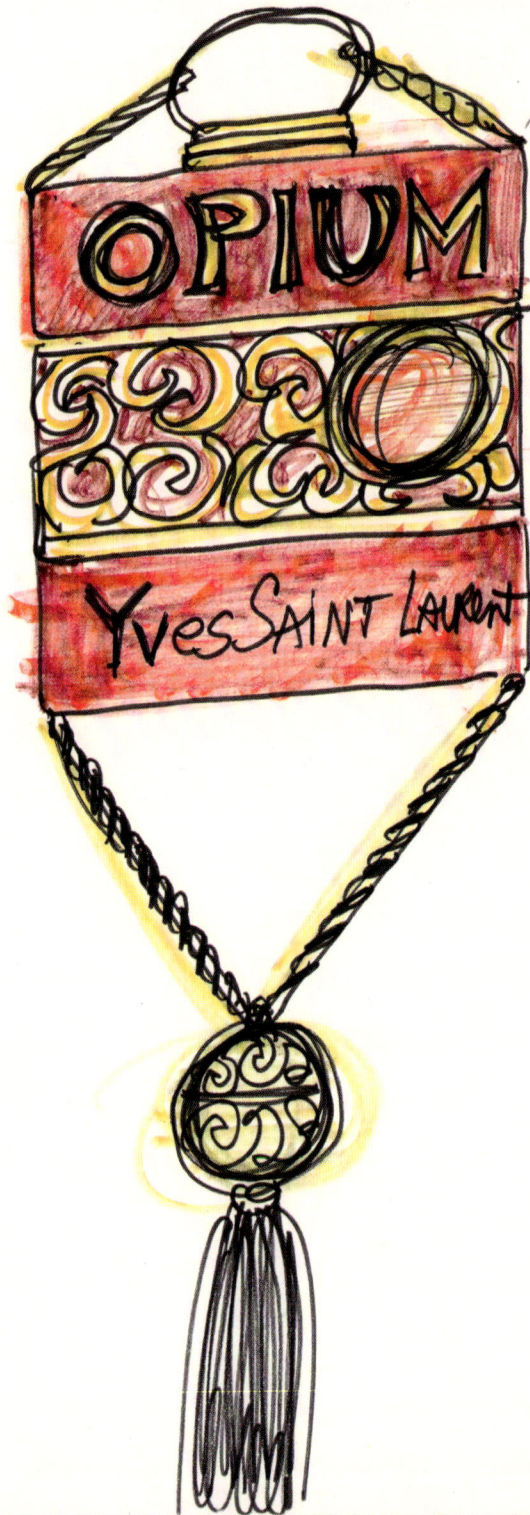

Research sketch for Opium perfume flask, circa 1977.
Musée Yves Saint Laurent Paris.

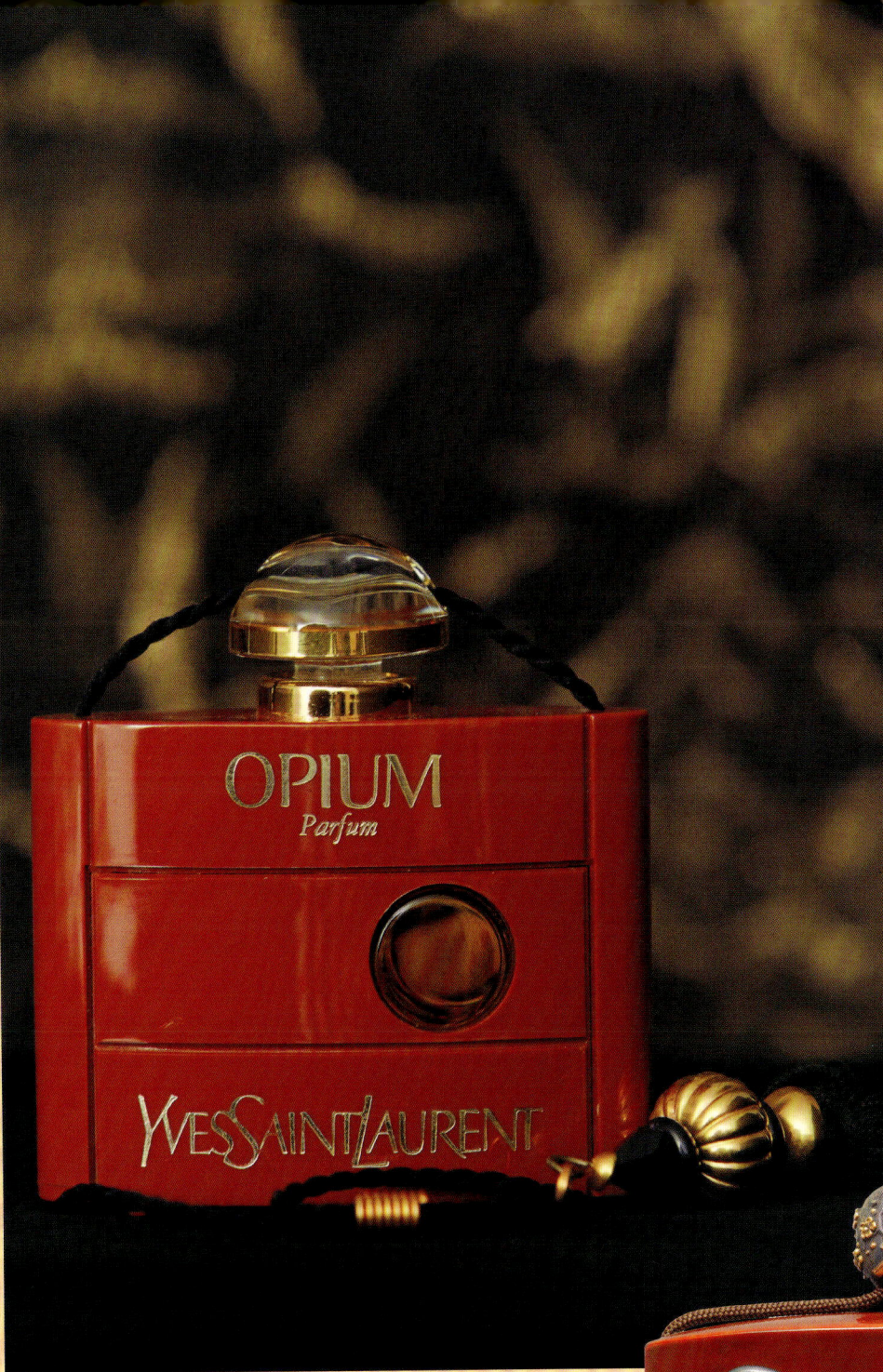

more seductive manner. The stopper is fashioned on Japanese *netsuke* and the bottle is inspired by the *inrô* (*in*: seal; *rô*: box), a small portable Japanese lacquered wood case with drawers. It was closed by a cord and topped with a sculpted ball (the *netsuke*) depicting a person or animal, and used to carry medicinal herbs and aromatics, precious objects or opium for pain relief. The *inrô* was slipped under a samurai's kimono and attached by a silk cord.

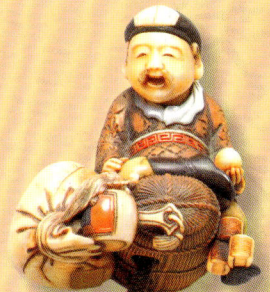

OPIUM BY YVES SAINT LAURENT

In eighteenth-century China, opium dens were much frequented by Westerners, who consumed excessive quantities of the drug, as a means either of cultural immersion or escapism. This perfume (1977) embodies Yves Saint Laurent's fascination with the East: 'Opium is the *femme fatale*, the pagodas, the lanterns.'

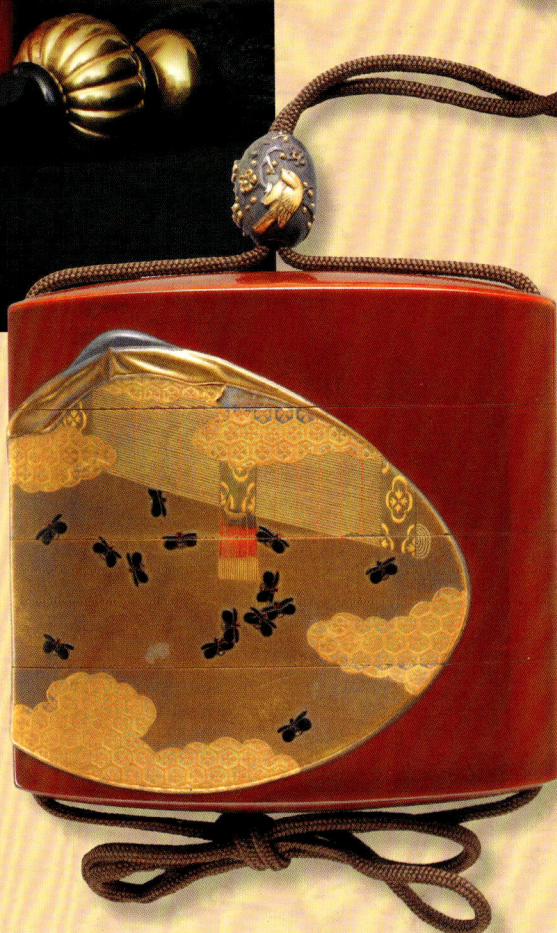

An *inrô* (small lacquered case) decorated with shells and fireflies, Japan, late eighteenth century.

PERFUME AT VERSAILLES

THE PALACE OF LOUIS XIV, THE SUN KING, WAS BUILT TO RADIATE SPLENDOUR AND BECAME A MODEL FOR OTHERS THROUGHOUT EUROPE. CONSTRUCTION BEGAN IN 1661. EACH DAY, BETWEEN THREE AND TEN THOUSAND PEOPLE FLOCKED TO VERSAILLES, BUT SANITARY FACILITIES WERE RUDIMENTARY AND PERFUMES WERE USED PRIMARILY FOR HYGIENE AND MEDICAL PURPOSES. THAT SAID, THEIR SCENT DID ADD A TOUCH OF ELEGANCE AND SOPHISTICATION!

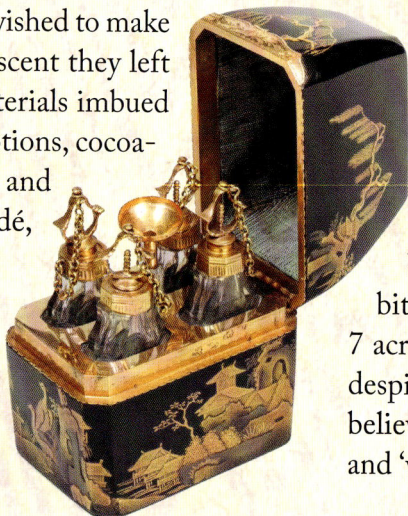

Seventeenth-century drawing depicting Madame de Montespan at the Château de Clagny, which once stood in Versailles.

LOUIS XIV

Louis XIV was a great patron of the arts and literature and turned the French court into a playground of luxury and pleasure. During his reign, perfume arrived at Versailles as a royal privilege reserved for the elite, in much the same way that it was the preserve of the gods in ancient times. In 1693, the Parisian perfumer Simon Barbe, in his manual *The French Perfumer*, described Louis XIV as 'the sweetest-smelling king of all'. This referred to his role as absolute monarch ruling by divine right – rather than his body odour which, if we are to believe the memoirs of the Duke de Saint-Simon, was not very fragrant at all.

Perfumers created personalized scented waters for famous clients who wished to make an impression at court by the scent they left in their wake. People used materials imbued with fragrant essences, body lotions, cocoa- and vanilla-scented creams … and some, like the Prince de Condé, even flavoured their tobacco.

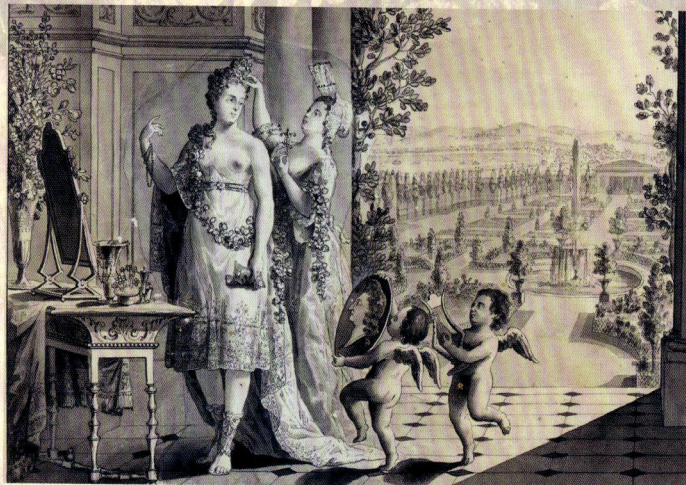

Perfume case containing four crystal bottles with gold stoppers and a perfume funnel, also gold, by Antoine Jan de Villeclair, circa 1755–6.

THE KING'S PERFUME FOUNTAINS

To please his favourites, the most famous being Louise de La Vallière, Marie-Angélique de Fontanges and Françoise Athénaïs de Montespan, the king developed a liking for strong perfume. He also commissioned the architect Louis Le Vau to have a small castle nicknamed the Palace of Flora, later the Porcelain Trianon, built in the grounds of Versailles for the Marquise de Montespan. It was surrounded by rare flowers with the strongest fragrances, filling the air with heady aromas. At Versailles, jasmine grew in the flowerbeds designed by landscape architect André Le Nôtre, and the varieties were often chosen for their strongly scented blooms. In *The French Perfumer*, Simon Barbe described the court's use of perfume, saying that the flowers chosen were orange blossom, rose, nutmeg, tuberose and jasmine, which all have heady smells and were selected because of the use of skins to cover women's bodies, boxes and other similar items.

By the end of his reign, the only fragrance Louis XIV liked was orange-blossom water, which he even used to scent the fountains of Versailles. This water was made from the bitter oranges grown in the Orangery built by Jules Hardouin-Mansart between 1684 and 1686. The king had some 2,000 bitter orange trees planted in the vast 3-hectare (over 7 acres) space. In the latter years of his life, Louis XIV despised all perfumes and banned them from the court, believing that they were responsible for the headaches and 'vapours' which beset him until his death in 1715.

According to Diderot and d'Alembert's *Encyclopedia* (1751), both men and women were now expected to be 'light insects in ephemeral, alluring attire who flit about and shake their powdery wings'. Heavier animal scents would soon be replaced by volatile balsamic and floral fragrances. Having embraced the idea of hygiene that had first appeared in England, the French were now open to subtler fragrances. Perfume was no longer used to guard against unpleasant smells. Its purpose was seduction. Whether it was an essential prerequisite of gallantry or not, it was very much part of a man's grooming habits.

Eau de Cologne was first introduced to Versailles by soldiers returning from the Seven Years' War. The king, Louis XV, began to use it for its revitalizing and invigorating properties.

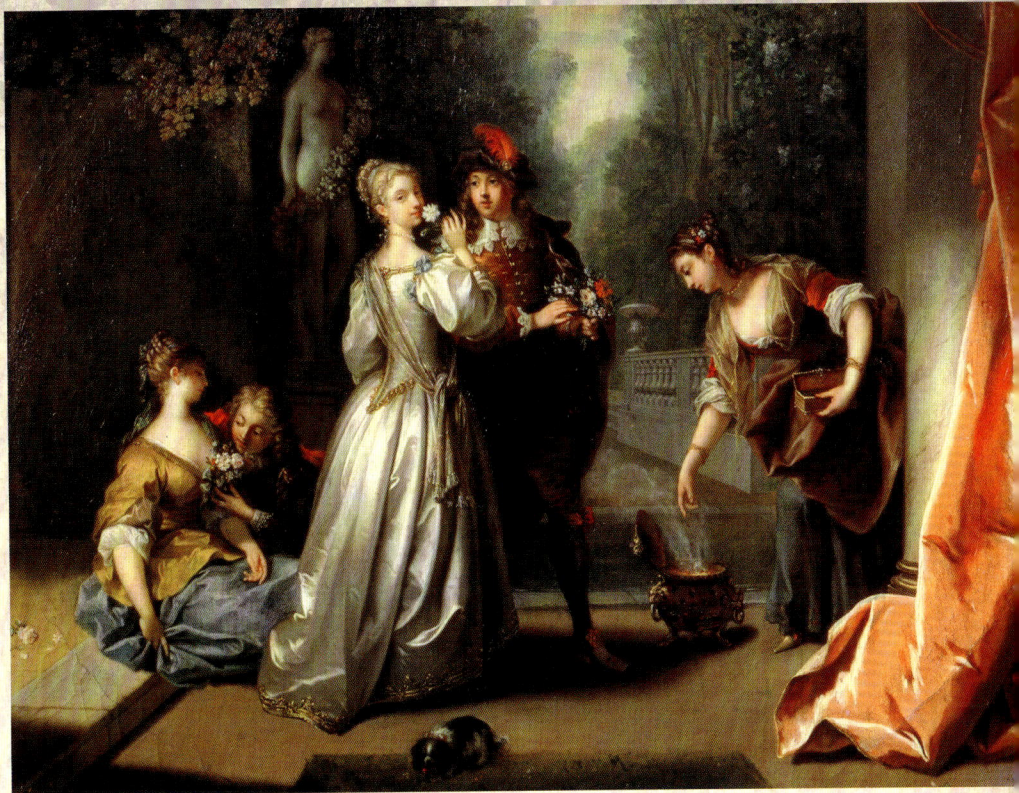

'Smell', from *The Five Senses* series of paintings by Jean Raoux, circa 1720–30.

LOUIS XV AT THE PERFUMED COURT

Under Louis XV, whose reign began in 1722, the elite learned to smell nice again, and the concept of hygiene gradually returned to Versailles. After the turbulent regency of Philippe I, Duke of Orléans, nonchalance reigned supreme at court, nicknamed the 'perfumed court' because it was fashionable to perfume everything and to wear a different fragrance every day, and even at different times of day. Everyone at the time wore perfume, except the philosophers, who condemned it and used their unpleasant odour to try to stand out from the crowd. In 1768, the society chronicler Louis-Antoine Caraccioli wrote that all the veneers were perfumed, from the panelling to the minds. Indeed, on 1 January, the king himself gifted his own fragrant creations to the ladies of the court. Makeup and perfume lover Madame de Pompadour, who spent no fewer than 100,000 livres each year on scent, was prominent in the creation of the perfumed court. She supported the manufacture of porcelain and biscuit-porcelain perfume bottles at the Sèvres factories and gave visiting diplomats small bottles of rose essence, allegedly distilled by the king himself in his chambers. The gardens of the Grand Trianon had an area given over entirely to plants or flowers grown specifically for the production of royal scented waters.

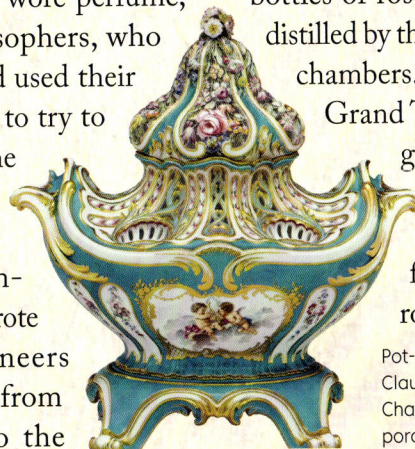

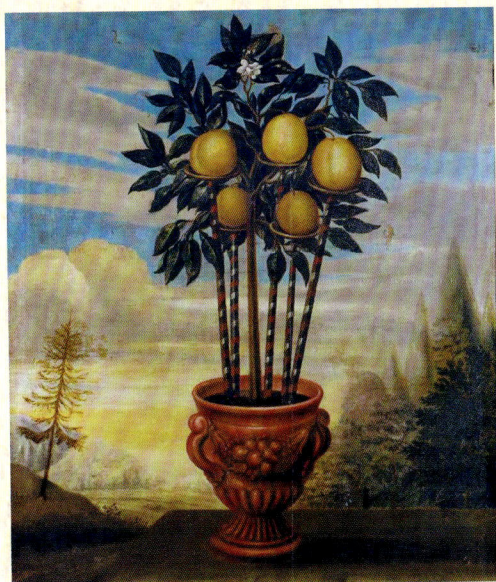

Pot-pourri holder by Jean-Claude Duplessis, decorated by Charles Nicolas Docin. Sèvres porcelain, eighteenth century.

JEAN-LOUIS FARGEON, MARIE-ANTOINETTE'S PERFUMER

Merchants welcomed the 1770 marriage of Marie-Antoinette and the Dauphin, the future King Louis XVI, as positive for the capital's luxury trade. Like many others, Jean-Louis Fargeon, who belonged to a long line of perfumers, began to dream of serving the Dauphine. In 1773, he decided to go to Paris with the aim of becoming perfumer to the future queen. She, to set the right tone, was said to have wanted only Parisian suppliers because, since the Regency, they had become much more creative than those in Versailles. Fargeon was hired as an apprentice by widow Vigier, whose husband had been the perfumer of Louis XV, and in 1774 he became a master glover–perfumer. The same year, Louis XV died and the 18-year-old Marie-Antoinette was crowned Queen of France alongside her husband Louis XVI, who was only two years her senior. Eighty-seven merchants attended the court and created thousands of objects to flatter the young queen, whose beauty charmed all who met her. Now one of the queen's suppliers, Jean-Louis Fargeon collaborated with both her hairdresser, Léonard, supplying him with floral oils and jasmine-scented hair pomades, and her dressmaker, Rose Bertin, perfuming the fabric flowers she sewed on the queen's gowns. Over time, he could count almost all court members among his clients, including Louis XV's daughters and the king's brothers.

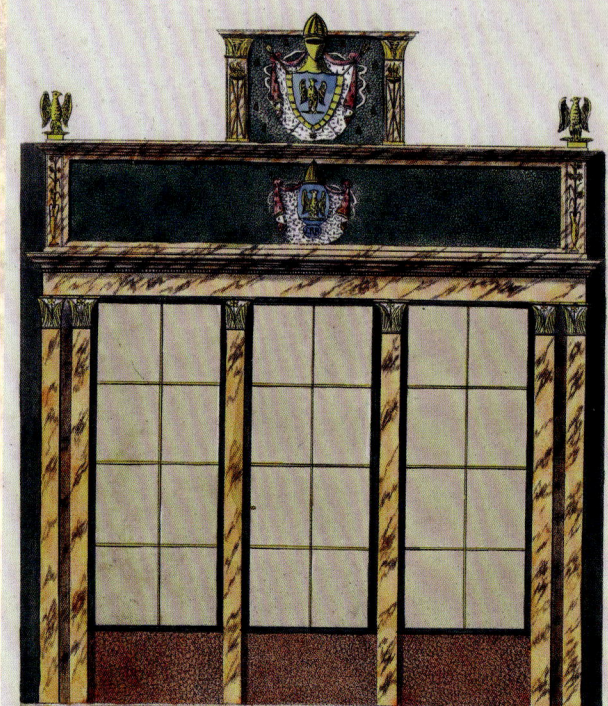

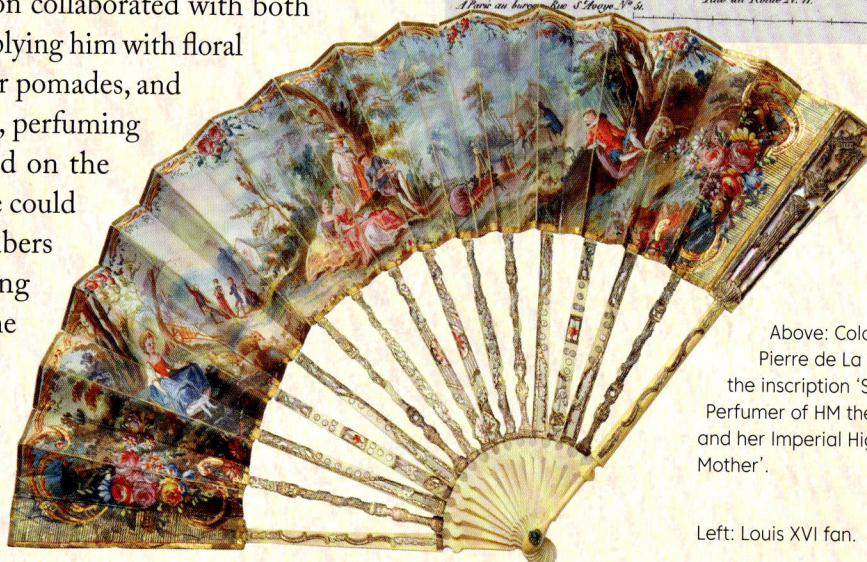

Above: Coloured etching by Pierre de La Mésangère, bearing the inscription 'Shop of Mr Fargeon, Perfumer of HM the Queen–Empress, and her Imperial Highness, the Queen Mother'.

Left: Louis XVI fan.

Technological advances

Since the reign of Louis XV, perfume making had been making giant strides. At his rue du Roule workshop in Paris, Jean-Louis Fargeon set out to improve the distillation technique. He now began using water distillation, distilling the raw materials several times and then separating the essential oils from the distilled water to obtain what were called ardent spirits. Enfleurage, a process developed in the city of Grasse at the time of Louis XV, was used to extract olfactory 'molecules' from flowers referred to as 'silent' because they were too delicate to yield anything by distillation. These technological advances injected a new-found creativity into the process because perfumers now had access to a wider range of scents and were no longer dependent on what was available seasonally. This was the origin of the floral *aux mille fleurs* (thousand flowers) bouquet, so called because the scent was made with flowers from every season.

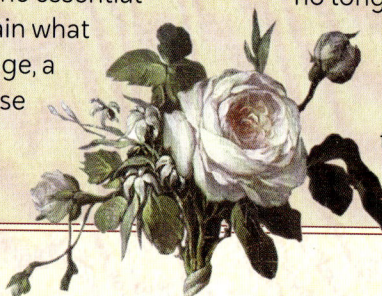

MARIE-ANTOINETTE AND ALL THINGS FRAGRANT

Marie-Antoinette bathed several times a week. Her ladies in waiting gave her 'modesty baths', rubbing her with soaps and sachets of plants to perfume and disinfect the bath water and turn it opaque to preserve her modesty. This dispensed with the need for her to use heavy, intoxicating scents to mask her body odour. The perfumer delivered to the queen's residence several dozen pairs of white gloves, dogskin mittens, bottles of lavender, litres of spirit of wine, pots of orange blossom and almond paste pomade, orange-flower powder, and taffeta-lined baskets scented with violet powder and cypress leaf, together with a myriad of accessories. Marie-Antoinette particularly loved Fargeon's scented fans which, after the death of her children and during the initial revolutionary unrest, she used increasingly to hide her tears rather than to conceal a mocking smile. Fargeon created for her a radical vinegar, known as spirit of Venus. She also enjoyed his lemon, double orange flower and cucumber pomades, *aux mille fleurs*-scented sticks, lavender spirit waters, jasmine pomades, Eau de Cologne and scented sachets. Fargeon chose contemporary names for his perfumes, such as Bouton d'Or (buttercup), Prés Fleuris (flowering meadow) and Eau de Bouquet de Printemps (spring bouquet).

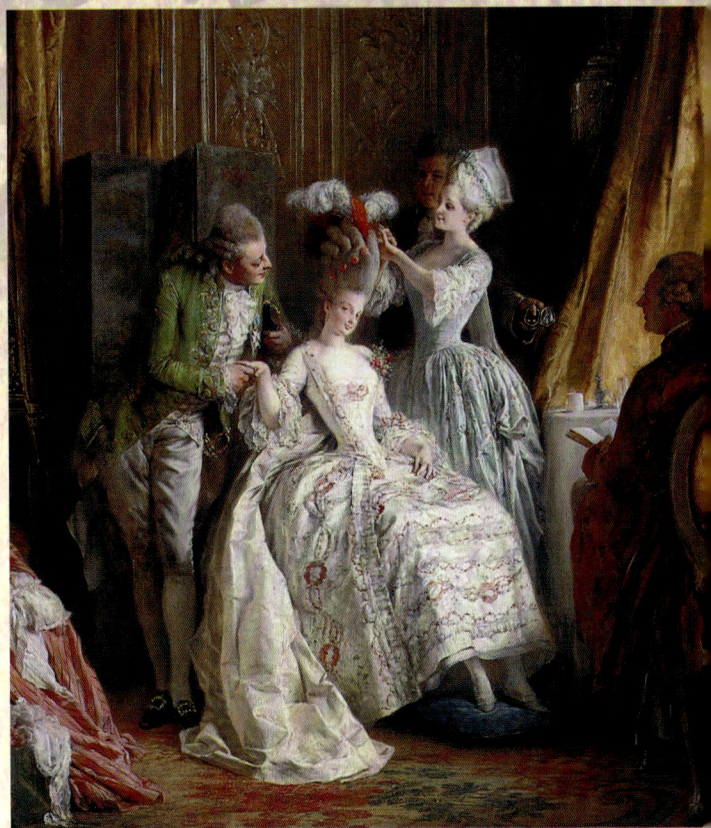

Heinrich Lossow painting depicting Marie-Antoinette having her hair done, nineteenth century.

JEAN-FRANÇOIS HOUBIGANT, FARGEON'S RIVAL

In 1775, Jean-François Houbigant, who benefited from the patronage of the Duchess of Charost, opened a boutique called À la Corbeille de Fleurs at 19, rue du Faubourg-Saint-Honoré in Paris. It was an immediate success. He married Adélaïde Nicole Deschamps, the daughter of a Faubourg-Saint-Honoré perfumer for whom he had worked as an apprentice. The Marquis de Polignac, Comtesse de Pontchartrain, Marquise de Grammont and Bishop Antoine-Eustache d'Osmont … aristocrats and the local bourgeoisie, both men and women, and even the clergy, were among his clients and bought perfumes, gloves, powders and pomades from him. He launched a refreshing, soothing floral water, Eau d'Houbigant, and also sold wig powder, *aux mille fleurs* extracts, gloves and fans, incense bricks and, in honour of his patron, a 'Duchess pomade'. Eighteen years later, on 16 October 1793, Queen Marie-Antoinette was sentenced to death for high treason by the revolutionary court

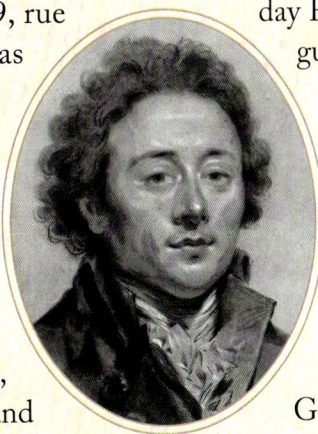

and beheaded. Imprisoned under the Reign of Terror, Jean-Louis Fargeon was released on 27 July 1794, the day Robespierre fell from power, and escaped the guillotine. He died in his apartment in 1806 at the age of 58. His widow and two sons then founded a company to carry on his work. The following year, on 22 October 1807, Jean-François Houbigant also died. His son, Armand-Gustave Houbigant, took over the business and the Maison Houbigant name continued to perfume elegant society. Today, Houbigant perfumes are still produced in Grasse, where Jean-François Houbigant developed his first creations. The Fargeon perfume dynasty, on the other hand, came to an end when his sons sold the family business to Jean-Baptiste Gellé, who, for centuries to come, was famous for his 'science-based products'.

Portrait of perfumer Jean-François Houbigant (1752–1807) by Claude Hoin (1750–1817).

THE GLOVER–PERFUMER COMMUNITY

FROM THE RENAISSANCE UNTIL THE END OF THE EIGHTEENTH CENTURY, IT WAS THE GLOVER–PERFUMERS, AND NO LONGER APOTHECARIES, DISTILLERS, DRUGGISTS OR CHEMISTS, WHO MONOPOLIZED THE PERFUME INDUSTRY. PERFUMER WAS A COMMON TERM FOR SEVERAL OTHER ACTIVITIES THAT WERE CONDUCTED BETWEEN PARIS, MONTPELLIER AND GRASSE, EARNING FRANCE A REPUTATION AS PERFUME'S ELECTED HOME.

A female glover–perfumer in the eighteenth century. Etching by Pierre Vidal from an illustration by Nicolas Edme Restif de La Bretonne.

AN EXACTING, METICULOUS PROFESSION

The guild of glover–perfumers had its origins in the tanning industry, which used heavy perfume to mask the unpleasant smells that clung to tanned leather. Philippe II of France granted a charter to the first guild of master glovers and perfumers in 1190. In 1387, John the Good confirmed the privileges granted and the community's coat of arms. The guild was based at the Église des Innocents and chose Saint Anne as its patron saint. Henry III drew up a charter in 1582 and Louis XIII issued letters patent in 1614 authorizing the glovemakers of France to 'call themselves and describe themselves as both glovers and perfumers'. In his 1656 statutes, expanded by the Community of Glover–Perfumers, Louis XIV declared that no one could be admitted as 'marchand maître gantier parfumeur' (master glover–perfumer and merchant) unless they had completed an apprenticeship with the masters and produced a masterpiece. The aspiring apprentices were then taken to the King's Procurer at the Châtelet in Paris to swear an oath and be received as master. As the qualities required for the glover–perfumer profession were cleanliness and attention to detail, rather than physical strength, it was open to women, who were themselves often seamstresses.

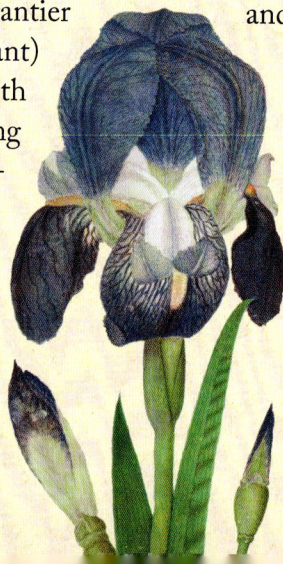

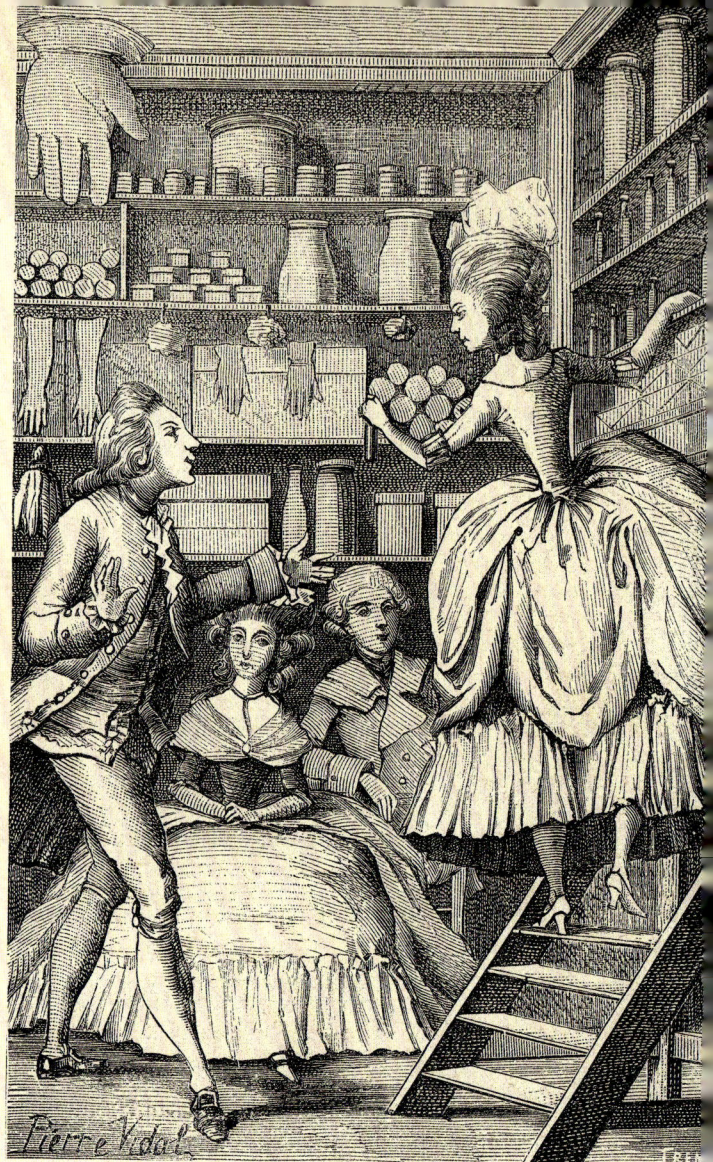

PARIS: THE EPITOME OF LUXURY AND ELEGANCE

In 1725, there were 250 glover–perfumers working in Paris and sourcing their materials from Grasse or Montpellier. From the Regency period, when a young Louis XV was on the throne, the profession of perfumer had become the most lucrative in the capital. In the nineteenth century, Paris and Grasse joined forces to form a profitable international trade network for the industry. Grasse harvested, traded and processed the raw materials, while the perfumes were created, manufactured and packaged in Paris. At the Great Exhibitions of the nineteenth and twentieth centuries, and the 1925 Exhibition, where Paris shone as a beacon of progress, it opened its doors to perfumers and couturiers.

Blue and white iris, drawing, 1608.

MONTPELLIER: CITY OF APOTHECARIES

In the Middle Ages, from the twelfth century onwards, the trading city of Montpellier had a renowned faculty of medicine, where merchants prepared and sold scented powders and waters. In the thirteenth century, most spices and aromatics entered France via the city's port. Apothecaries had two roles: they imported and manufactured drugs for the sick and also created and sold perfumes known as 'elixirs', which translates as 'the most precious medicines'. Because of Montpellier's *garrigue* (shrubland), where a variety of aromatic plant species grows, Queen of Hungary's Water (see page 40) became its speciality, around 1370, and was sold throughout Europe. The city was also home to glovers from 1551 onwards. They became glover–perfumers in 1750 and two local families, the Deloches and Fargeons, were the oldest and wealthiest in the trade. However, by 1750, the city's perfume trade was in decline, with Grasse taking over.

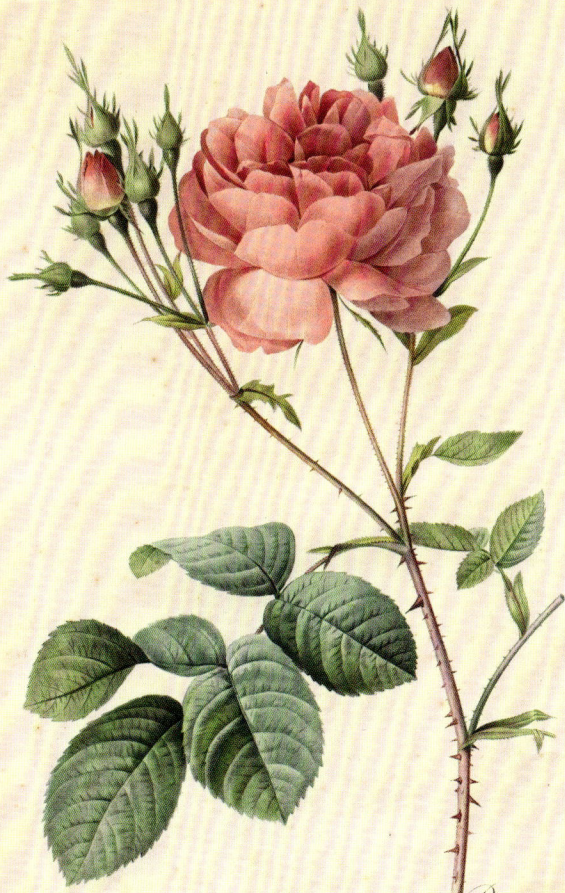

Rose of Cumberland (*Rosa centifolia Anglica rubra*) and Yellow and White Iris (*Iris ochroleuca*) by Pierre-Joseph Redouté (1759–1840) in *Les Liliacées*.

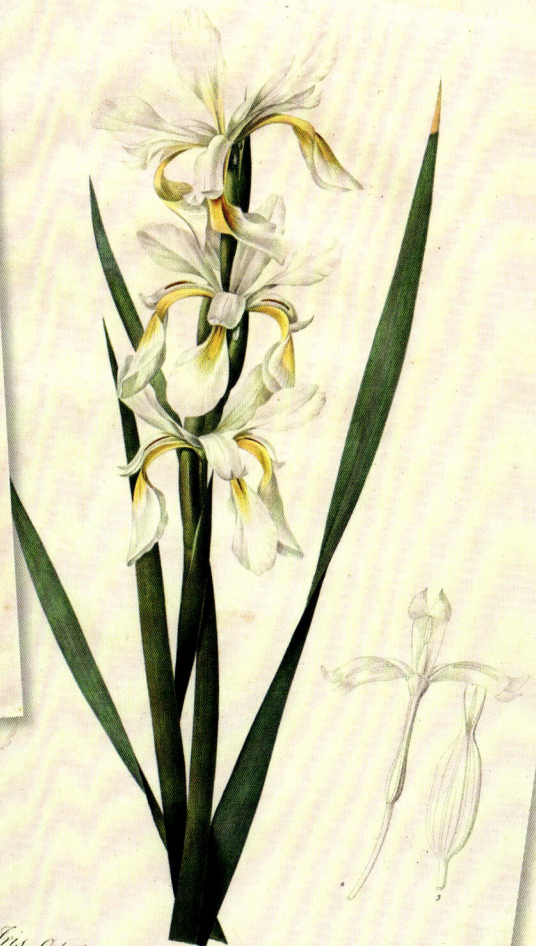

59

Advert for jewellery and 'all sorts of perfumes and generally all things concerning a Lady's *Toilette* at a boutique on Place des Terreaux, Lyons, 1730.

GRASSE: TOWN OF TANNERS AND FLOWERS

The Grasse perfume industry developed because of its tanneries, which had been in the town since the Middle Ages, its trade route with Italy and Europe, its Provençal microclimate and a large plantation of bitter orange trees. Grasse specialized in leather tanning and the tanners devised scented waters to mask the stench given off by the tanned leather. In the seventeenth century, because of taxes on leather and competition from Nice, the leather industry declined and perfumery took its place. Famous for its cultivation of perfumed plants, such as jasmine and cabbage roses, Grasse became the perfume capital of the world. From the nineteenth century onwards, the town developed into an international hub where raw materials were harvested, traded and processed, while the actual manufacture of the perfumes was left to companies in Paris. From 1900, French perfume production expanded rapidly and the Grasse manufacturers took charge of the lucrative activity of importing the raw materials, primarily exotic essences. Now, in the early twenty-first century, perfume is still Grasse's main business and the town continues to play a leading role in the industry.

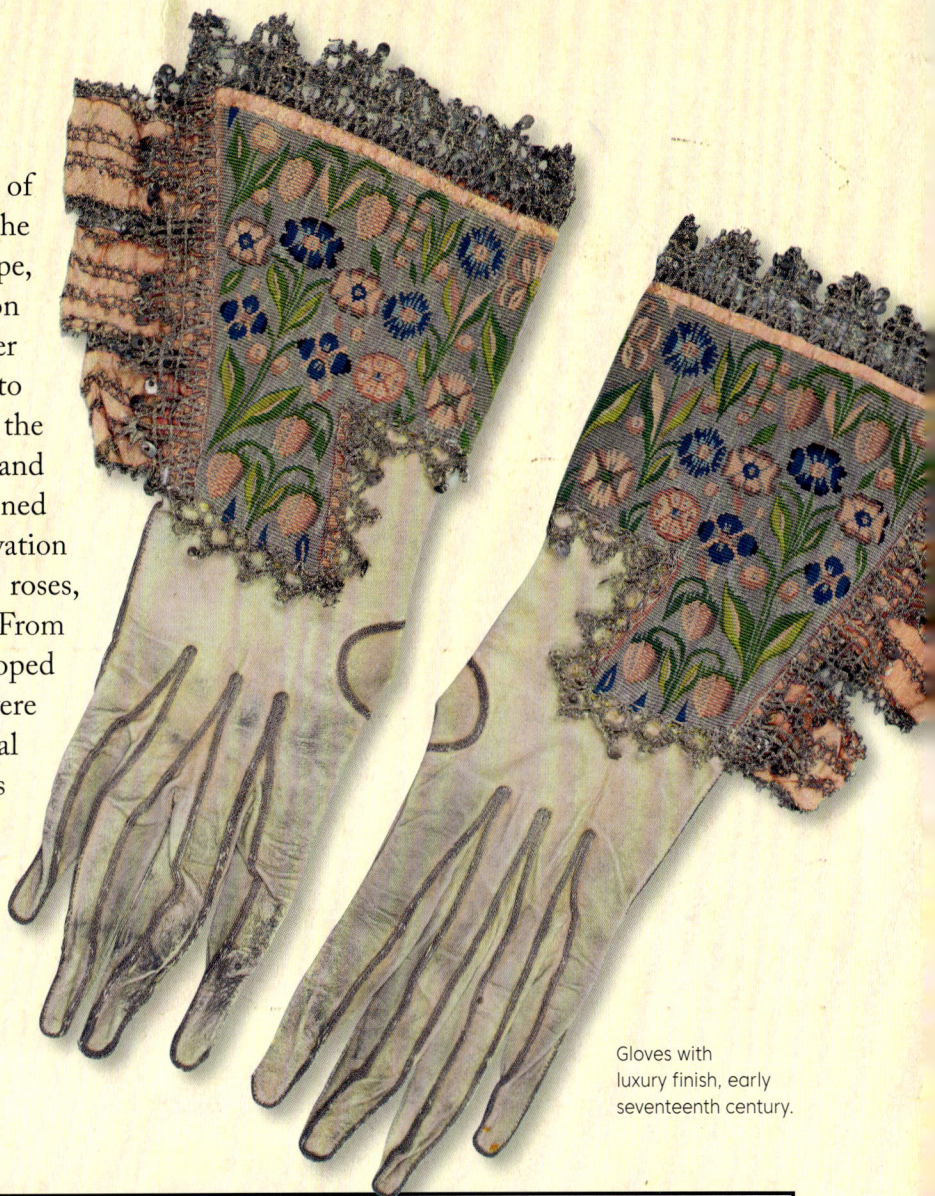

Gloves with luxury finish, early seventeenth century.

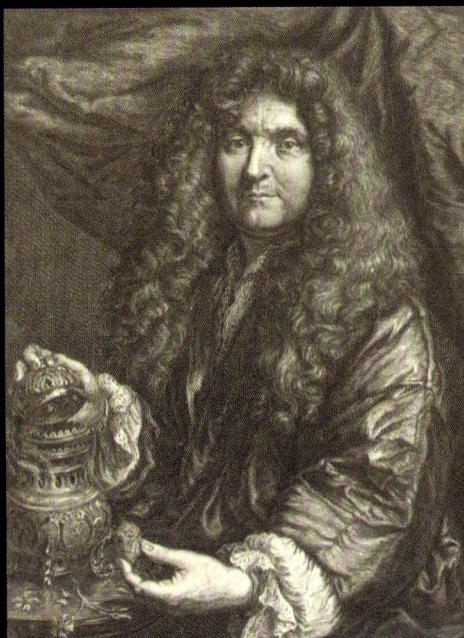

Court connections

In 1533, Catherine de' Medici arrived in France from Italy betrothed to the future Henry II, bringing with her René le Florentin, her personal perfumer. He opened an elegant boutique on the Pont-au-Change in Paris. Immediately, French perfumers began to follow the example of this former student of the Florence school, who excelled in the art thanks to the new aromatic substances brought back by the explorers of the time: Vasco de Gama, Ferdinand Magellan and Marco Polo. During Louis XIV's reign, the king's valet, Martial, was also an apothecary and perfumer. In 1699, the glover–perfumer Simon Barbe published a famous treatise on perfumery entitled *The Royal Perfumer*. Colbert's (see page 27) trade policy granted the perfume industry considerable privileges with a view to promoting French arts and crafts, and ultimately securing the exports that would bring into the kingdom the gold it could not produce because it had no gold mines. In the eighteenth century, the perfume industry took over from glove making and in March 1791, the Paris Community of Glover–Perfumers was disbanded and a free market established.

Portrait of perfumer Jean Chabert by Jacques Buys, in the style of Adriaen van der Kabel, circa 1675–1700.

THE BIRTH OF EAU DE COLOGNE

SINCE ITS INVENTION IN 1695, EAU DE COLOGNE
HAS BECOME A UNIVERSALLY POPULAR PERFUME.
UNTIL THE 1960S, IT WAS SAID THAT IF YOU RUBBED
YOURSELF LIBERALLY WITH EAU DE COLOGNE
EACH MORNING YOU WOULD HAVE A GOOD DAY.
DESCRIBED AS FRESH, INVIGORATING, LIGHT,
SOOTHING AND BENEFICIAL, IT IS THE HEALTH AND
WELL-BEING STAR OF THE PERFUME INDUSTRY.

ITS ORIGIN STORIES

Health, hygiene, beauty … Eau de Cologne is at the crossroads
of these. According to legend, but also backed by written histo-
rical evidence, a young Italian named Giovanni Paolo Feminis
invented the citrus-based formula around 1695, calling it 'aqua
mirabilis'. He then passed it on to Giovanni Maria Farina and
Giovanni Antonio Farina, brothers who were probably apothecaries in Cologne, in 1709. According to other sources, including
the Roger&Gallet archives, Giovanni Paolo Feminis set off on
a mule for Cologne, where he is thought to have invented aqua
mirabilis from scratch. He is said to have passed the formula on
to his son-in-law, Giovanni Antonio Farina, who in turn left it
to his grandson, Jean-Marie Farina, when he died in 1788.
However, according to a different document belonging
to Roger&Gallet, Giovanni Paolo Feminis ran a
grocery business between Lombardy and Piedmont,
and moved to Cologne, where he sold 'sugar, citron
fruit, oranges and candied fruit'. Once there, he
distilled aqua mirabilis using a recipe he received
from an English officer who had returned from the
Indies, where he had allegedly cured a monk with
the miracle water. Whatever the case, a document
establishing the Eau de Cologne business corroborates
the link between the two family names: 'Feminis creator and
Antoine [Antonio] Farina distiller, at the Balance d'Or ['gold
scale' street] in Cologne.'

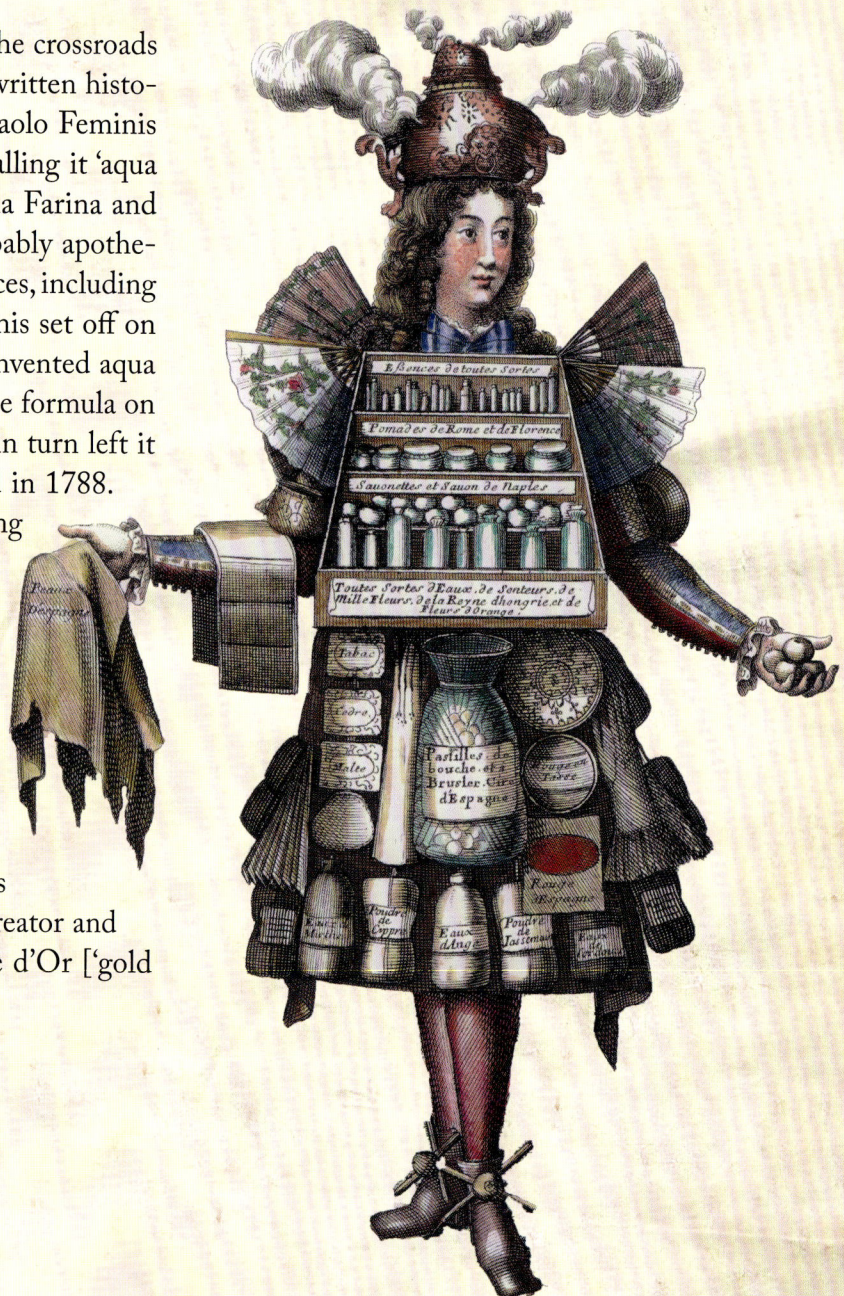

L'habit du parfumeur (The Perfumer's Costume),
from the series 'Les Costumes grotesques: habits
des métiers et professions' (Grotesque Costumes:
Uniforms of Trades and Professions), 1695.

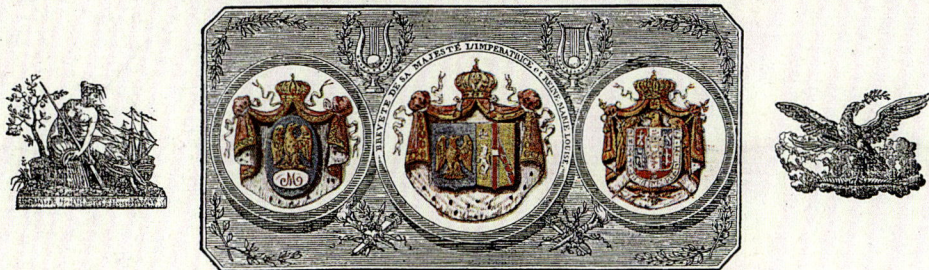

Eau de Cologne patent issued to Jean-Marie Farina, collection Roger&Gallet, published in *La Revue des marques de la parfumerie et de la savonnerie* (Review of Perfume and Soap Makers), 1925.

EAU DE COLOGNE AT VERSAILLES

Louis XV's army introduced what they called 'Eau de Cologne' to the court of Versailles at the end of the Seven Years' War. More of a medicine than a sophisticated fragrance at the time, its initial composition was spirit of wine, rosemary, lemon balm, bergamot, neroli, citron and lemon. In 1727, its health-giving properties were recognized by the Cologne Academy of Medicine. Many versions were made and competition became fierce, leading to a number of different eaux de Cologne (de Venise, Couronnée, Superbe, Sensuelle, Vigoureuse, Divine, Cordiale and others). It was a panacea with a fresh, light fragrance used both for healing, because of its high alcohol content, and for personal grooming. At the time, doctors in Europe still considered it dangerous to use water on the skin, so cloths soaked in lotions and vinegars were rubbed on the body.

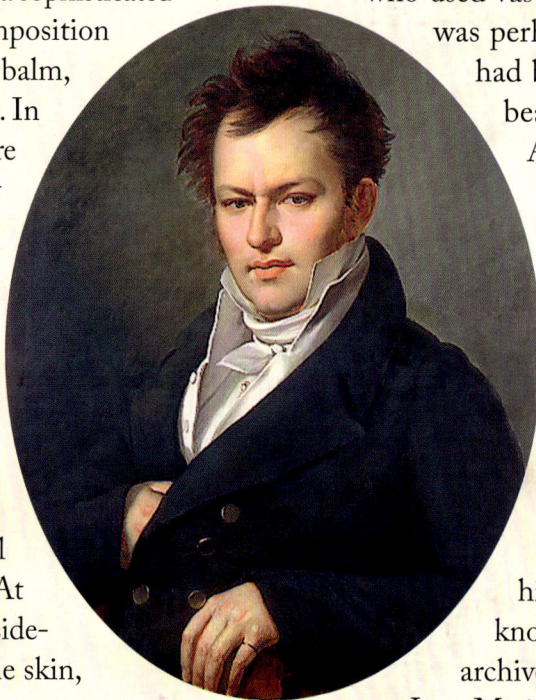

NAPOLEON AND EAU DE COLOGNE

At the age of 20, Jean-Marie Farina moved to Paris and in 1808 was awarded a warrant to supply Napoleon I, who used vast quantities of Eau de Cologne. This was perhaps not so surprising given that he had been born in Corsica, known for its beauty and sweet-smelling scrubland. As a student at the Brienne Military Academy in the Aube, far from his fragrant homeland, Napoleon wrote: 'Eyes closed, in the darkest night, if by some miracle I were transported to Corsica, I would recognize it immediately by its smell.' He had discovered the benefits of Eau de Cologne during his Italian campaign, but it was during his Egyptian campaign that he began to rub it on his body regularly. The wicker bottles known as 'Rouleau de l'Empereur' in the archives of Roger&Gallet, the successors of Jean-Marie Farina, are an indication of how often Napoleon used this beneficial water for his ablutions, as their oblong shape made it easy to slip one into his boot. As he suffered from liver disorders, he would have appreciated its invigorating and health-giving properties but also enjoyed its pleasant, but not overpowering, fragrance.

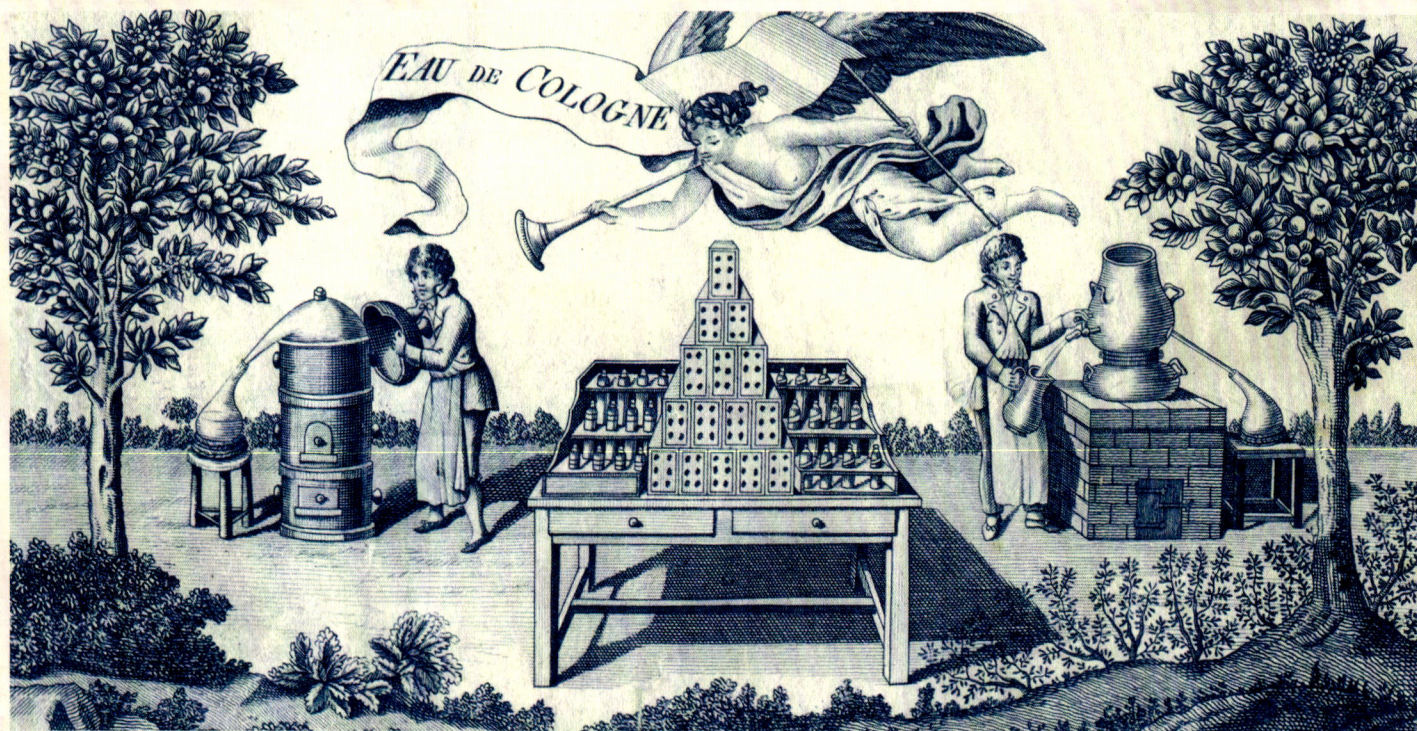

Above: Portrait of Jean-Marie Farina.

Below: Eau de Cologne, drawing from a medical and pharmaceutical leaflet.

A particularly hygiene-conscious emperor

Napoleon I is said to have used a bottle of Eau de Cologne a day, his consumption averaging 36–40 bottles a month in 1810. He also allegedly drank a few drops before going into battle. Constant, the emperor's first valet, recounts in his memoires that 'day and night, we kept water hot for his bath because he often decided to indulge in one at any hour of the day or night'. Napoleon loved bathing, which could take him several hours. The grooming regime that followed his very hot bath was meticulous and undertaken by four valets and a mamluk. During early morning conversations, he shaved then carefully washed his face, hands and nails, and Constant rubbed him with Eau de Cologne. He cleaned his teeth each day, using a wooden toothpick and a brush dipped in opium. Napoleon was a lifelong fan of the famous water and even had his mamluk, Ali, make him some using local ingredients while he was in exile on the island of St Helena.

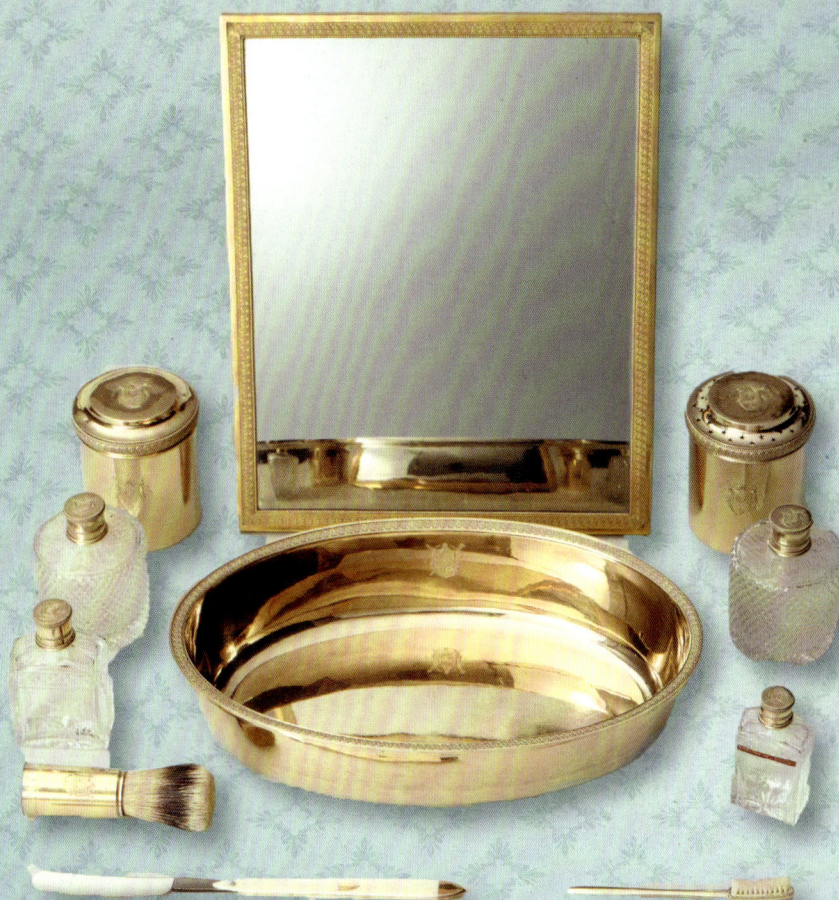

Travel kit belonging to Napoleon I and, later, Alexander I of Russia, 1807.

THE PERFUME ROUTE III

IN THE NINETEENTH AND TWENTIETH CENTURIES, FRANCE COLONIZED COUNTRIES IN NORTH AND EQUATORIAL AFRICA, SOUTHEAST ASIA, CENTRAL AMERICA AND MANY ISLANDS IN OCEANIA. THIS LED TO THE DISCOVERY AND CULTIVATION OF FRAGRANT SUBSTANCES NEW TO FRANCE, AND THE COUNTRY NO LONGER HAD TO RELY ON FOREIGN IMPORTS.

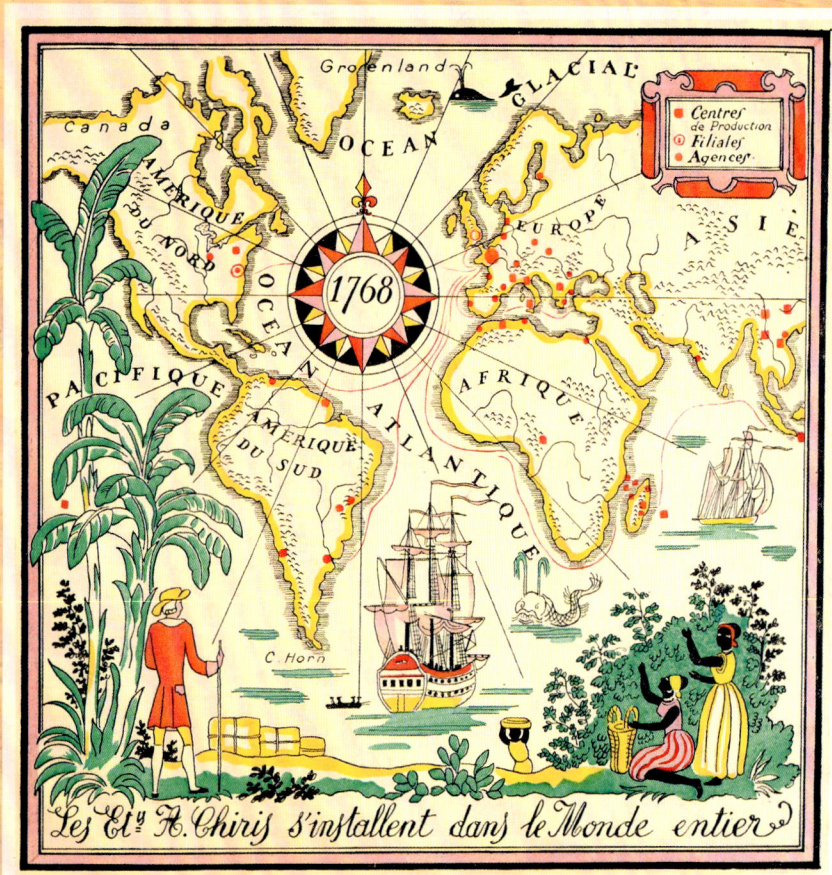

The Perfume Makers, by Rudolf Ernst, nineteenth century.

MADAGASCAR

France had control of the whole region from 1896 and farming, long abandoned by the locals, became one of the main industries. Initially, the focus was on sugar cane and sisal but gradually what were known

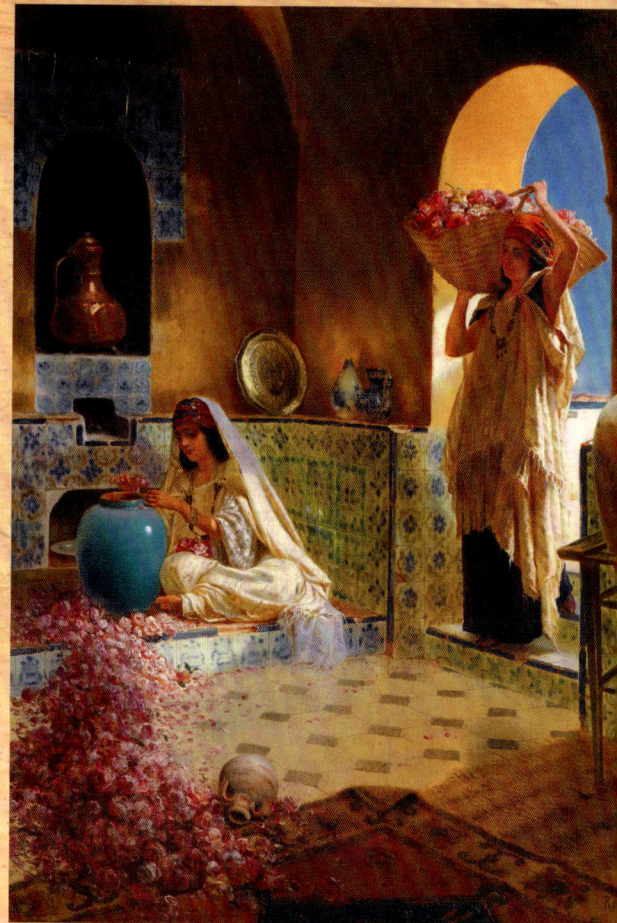

Établissements Antoine Chiris companies worldwide, 1931, Grasse.

as 'tropical crops' were grown. Some of these, including ylang-ylang, vanilla, clove, cinnamon, vetiver and patchouli, were of interest to the perfume market in Grasse. Around 1906, colonial companies such as Millot, created by Lucien Millot, established the first farms along the Sambirano River in the north of Madagascar. At the same time, the first semi-industrial plantations of ylang-ylang were introduced to the islands of Nosy Be, and later Nosy Komba, by the missionary Clément Raimbault. The Comoro Islands owe their perfume-plant plantations to the colonial company Bambao, owned by Établissements Antoine Chiris, who headed a Grasse perfumery.

ALGERIA

In the very early days of France's colonization of Algeria, Grasse perfumer Antoine Chiris bought the Sainte-Marguerite estate in Boufarik, where he built a factory of 3,000 square metres 9 (roughly three-quarters of an acre). Other 'perfume capital' companies followed suit, notably Roure-Bertrand, which also set up there. From the second half of the nineteenth century, the Grasse perfumers and a number of other settlers tried and successfully managed to acclimatize species of plants and trees for perfume making, such as geranium, eucalyptus, camphor, white lily, tuberose, acacia, lemongrass, rose, jasmine, lavender, petitgrain, mandarin, lemon and cypress in Boufarik and in the Oran and Constantine regions. Mignonette, violet, myrtle, pennyroyal, thyme and rosemary, as well as cedar, Aleppo pine and olive trees, could also be found in the surrounding countryside. Gradually, production in Algeria was narrowed down to geranium, eucalyptus, mint, rue, petitgrain, neroli and thyme.

EQUATORIAL AFRICA

Here, the soil and climate offered one major advantage. The natural raw materials could be harvested several times a year, whereas in Grasse, for example, only one harvest was possible. Roger&Gallet, Coty, Jeancard and Chiris trialled plantations in Equatorial Africa, primarily in Guinea, which was renowned for the quality of its orange essential oil.

ASIA

French perfume companies came to Indochina and the Dutch East Indies in search of star anise, benzoin, citronella, lemongrass, vetiver, cajeput, Annam heather, camphor, grapefruit, ylang-ylang, patchouli, cardamom, fragrant woods and musk. These species were grown across the region depending on the local climate. In Indochina, Établissements Antoine Chiris opened a factory in the 1920s in Tonkin (northern Vietnam), primarily for refining the star anise essence produced by Indochinese distillers and for Tonkin musk, which is similar to Chinese musk (known as true musk in some provinces of China).

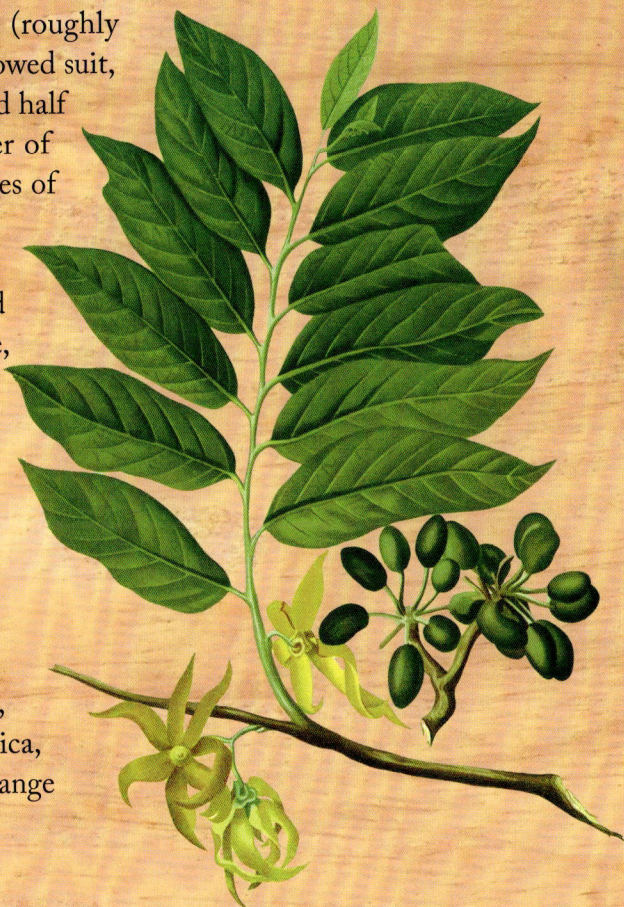

Ylang-ylang (*Cananga odorata*) leaves, flowers and fruit.

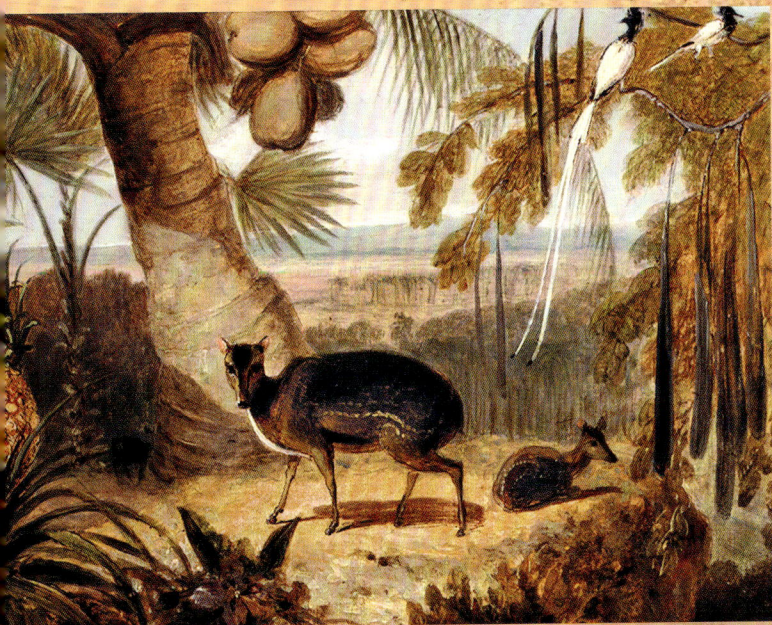

LATIN AMERICA AND OCEANIA

In the twentieth century, some French colonies, including French Guiana, Tahiti, Guadeloupe and Martinique, joined the international network of producers of fragrant, aromatic and medicinal plants. Towards the end of the nineteenth century, vast quantities of rosewood were brought back from French Guiana. In the first half of the twentieth century, Martinique and Guadeloupe produced a lot of vanillin, pepper, cloves, cinnamon and nutmeg and, at the same time, Tahiti specialized in vanilla production, specifically the variety *Vanilla tahitensis* 'Moore', which has warm, slightly smoky notes.

Musk Deer and Birds of Paradise, painting by William Daniell. Musk, which is nowadays mainly reproduced synthetically, used to be extracted from the abdominal glands of musk deer in Central Asia.

GUERLAIN, ONE OF FRANCE'S GREATEST PERFUMERS

ALMOST TWO CENTURIES HAVE PASSED, AND MANY PERFUMES HAVE BEEN CREATED, SINCE THE DAY IN 1828 WHEN EXPERT NOSE AND ASTUTE BUSINESSMAN PIERRE FRANÇOIS PASCAL GUERLAIN DECIDED TO FOLLOW HIS CONVICTIONS AND FIND SUCCESS. AFTER ALL, WOMAN OF LETTERS MADAME DE STAËL HAD PREDICTED THAT 'MODERN PERFUMERY IS THE MEETING POINT OF FASHION, CHEMISTRY AND BUSINESS.'

Pierre François Pascal Guerlain, purveyor to the Imperial Court.

THE RISE OF ONE OF THE GREATEST PERFUMERS IN HISTORY

Pierre François Pascal Guerlain was born in Abbeville, northern France, in 1798 to a pewterer and spice merchant. At the age of 19 he signed up as a travelling salesman and representative for some of the major perfume houses of the time. But he wanted to work for himself so he took a course in chemistry and soap making in England, where France's favourite perfumes, for example ones made by Yardley, were being produced, while continuing with his business commitments. Once he had perfected the art of perfumery, he returned to Paris and in 1828 established himself as a 'perfumer and vinegar maker, doctor and chemist', opening a shop on rue de Rivoli, which would subsequently relocate to rue de la Paix. In his factory next to the Arc de Triomphe, he would work in his laboratory, creating perfumes such as 'Bouquet Queen Victoria'. His quality products were popular with elegant Parisians.

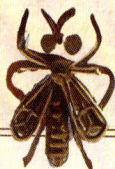

The Man Behind Eau De Cologne Imperiale

Guerlain was the official supplier of Eugenie de Montijo when she was still a mere countess. After she married Napoleon III, she did everything within her power to have Guerlain recognized as the 'Prince of Perfume' in the eyes of the court and the wider world. To thank her, he created Bouquet de l'Impératrice and, in 1853, dedicated his Eau de Cologne to her, which became known as Eau de Cologne Impériale. Having tired of the heady scents of cheap perfumes, the empress loved this extremely delicate blend of bergamot, lemon, rosemary and orange blossom. To honour the Empire, the bottle was a feat of technology made from semi-manufactured glass by French glassmaker Pochet. The current version is adorned with 69 bees in relief and has a gilded Guerlain label. The bees symbolize not only the Empire but also immortality and resurrection, reflecting the extent of Napoleon III's sovereignty at the time.

Eau de Cologne Impériale by Guerlain in its iconic gilded bee bottle.

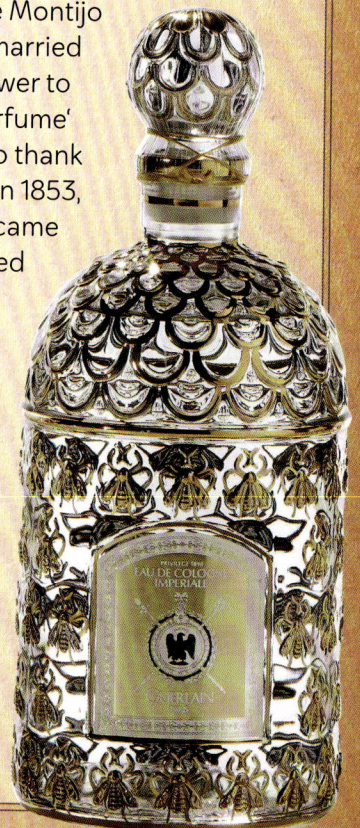

GUERLAIN: HER MAJESTY'S OFFICIAL PERFUMER!

On 11 May 1853, a letter signed by the Ministry of State on behalf of the empress and written by her secretary, Damas-Hinard, was sent from the Tuileries to inform Pierre François Pascal Guerlain that he had been appointed Her Majesty's official perfumer on account of the Eau de Cologne he had created in her honour. Subsequently, he received great acclaim in articles in *La Mode*, *La Corbeille* and *Le Petit Courrier des Dames* magazines.

The perfumer cleverly capitalized on his royal warrant by displaying the imperial coat of arms above his magnificent boutique on rue de la Paix in Paris. He also had it printed on his letterhead and all his sales documentation. As an added bonus, the title earned him an extraordinary reputation with foreign courts. He became supplier to the Grand Duchess of Baden and Her Majesty the Queen of Belgium, and expanded his business to some 50 cities outside France – Vienna, Geneva, Florence, Moscow, New York and Boston to name a few. Guerlain perfumes could be bought almost anywhere in the world and, little by little, he added makeup and cosmetics to his range.

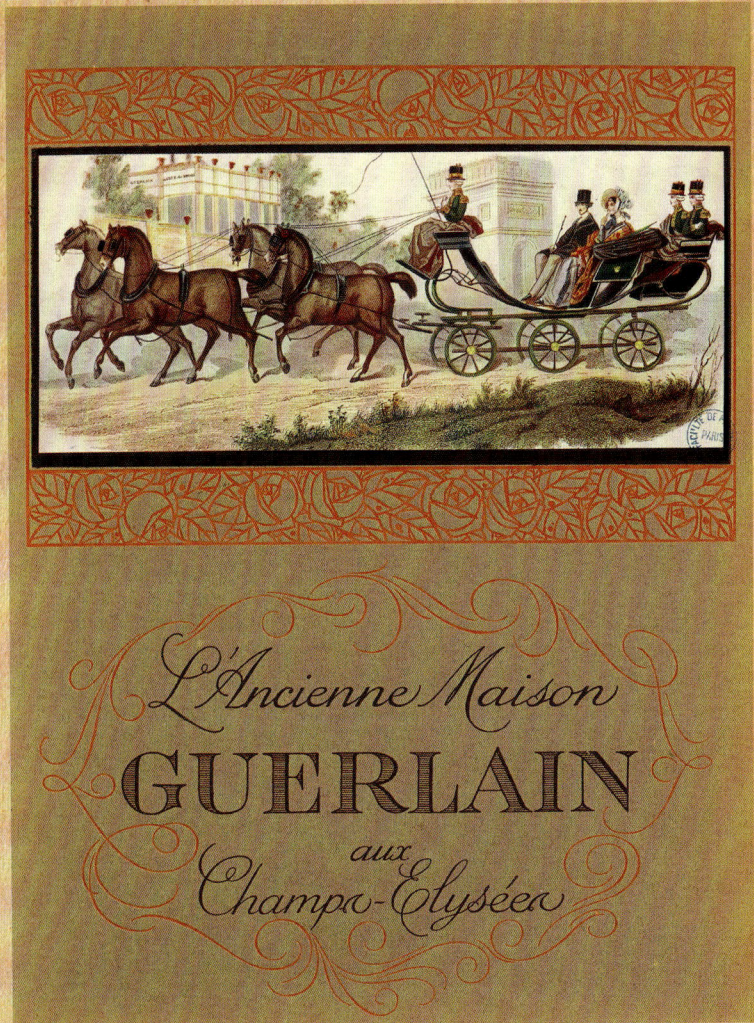

L'Ancienne Maison GUERLAIN *aux Champs-Élysées*

The old Maison Guerlain on the Champs-Élysées, page from the book *La parfumerie française et l'art dans la présentation* (French Perfume and the Art of Presentation), 1925.

KEEPING IT IN THE FAMILY

When Guerlain died, in 1864, the business stayed in the family with his two sons, Aimé and Gabriel, who shared the tasks of creation and management. They inherited a motto from their father: 'Make good products, never compromise on quality. Have simple ideas and apply them to the letter.' Aimé created Jicky in 1889 and founded a perfume union in 1890. Jacques Guerlain, who had been taught the ropes by his uncle Aimé, succeeded him as co-proprietor in 1897. When Jacques died in 1963, his grandson Jean-Paul Guerlain took over the creative side of the business, having learned the perfumer's art and inherited a love of beautiful things from his grandfather. The very essence of the Guerlain name rests on Pierre François Pascal Guerlain's legacy, which is the cornerstone of the brand: expertise rooted in audacity, quality and know-how, the merest hint of a fragrance marrying spices and Eau de Cologne, a cosmopolitan clientele, luxury and truly unique compositions.

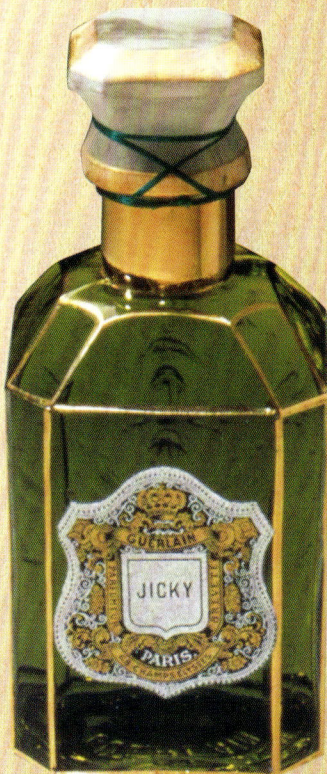

Jicky perfume by Guerlain.

Oriza L. Legrand

The story of the Oriza L. Legrand perfume brand began in 1720, during the reign of Louis XV, before Louis Legrand became the sole owner of the company Parfumerie Oriza in 1811 and set up shop at 207, rue Saint-Honoré in Paris. With panache and elegance, its innovative creations have spanned the centuries, earning the brand a central role in the history of perfumery.

Fargeon the Elder, purveyor to the French court

The founder, Fargeon the Elder, was a member of the brilliant family of perfumers from Montpellier (for his descendant Jean-Louis Fargeon, see page 56). He claimed to have been given his perfume and cosmetics formulas by Ninon de Lenclos, the famous courtesan who died in 1705, but whose beauty and eternal youth were still the envy of all the ladies of the court of Versailles. Fargeon the Elder was appointed 'Purveyor to the French Court' by Louis XV, his first client. His reputation was established and the story of the iconic Maison Oriza was born. His successors, Louis Legrand and Antonin Raynaud, would continue this legacy but bring it into a modern age of industry, scientific progress and increasingly innovative products. From simple craftsmen and shopkeepers, they became powerful industrialists and applied their astute skills and noses to establish perfume as a sensuous product on the luxury market.

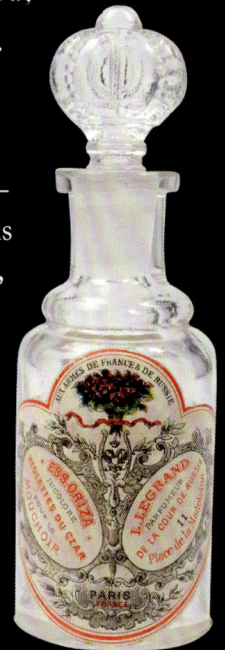

Violettes du Czar, a perfume by Oriza L. Legrand, 1862.

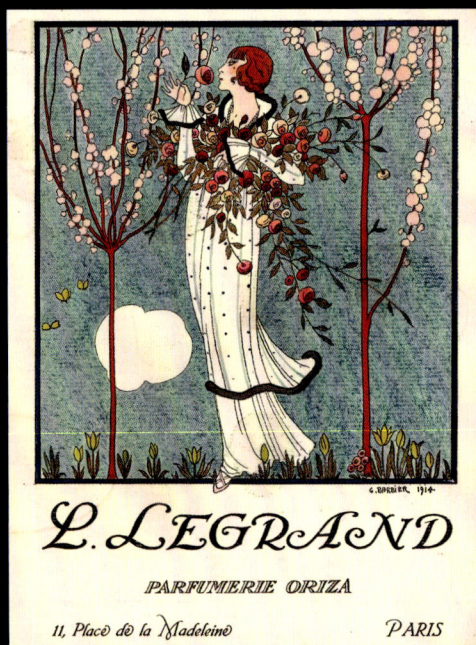

1914 advertising brochure for L. Legrand perfumes. Illustration by Georges Barbier.

Antonin Raynaud

Antonin Raynaud was born in Grasse in 1827. The young hopeful, whose father was a butcher, arrived in Paris seeking work. In 1857, he joined L. Legrand, the successor of Fargeon the Elder, as an 'employee with a stake in the business'. In 1860, he took full ownership of Oriza L. Legrand, which was the purveyor of perfume to the French court until Napoleon III, and also supplied the most prestigious courts outside France. In the same year, he built a steam-powered factory in Levallois, which was held up as a model and garnered interest because of its ultra-modern powerful machinery. The press sang the praises of the company's elegant bottles, delicate fragrance compositions and sumptuous showroom, which moved to 11, boulevard de la Madeleine in 1890.

An 1887 advert announced a new discovery – 'solid perfumes, or *concretes*, named Essence Oriza', of a hitherto unknown concentration and smoothness. Oriza L. Legrand was present at World's Fairs in France and abroad, where it won the highest accolades for the exceptional quality and innovation of its creations. The company has been a leading light in the luxury perfume industry for almost 300 years.

Advert for the perfumer Oriza L. Legrand, showing a view of the Legrand factory, print, seventeenth century.

Gellé Frères

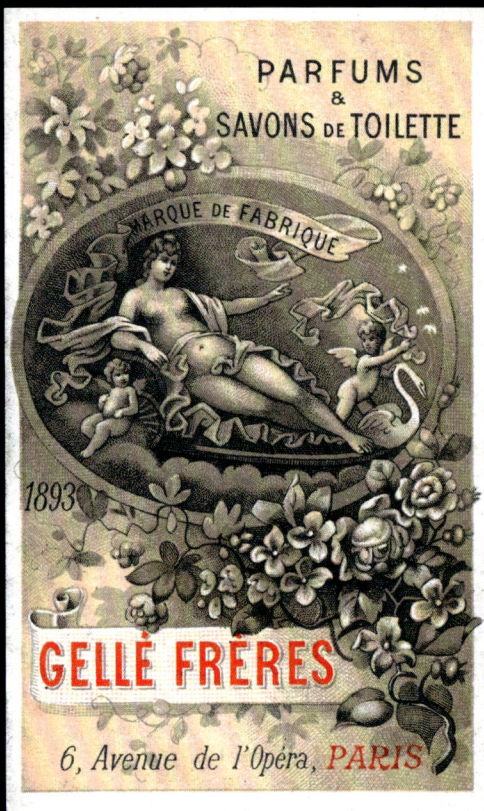

1893 Gellé Frères advertising postcard.

Gellé Frères was founded in 1826 when it took over the company of Jean-Louis Fargeon, Marie-Antoinette's perfumer. It helped pioneer change in the perfume industry in the early nineteenth century as one of the first companies to use steam to manufacture its products, mainly its toilet soaps.

Brothers in business

Jean-Baptiste Augustin Gellé was born in Abbeville on 28 August 1801. The son of a currier (someone who stretches leather in the tanning industry), he was, just like Pierre-François-Pascal Guerlain who also hailed from Abbeville, new to the perfume trade. Yet in buying Maison Fargeon from the sons of Jean-Louis Fargeon he took on a professional and aristocratic legacy.

In 1827, Gellé Frères were operating from an Eau de Cologne warehouse at 8, rue Jessaint in what was then La Chapelle (now a part of Paris). On 1 November 1831, Jean-Baptiste went into partnership with Nicolas Wilborde, who was already working for him, and they declared themselves to be 'wholesale perfumers, inventors of the Gellé Frères regenerator for hair care and growth, suppliers to several French and foreign princes'. In 1851 their steam-powered plant, close to the Porte Maillot in Neuilly-sur-Seine, was described as a factory making soaps, perfumes and brushes for personal grooming. This state-of-the-art manufacturing plant produced superior quality health and hygiene products such as their Vinaigre d'Albion, an elixir made from the concentrated sap of the most invigorating and fortifying alpine plants. The factory was destroyed by bombing in the 1870 Franco-Prussian war and rebuilt at Levallois.

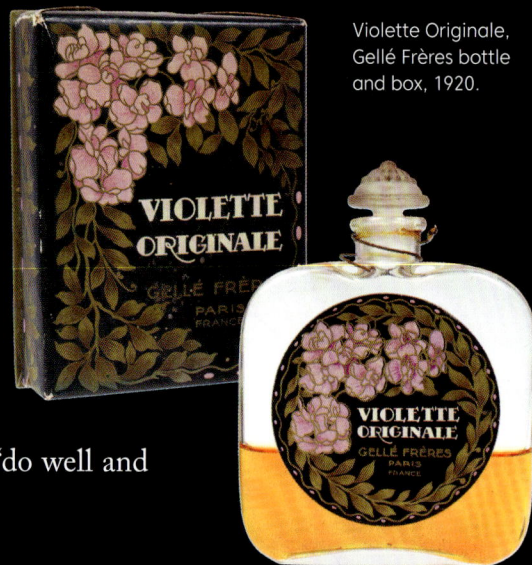

Violette Originale, Gellé Frères bottle and box, 1920.

GELLÉ-LECARON COLLABORATION FROM 1855

In 1855, Jean-Baptiste Gellé began a collaboration with his son-in-law Jean-Émile Lecaron, who would later teach his own sons Maurice and Paul-Émile the trade. The latter took over the company in 1891, moving it to 6 avenue de l'Opéra and setting up stores abroad. The Gellé Frères brand won awards and distinctions at World's Fairs for their subtle fragrances and cosmetics. Jean-Baptiste Gellé died in Neuilly-sur-Seine in April 1895. He had written a treatise on perfume in 1861 entitled 'A Treatise on Cosmetics from the Point of View of Hygiene and the Preservation of Beauty'. Celebrating women, the company motto was: 'do well and excel for the best market of all'.

BREVETS ETRANGERS

BREVETS FRANÇAIS

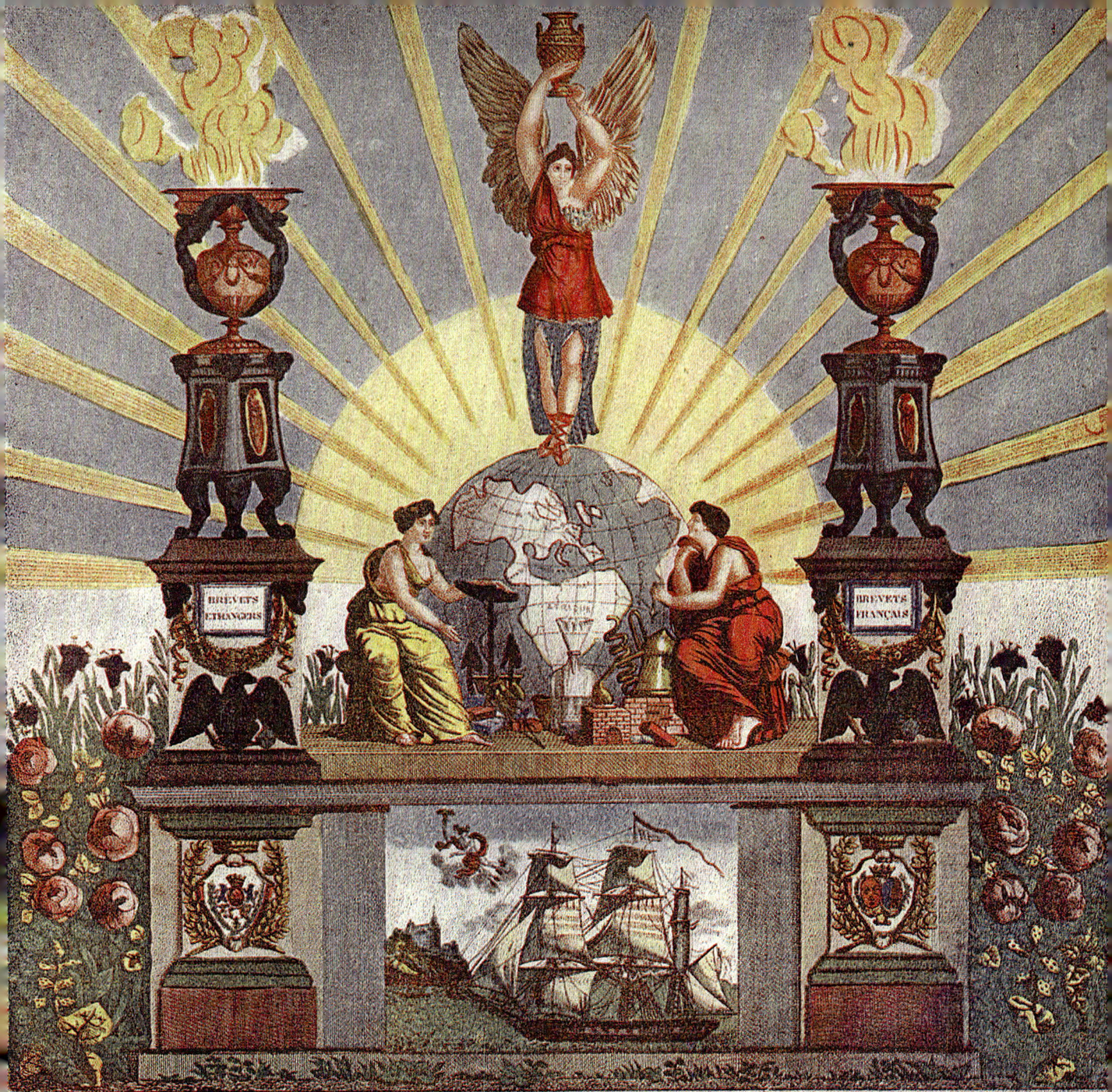

DOUBLE EAU DE COLOGNE
ROYALE RECTIFIÉE
de
GELLÉ FRERES
Successeurs de FARGEON jeune
PARFUMEUR DISTILLATEUR BRÉVETÉ et
FOURNISSEUR DE S. A. R. MADAME,
DUCHESSE DE BERRY,

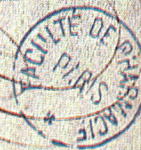

Nous garantissons cette Eau de Cologne pour être la Seule Soumise aux procédés de la Rectification, la Sage Combinaison des Plantes, et des Aromates qui la composent la rend Suave Spiritueuse et la plus efficace on peut s'en convaincre on Délivre ici des echantillons Gratis pour essai un flacon de notre Eau de Cologne Royale, fait plus d'effet par sa force que deux de celle qui est la plus en renommée, et à toujours un an de mise en flacon.

L'ENTREPÔT GÉNÉRAL est Chez GELLÉ FRERES Parfumeurs Distillateurs Rue des Vieux Augustins N.º3ŋ.

À PARIS

L.T. Piver

The company was founded in 1774, but it was Louis Toussaint Piver who really set it on the road to success when he took over in 1813. Inspired by creativity, quality and technological progress, L.T. Piver is one of the oldest perfume houses still in business today.

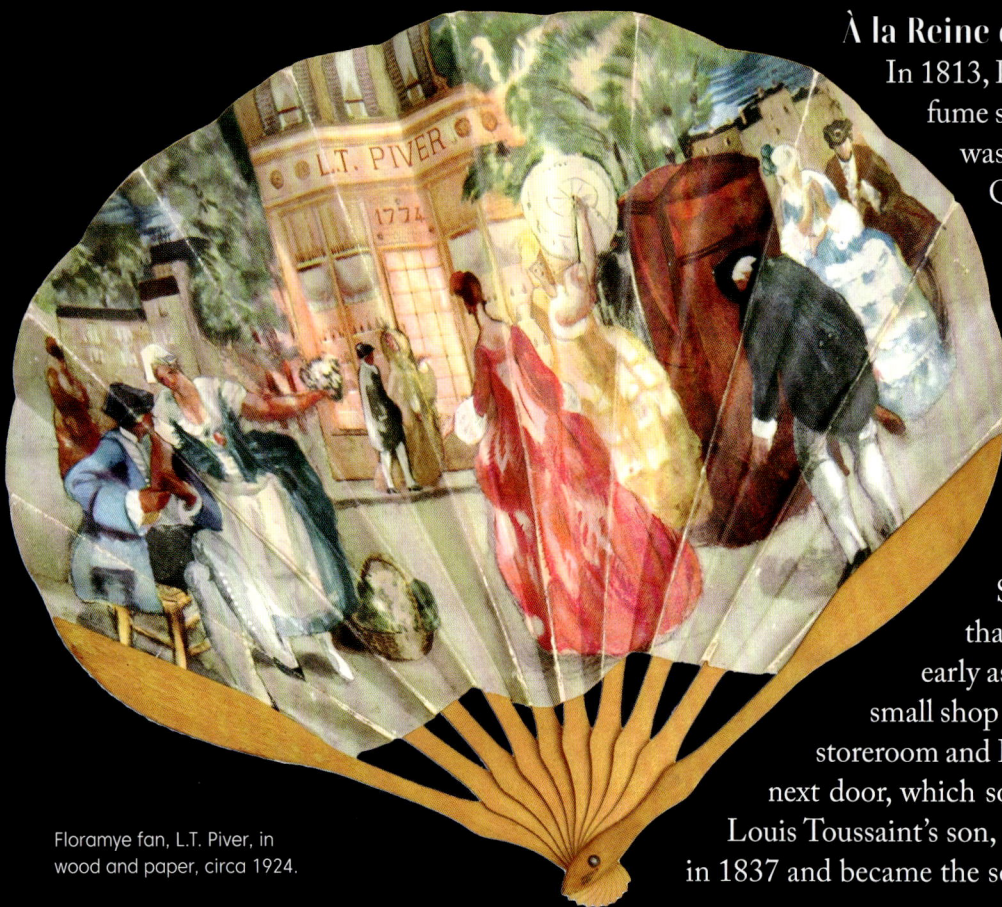

Floramye fan, L.T. Piver, in wood and paper, circa 1924.

À la Reine des Fleurs!

In 1813, Louis Toussaint Piver took over a perfume shop that had been opened in 1774 and was called À la Reine des Fleurs (At the Queen of Flowers). It supplied perfumes, floral waters and scented products to the court of Louis XVI and foreign courts. Piver joined as an apprentice to the perfumer Pierre-Guillaume Dissey. He married the owner's sister-in-law and the two men became partners in 1813, the company being known as 'Dissey-Piver, wholesale perfumers, 103, rue Saint-Martin'. Business grew so rapidly that they opened stores outside France as early as 1817. After Dissey died, in 1823, the small shop in rue Saint-Martin was turned into a storeroom and L.T. Piver opened a beautiful boutique next door, which soon thrived. Alphonse Honoré Piver, Louis Toussaint's son, decided to join his father as a partner in 1837 and became the sole director in 1844.

Alphonse Honoré Piver, the inventor in the family

Alphonse Honoré Piver experimented with enfleurage and invented what is known as the pneumatic method. With Eugène Million, he devised an extraction process that used volatile solvents, which was considered groundbreaking for the perfume industry at the time. Alphonse Piver was hailed as an industry pioneer when he used the Million process for perfumes, using carbon disulphide in the distillation process to extract fragrances from iris roots and heliotrope flowers, two essences that were very much in vogue at the time. However, this process was difficult to put into practice because of the cost and the risk of explosion. Extraction came into common use at the end of the nineteenth century. Alphonse Piver also made synthetic products and, simultaneously, created a hugely popular range of perfumes and beauty products.

L.T. Piver expands beyond France

In 1846, L.T. Piver opened boutiques in London and Brussels. With its appointment as purveyor to Napoleon III in 1858, the company gained international renown and had up to 120 branches outside France. It was awarded a medal at the 1862 International Exhibition in London, which was attended by many French perfumers. L.T. Piver continued to expand. It opened flower-processing plants, including one in Grasse and another in Aubervilliers, which specialized in cosmetics manufacturing. And to further its contribution to technological progress, the directors hired two chemists, Georges Darzens and Pierre Armingeat. The company is particularly well known for its perfumes Trèfle Incarnat (1896), Parfum d'Aventure (1931) and Cuir de Russie (1939).

One of the oldest perfume houses still in business

L.T. Piver was never short of imagination. To accompany its many perfumes made from rare and precious ingredients, it launched comprehensive ranges of beauty and body cleansing products, such as perfumed gloves, rice powders, lettuce juice and marshmallow soaps, almond cream and iris milk. It is today reputed to be one of the oldest perfume companies still in business and has its own workshop in Grasse, where it creates cutting-edge formulas.

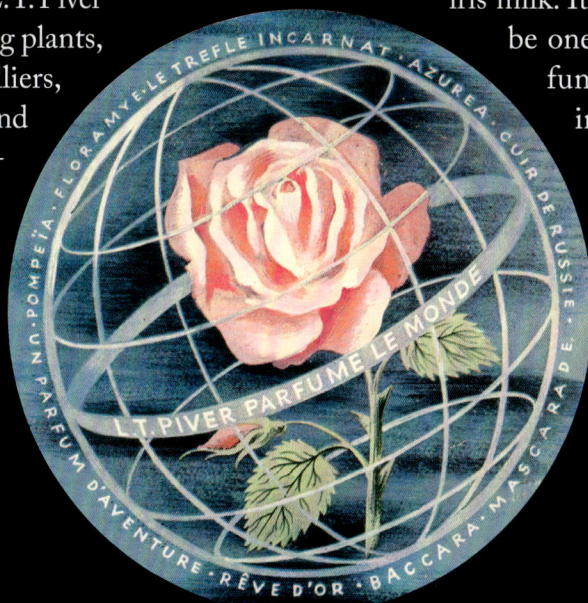

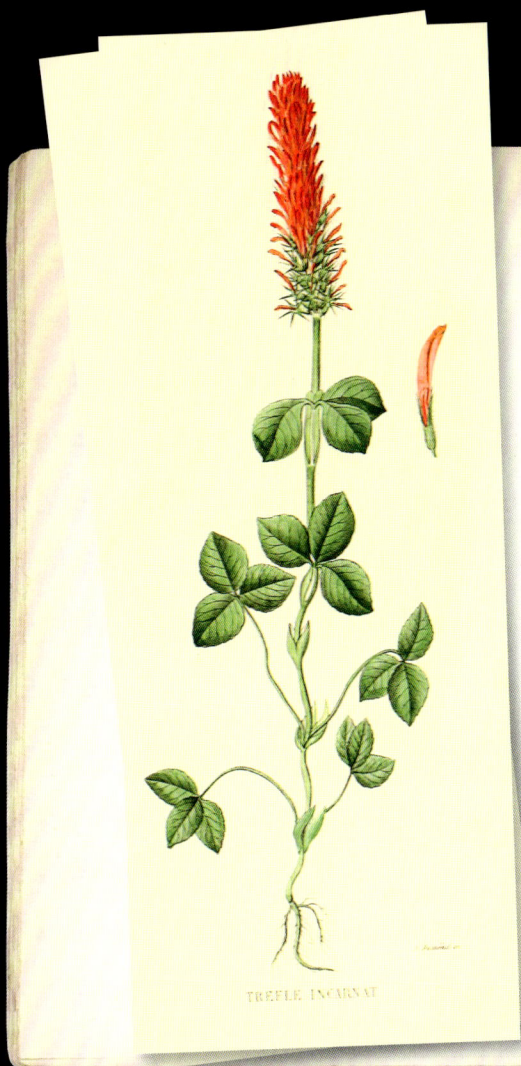

The clover accord

With Trèfle Incarnat, perfumery really did make its entrance into the modern world. It was the first perfume based on an accord known as 'trèfle' ('clover' in English), which married floral notes with fougère, a perfume family that takes its name from the French word for 'fern'. Its standout feature was Darzens' new discovery, amyl salicylate. Subsequently, some old formulas were reworked to incorporate synthetic notes and many other perfumers followed suit. Some of the resulting creations were presented in high-end crystal bottles made by famous artists such as Lalique and Baccarat.

Botanical drawing of *Trifolium incarnatum* (crimson clover).

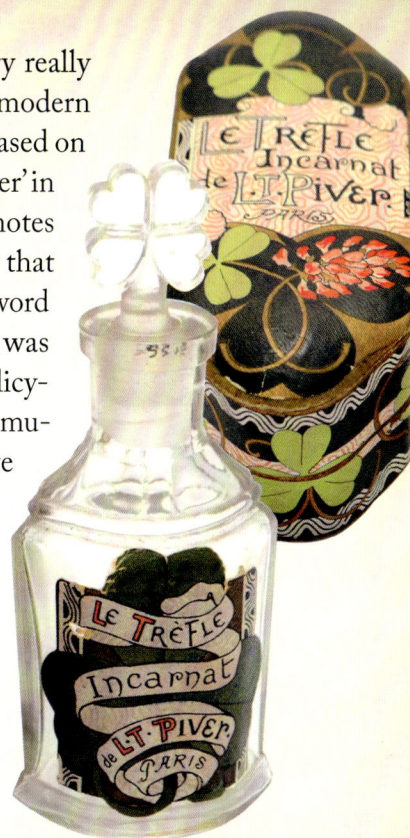

Roger&Gallet

Roger&Gallet carried on the work of Jean-Marie Farina (see page 62). Known for Eau de Cologne, having inherited authentic formulas from its predecessor, it very quickly established itself as a player in the perfume industry, not only in France but in England too. With one eye on innovation, Roger&Gallet has managed to keep tradition alive, marking it out as one of France's great perfume houses.

Two families: Roger and Gallet

The house was established in Paris in April 1862, when Léonce Collas sold his business to Charles Armand Roger and Charles Martial Gallet, who were brothers-in-law. The former was a hat maker in Paris and then Chile, where he made his fortune. He was also a representative for Parisian perfumers in Latin America. When he married Léonce Collas' cousin, Coralie Collas, in 1844, he was thinking about setting up a business. Charles Martial Gallet, a banker in Vire, married Coralie's sister, Octavie Collas, in 1847. Léonce Collas, the wives' cousin, was struggling to develop the business established in Paris by Jean-Marie Farina in 1806, which his father had bought in 1840.

The two brothers-in-law joined forces to establish a family business and shared the task of running it. Their wives, Coralie and Octavie, took it in turn to man the shop in the first year. Roger and Gallet moved the company head-quarters to 38, rue d'Hauteville in Paris and converted the rue Saint-Honoré premises into an ultra-chic boutique. In 1863, they had a 3,000 square metre (three-quarters of an acre), steam-powered factory built at rue Valentin in Levallois-Perret.

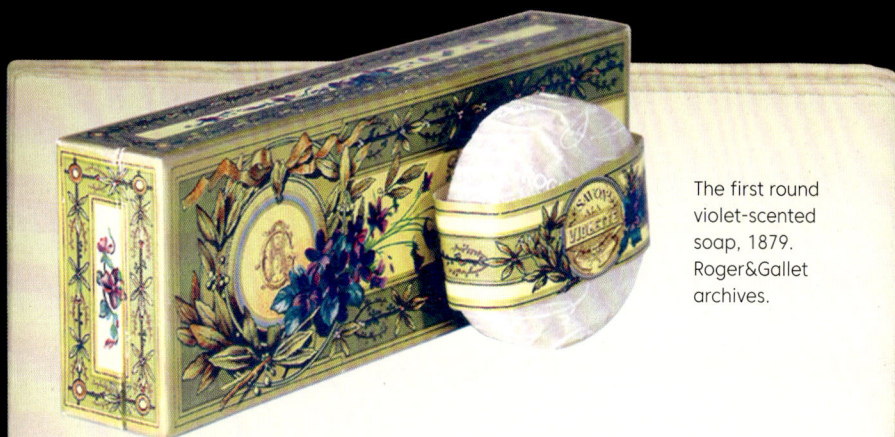

The first round violet-scented soap, 1879. Roger&Gallet archives.

Soap as soft and fragrant as its English counterpart

Roger&Gallet's were the only French soaps that could rival English soaps, reputed to be the softest, most fragrant and luxuriant in the world, to garner favour with Queen Victoria. The secret to this success was threefold. They used only the finest raw materials, the most natural essences (with a 100% plant base rich in essential oils) and the traditional cauldron method. Scented to the core, the soaps were soft on the skin and came in a distinctive round shape, first developed in 1879 for the original violet version. The lavender, tea rose, sandalwood, jasmine, hyacinth, lilac, ylang-ylang and carnation soaps were also very popular in Great Britain for their French-style presentation: the company seal embossed in the soap, exquisite packaging, tissue paper wrapping and wraparound label in the colour of one of the ten fragrances available in the 1900s. Adopting English-style grooming rituals, Roger&Gallet made pots of smelling salts (1880), perfumed talcum powder (1904) and a range of shaving sticks.

Parfumerie

ROGER & GALLET

Paris

First official advert of Roger&Gallet, Roger&Gallet archives, circa 1895.

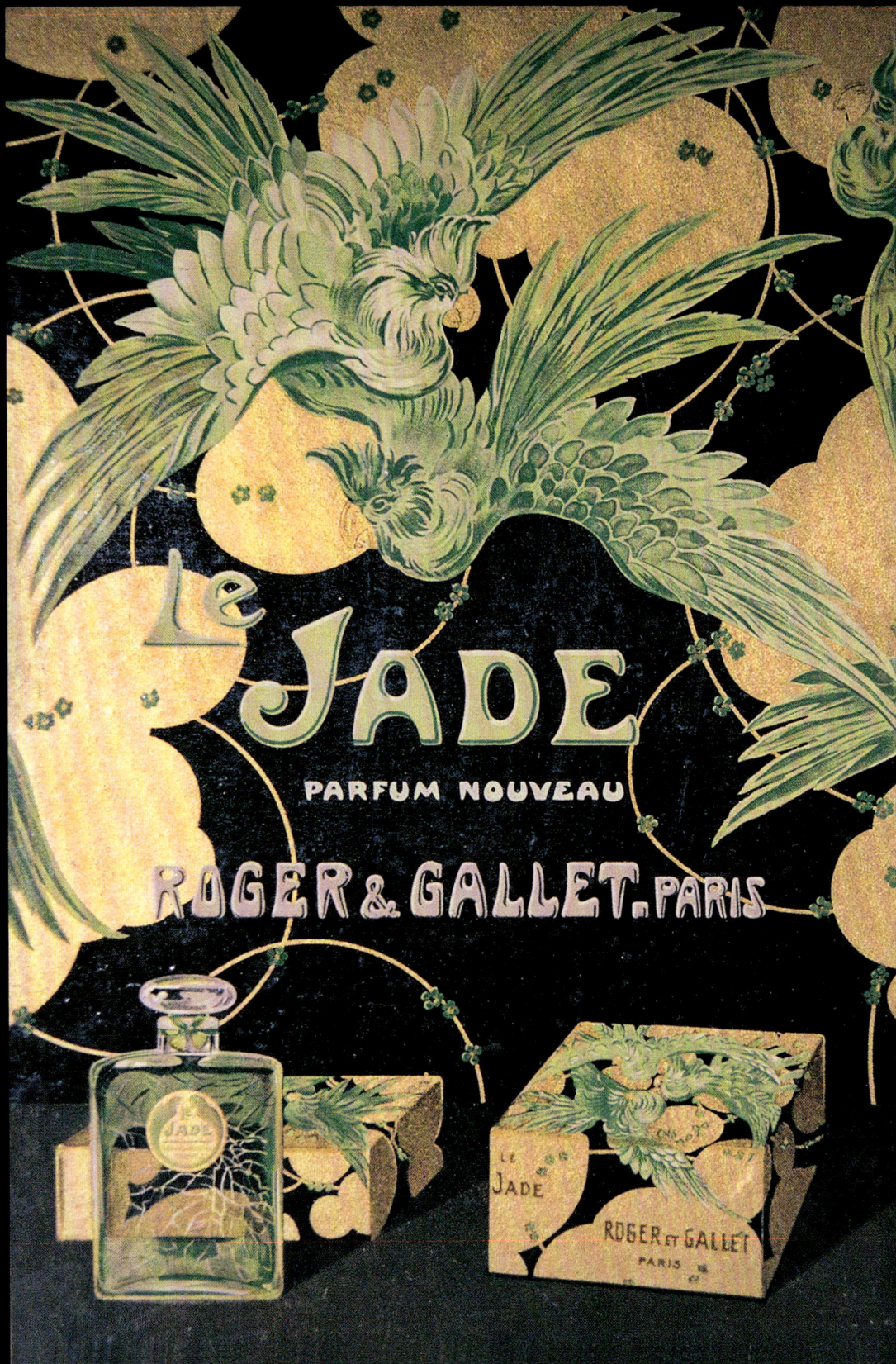

Advert for the perfume Le Jade by Roger&Gallet, Roger&Gallet archives, 1923.

Best-selling perfumes

Paul Pellerin, Armand Roger's son-in-law, took the reins in 1885 and Roger&Gallet stopped producing makeup and body-care items to focus on perfumes and luxury goods. The first of these were Violette de Parme (1880), Violette Ambrée (1891) and Vera Violetta (1893), the company's most successful perfume. The full range of accompanying products varied and might include rice powder, lotion and soap. From 1908, René Lalique made coloured patinated glass bottles for Narkiss and Cigalia in the classic Art Nouveau naturalist style.

Roger&Gallet was lauded at the 1925 Paris Exhibition for the luxury and artistic quality of its creations. Business was thriving. The company expanded to all five continents and regularly released new lines, even at times of financial crisis when production slowed down. After the war, and a few commercial failures, the company's image suffered, so they decided to concentrate on Eau de Cologne and related products.

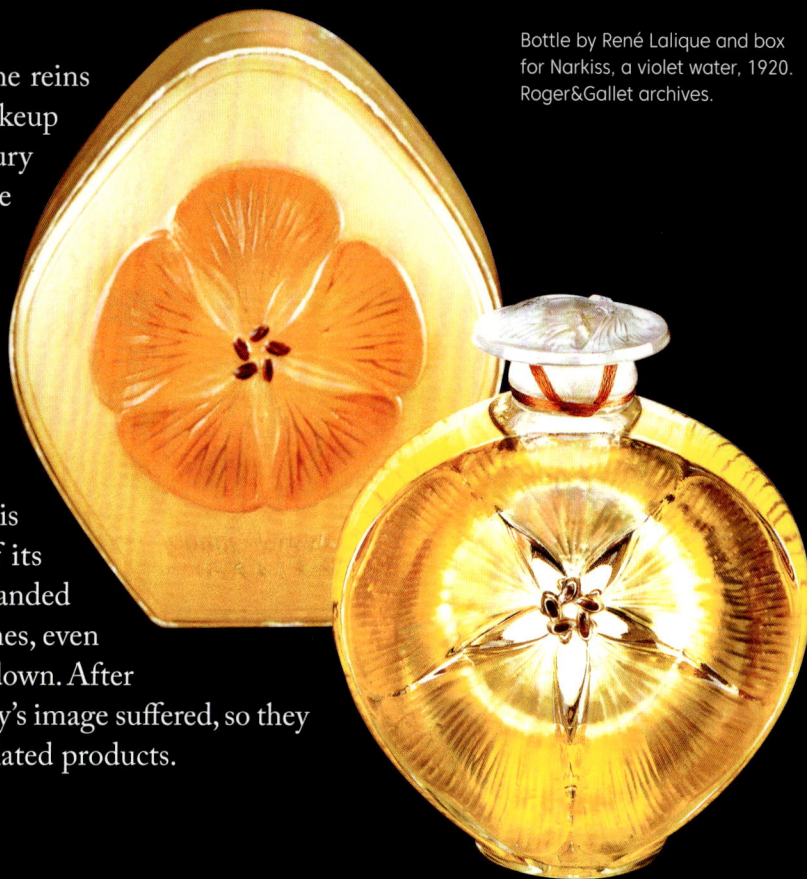

Bottle by René Lalique and box for Narkiss, a violet water, 1920. Roger&Gallet archives.

Marghoubi advertising sign, 1926. Roger&Gallet archives.

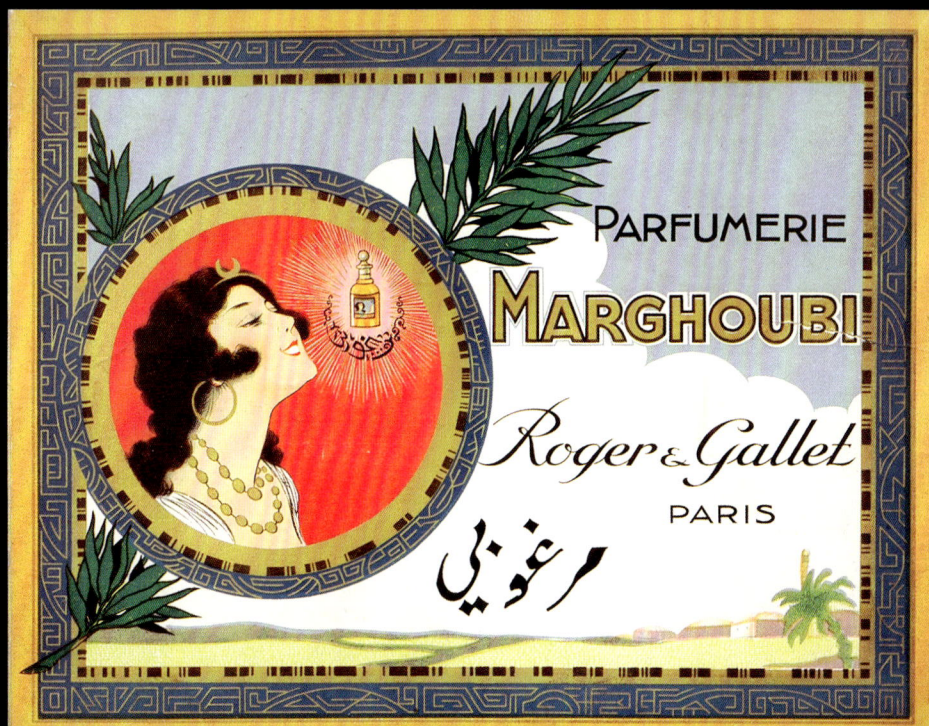

PARFUMERIE

MARGHOUBI

Roger & Gallet

PARIS

مرغوبي

Roger&Gallet in the twenty first century

In the 2000s, the company launched new perfumed waters, first Thé Vert in the year 2000 and then Eau de Gingembre in 2003. In 2007, they reinvented their range of colognes and perfumes, giving them a pared-back contemporary feel. The delicate scents were inspired by private gardens in faraway places, the beautiful grounds of the Alhambra for Cédrat de Calabre, Rose du Bengale and Bois d'Orange, for instance. Their 2013 releases – Fleur de Figuier and Gingembre Rouge – were aimed at the contemporary young woman, while in 2017 another invention, extrait de Cologne, offered eau de toilette strength in a signature cologne. Proof, if it were needed, that Roger&Gallet could innovate without losing sight of its heritage.

François Coty

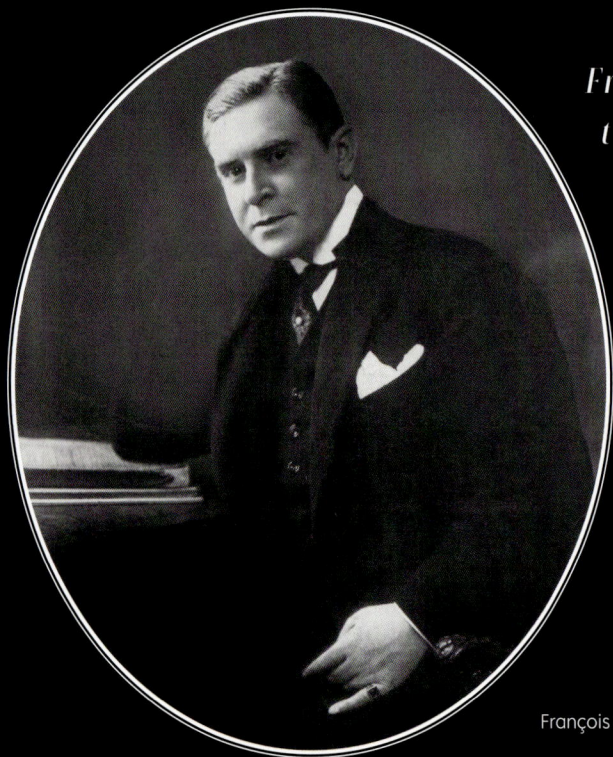

François Coty's arrival on the scene at the beginning of the twentieth century rocked the perfume industry to its core. He was an extraordinary man with a burning ambition, an exceptional nose and great organizational skills. Modelling himself on the American self-made man, he shaped the olfactory landscape, distribution, advertising and export trade of modern-day perfumery.

François Coty in August 1932.

But first, some chemistry lessons

Corsican-born Joseph Marie François Spoturno was never destined for a career in perfume. He was orphaned at a very young age and brought up by his grandmother. Due to a lack of money, he had to leave school at the age of 13, but that did nothing to dampen his ambition – quite the contrary. In 1900, he arrived in Paris to work as secretary for the politician Emmanuel Arène, who had been his commander in the army. He also worked as a fashion-accessories salesman and, the same year, married Yvonne Le Baron, the daughter of an artist.

The 1900 Paris Exhibition was in full swing and François Spoturno happened upon perfume classes on offer at the event while visiting his pharmacist friend Raymond Goery at his premises on Champ-de-Mars at the foot of the Eiffel Tower. He had no training

in chemistry or perfumery but spent his free time with his friend, who was making an artisan Eau de Cologne that did not stray far from the standards found in the pharmaceutical Codex. Spoturno likened it to all the perfumes of the time, which he found dull, old-fashioned and lacking in imagination, a discerning opinion that would later shape his reform of the perfume industry. He decided to study chemistry to cultivate his love of perfume and perfect his skills in this area. This he did in Grasse, where he learned about natural raw materials and synthetic substances, and spent some time at the laboratories of Chiris, which was to become Coty's first supplier.

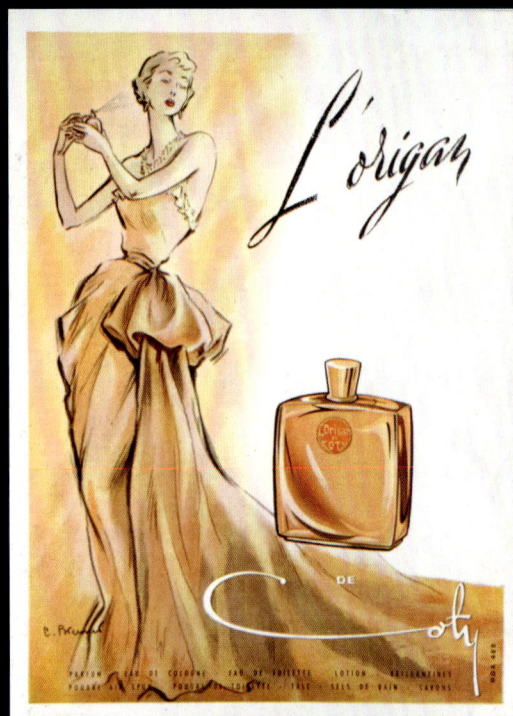

Advert for the Coty perfume L'Origan, 1905.

Coty, his mother's maiden name

Spoturno borrowed several thousand gold francs from his grandmother to get him started and launched his company under his mother's maiden name, Coty. In 1904, he took over modest premises on rue de la Boétie in Paris, which housed a shop, a manufacturing laboratory and a packing room at the back. François Coty certainly did not have the experience or the capital of leading perfumers of the day, but he had an ace card: innovation. As an unknown at the time, he had no reputation to maintain nor style constraints. His guiding principles were modernity and a desire to take perfume beyond the usual clientele, society women and coquettes, to the lower ranks of the bourgeoisie. Paris was the capital of pleasure, arts and literature and Coty believed that perfume should be part of this new dynamic. He wanted to create new fragrances for women. In 1904, he released a soliflore (single floral scent) named La Rose Jacqueminot, which was an immediate triumph, and François Coty became an overnight success. He went on to launch L'Origan and Ambre Antique in 1905, Chypre in 1917, and many more.

The bottle is just as important as its contents

In the belief that the look of a perfume was just as important as its scent, Coty revolutionized the industry by creating bottles that were decorative objects in their own right. He pioneered collaborations between glassmakers and perfumers when, in 1910, he commissioned René Lalique to make the crystal bottle for his perfume Cyclamen, which was decorated with dragonflies that had women's bodies. He said that a bottle should be reassuring and a reflection of good taste and self-esteem.

Coty's partnership with Lalique started the trend for creating a new and unique bottle for every perfume. For the label design and production and box printing, he worked with Draeger, a young art printer in Montrouge. Together they created gold prints on real gold paper and Draeger made the most of Coty's perfume boxes, frequently using fine gold. For the packaging, Coty commissioned paintings by Jean Helleu, such as the one of the young Parisian woman who became the figure on his powder box. The first Parfums Coty advertising poster, circa 1910, was a watercolour print signed by the artist.

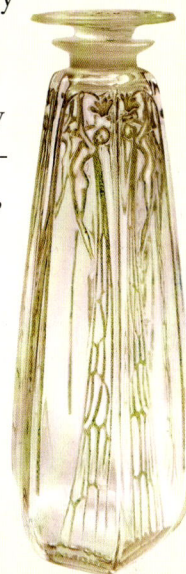

The Perfume Dance, colour lithograph by Sem (Georges Goursat), Angoville-sur-Mer album.

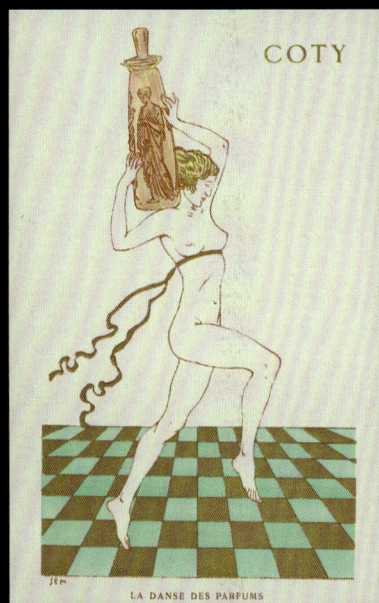

A resounding success

Products such as his powder compact brought Coty international renown. In 1914, 30,000 metal compacts were sold each day in the United States alone. His fortune was built on perfume but cemented by powders. As revenue continued to grow, he opened warehouses outside Paris and a luxury boutique and showroom on place Vendôme. He also established a position for himself on the export market, did business abroad and attended the International Exhibitions in Belgium in 1911 and Kyiv in 1913. He consolidated his success during World War I after he was demobilized because of injury in 1915. He had other buildings constructed in Suresnes and set up home in the adjacent Château de Longchamp. By 1923, François Coty was a powerful industrialist. His prosperous business became a limited company and ever-growing revenue delivered incredible profits. A hugely successful perfumer, politician and press tycoon (he bought *Le Figaro* newspaper in 1922), he was one of France's leading business owners. Coty died in 1934, having radically and decisively changed the world of perfume.

D'Orsay

Count Alfred d'Orsay, the man behind Parfums d'Orsay, was a true character and the archetypal nineteenth-century dandy. When he died in 1852, he left behind an impressive perfume legacy, which his family decided should not be forgotten. So, in 1908, they gave their blessing to the creation of a French company named Parfums d'Orsay.

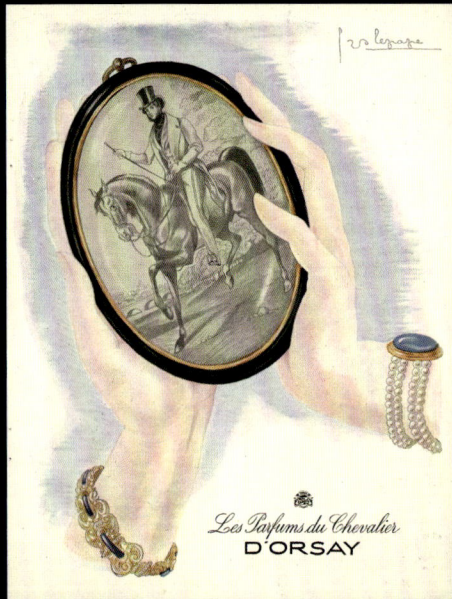

Les Parfums du Chevalier, advert by the fashion illustrator Georges Lepape, 1945.

Count Alfred d'Orsay, also known as 'the archangel of dandyism'

Parfums d'Orsay was established in 1908 by Dutch and German investors named Léon Fink, M. Van Dyck and the married couple Siegfried and Sally Berg to celebrate the life of the Count Alfred d'Orsay, a lovable, flamboyant dandy who was born in 1801. His father was a general, and his mother of noble descent. His grandmother, Mrs Crawford, regularly entertained the rich and famous. Count Alfred d'Orsay certainly knew how to use his charm and quickly won over London and Paris. He was a friend of the painter Gustave Doré and welcomed Hector Berlioz, Eugène Sue, Alfred de Vigny and Franz Liszt (for whom he arranged a concert at Buckingham Palace) to his Gore House residence in London. The 'archangel of dandyism', as French statesman Alphonse de Lamartine called him, created the first of his perfumes in 1830 to express his love for a married woman, the exquisite Lady Blessington. The perfume he gave her, a fresh, airy floral composition of orange blossom and rosewood with a simple blank blue label, marked the beginning of a beautiful story.

A success story

With bottles designed by Lalique, Baccarat or Daum, Parfums d'Orsay soared to success alongside Houbigant, Coty and Guerlain, in the early days of modern perfumery. Between 1908 and 1914, elegant women wore the sweet scents of perfumes such as Eau de Cologne d'Orsay, Chevalier d'Orsay, Tilleul, Le Chevalier à la Rose, Leurs Âmes and La Rose d'Orsay. In 1916, the distinguished perfume house was sold to a financial group. Despite changing owner many times in its history, and its activities ceasing between 1983 and 1995, the brand has made a name for itself internationally thanks to the perfumes inherited from Count Alfred d'Orsay.

Injecting new blood

In 2007, the Huet family took over the reins with a view to giving the company back its sparkle. Today, Parfums d'Orsay occupies a niche market, not only in its native France but also worldwide, in the United States in particular. Four of the company's iconic fragrances are still on the market: Étiquette Bleue (1830), Chevalier d'Orsay (1911), Tilleul (1915) and Arôme 3 (1943) . Quality ingredients such as iris, tonka bean, myrrh and precious woods have been added to the base to give the perfumes a more contemporary feel.

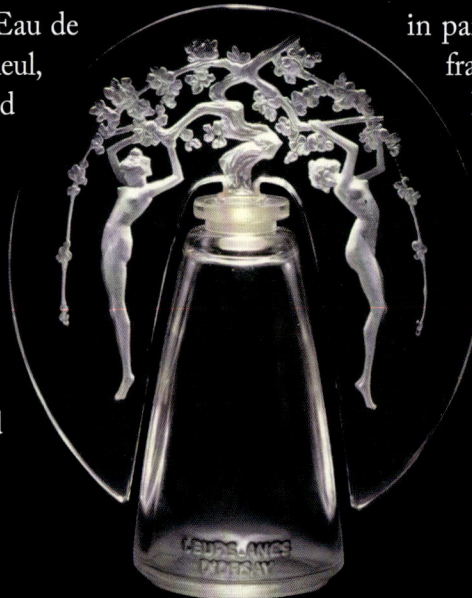

Leurs Âmes, René Lalique bottle for Parfums d'Orsay, circa 1913.

Lancôme

Behind this famous name was a woman, the Duchess of Lancosme. She was a well-known client of François Coty and her family was left without an heir. It was thought the name might bring the brand luck, and it was an overnight success. With its elegant fragrances, exceptionally beautiful boxes and contemporary bottles, Lancôme has for many years been a well-known international name.

The ex-MD of Coty creates Lancôme

Born into a family of distillers, the managing director of Coty, Armand Petitjean, founded Lancôme in 1935. He brought in the d'Ornano brothers to handle sales and marketing, the chemist Pierre Vélon and a legal expert named Édouard Breckenridge. To design the perfume bottles and boxes, he enlisted the help of the artist Georges Delhomme, who had been studio director for Coty from 1930 to 1934. Armand Petitjean's aim was to create a company to rival the American brands that had started to invade the French cosmetics market. 'I had seen that two American brands had taken control of the beauty industry. A French brand should be up alongside them,' he said at a course he gave at the Lancôme school, which opened in 1942. In 1935, he launched the perfumes Tropiques, Conquête, Kypre, Tendres Nuits and Bocages for the Brussels International Exhibition. They caused quite a stir and the new brand was among the prize winners. Two eaux de Cologne, a face powder and lipsticks were also launched the same year. He created Nutrix cream in 1936 to offer a complete skincare range. In 1938, the company brought out Rose de France, a pale pink, rose-scented lipstick. In its first four years, Lancôme launched nine perfumes, including Révolte with its cobblestone-shaped bottle, Flèches and Gardénia. Business grew rapidly on the French and international markets and, with the 1950 launch of Magie, followed by Trésor in 1952, the name Lancôme achieved worldwide fame.

Lancôme is bought by L'Oréal

In 1964, the company was sold to the L'Oréal group and became one of its flagship brands. Ô was launched in 1969 and, in 1990, a new and updated Trésor, the 'perfume of precious moments', with Isabella Rossellini as the first face of the globally successful perfume. Hypnôse Homme (2007) and Miracle Forever (2006), both launched on the back of the success of Miracle (2000) and Hypnôse Femme (2005), were two of the new releases in the 2000s. La Vie est Belle (2012) further reinforced its position as leader in the fine-fragrance market.

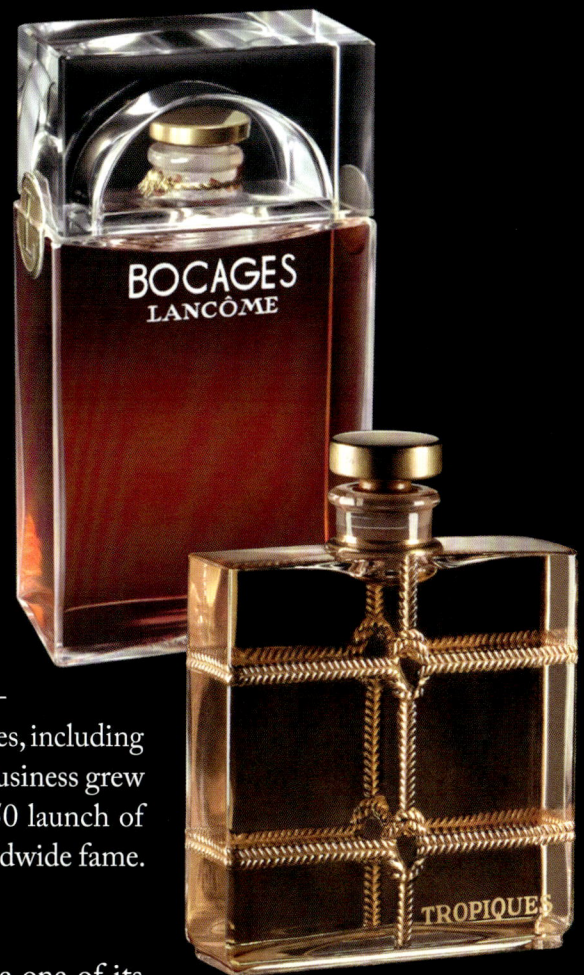

THE FIRST SYNTHETIC PERFUMES

THE FIRST SYNTHETIC PRODUCTS ENTERED THE PERFUME INDUSTRY BETWEEN 1830 AND 1889. UPTAKE WAS SLOW AT FIRST, BUT THIS INNOVATION WOULD LATER BECOME A KEY FACTOR IN THE INDUSTRY'S RAPID GROWTH AND CONSOLIDATED PERFUMERS' FORTUNES. CONSUMERS SCARCELY NOTICED A DIFFERENCE – BUT THE USE OF SYNTHETIC PRODUCTS WAS CONTROVERSIAL.

Portrait of Sir William Henry Perkin (1838–1907), British chemist and researcher who discovered the coumarin molecule, by Sir Arthur Stockdale Cope.

A MODERN ALCHEMY

Researchers began to take an interest in essential oils in the early nineteenth century and published works on three main topics: isolation, identification and synthesis. In 1833, Jean-Baptiste Dumas and Eugène Péligot isolated cinnamic aldehyde from cinnamon oil. In 1837, Justus von Liebig and Friedrich Wöhler introduced benzoic aldehyde in an important study they published on bitter almond oil. In 1840, Théophile Pelouze isolated borneol from pine oil, and Auguste Cahours discovered anethole, the principal constituent of anise oil, in 1842, followed by wintergreen in 1844. Charles Gerhardt's *Treatise on Organic Chemistry* (1853) was recognized as a benchmark reference work for the perfume industry. Organic chemistry became a science that focused on transforming organic substances, in other words making new substances from other substances.

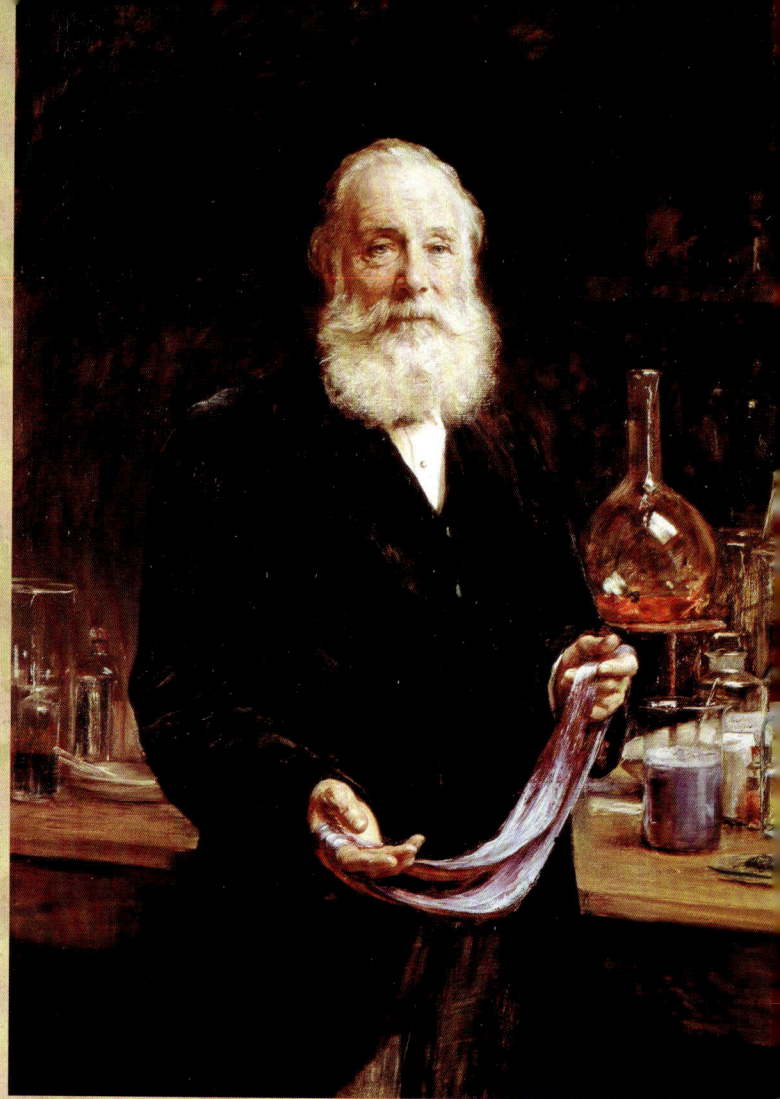

OLD SCHOOL VERSUS NEW SCHOOL

In the second half of the nineteenth century, the work of chemists involved learning and recognizing the various functions of complex molecules and, more importantly, finding ways to reproduce them synthetically. Industrial laboratories took over from university laboratories. However, nineteenth-century perfumers and society as a whole initially scorned and disparaged most of the first synthetic perfumes, believing them to be for the working classes, and merely for hygiene purposes. People also feared the damage artificial perfumes could have on health – causing behavioural disorders, for instance, or sterility in women. The considerably lower cost of synthetic raw materials could expand the market, but more conservative perfumers refused on aesthetic grounds to use manmade products in their compositions.

INITIAL SUCCESS FOR SYNTHETIC PERFUMES

In 1898, perfume finally entered the modern era with Trèfle Incarnat by L.T. Piver. This was the first perfume based on what was called the 'trèfle' or clover accord, a combination of floral and fougère (fern) notes, and the perfect base for Darzens' newly discovered amyl salicylate (see page 75). Gradually, perfumers began to update their old formulas to incorporate synthetic notes. One such example was British brand Atkinsons' Bouquet à la Maréchale, which was hugely successful until the start of World War I. Although it had started out as an entirely natural product, Atkinsons began to include vanillin and coumarin in its formula in 1915.

In 1900, Paul Parquet's L'Idéal contained just the right quantities of synthetic products to make it very much a perfume of its time. Immediately following the huge success of Rose Jacqueminot in 1904, François Coty, operating at the time from his 'Cité des parfums' in Suresnes, took an interest in perfume development and was extremely enthusiastic about the new synthetic bases. He and Jacques Guerlain were among the first to understand the incredible potential of these new materials. Coty's L'Origan (1905) comprised special methyl ionone, Dianthine (a carnation accord) and natural neroli, giving birth to a new, very important sub-family, spicy floral ambers, known today as the florientals. Guerlain, for his part, launched Après l'Ondée, with a hawthorn note obtained from aldehyde coated with appropriate crystals and citrus. In 1912, three hugely successful natural–synthetic hybrids – L'Heure Bleue by Guerlain, Caron's Narcisse Noir and Houbigant's Quelques Fleurs – paved the way for other fragrance creations that broke free from the classic floral structure.

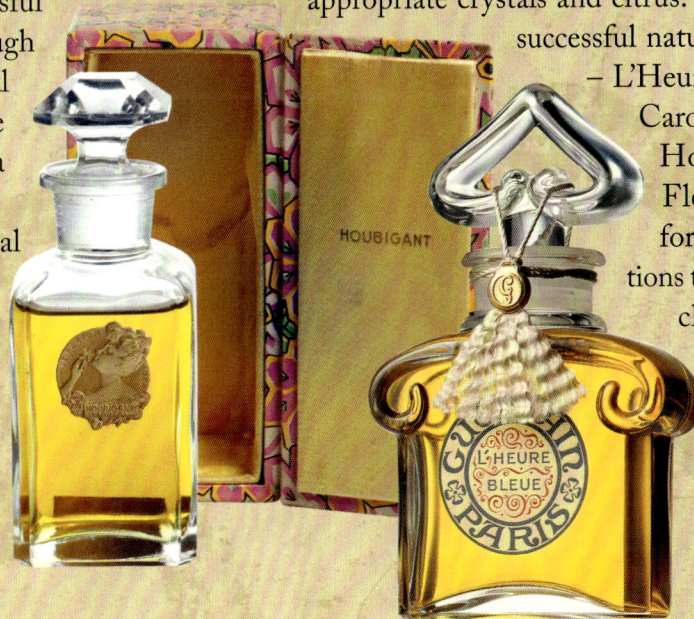

Far left: L'Idéal by Houbigant, 1900.

Left: L'Heure Bleue by Guerlain, 1912.

Below: François Coty, the Corsican industrialist who invented the modern perfume factory.

The 20-year rule

There are often 20 years or so between organic chemistry discovering a synthetic product and it being used in perfumery. Salicylic acid, for example, was discovered in 1860. It was the starting point for the manufacture of coumarin, synthesized by Perkin, and used in Houbigant's Fougère Royale from 1882. Likewise, in 1869, Fittig and Mielk discovered heliotropin, which was instrumental in the runaway success of amber-type perfumes (orientals), which had been in vogue since the early nineteenth century. Another vital discovery came in 1876, when Reimer made vanillin from guaiacol. Guerlain made the bold move of using it in 1889, together with coumarin, and confessed to using synthetic products in his famous Jicky perfume. In 1893, Tiemann and Krüger synthesized ionone from citric acid using citral extracted from lemongrass essential oil. The same year, Roger&Gallet negotiated an exclusivity contract for ionone with the company Laire, on the basis of minimum annual purchases. In 1904, François Coty used it in La Rose Jacqueminot, together with rhodinol, which had been discovered in 1891.

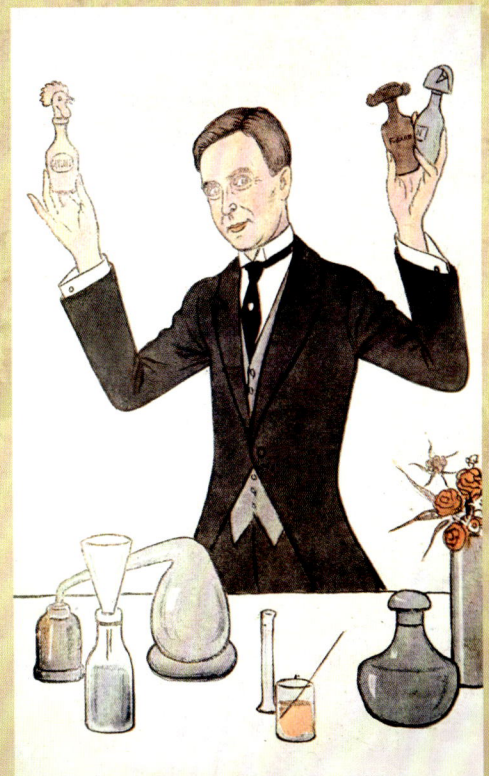

A PROFESSION IN ITS OWN RIGHT

THE FRENCH PERFUME INDUSTRY ESTABLISHED ITS NAME, AND THE WORLD MARKET, AT INTERNATIONAL EXHIBITIONS IN THE NINETEENTH CENTURY. PERFUMERS FROM OTHER COUNTRIES BEGAN TO COPY AND THE 1900 PARIS EXHIBITION MARKED A MAJOR TURNING POINT, WITH FRANCE WINNING 10 OF THE 17 GRAND PRIZES, 16 OF THE 27 GOLD MEDALS AND 19 OF THE 35 SILVER ONES.

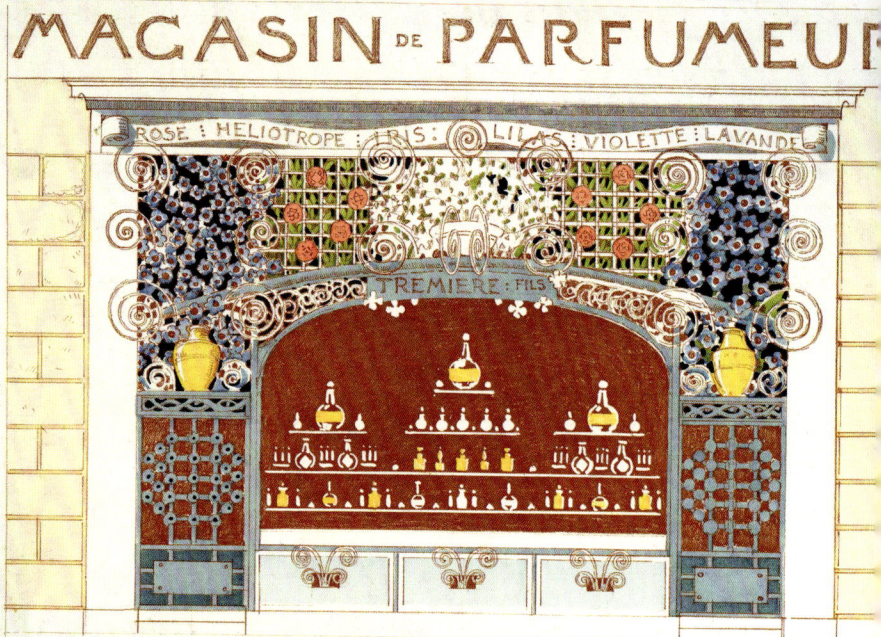

The Tremière et Fils shop front in Paris, early twentieth century.

KEEPING IT IN THE FAMILY

Despite their very different social and professional backgrounds, perfumers were treated like Parisian royalty. Some, the Houbigant and Chiris families for instance, had inherited family businesses established under the pre-Revolution Ancien Régime. Their strategy was therefore to make products from secret recipes and pass on the family tradition. The Chiris family of Grasse perfumers were notable figures in provincial business and public life. They operated like a dynasty, passing power from father to eldest son. This was a common strategy in the perfume industry and had been instrumental in some amazing success stories. Other perfumers might have been shop assistants who had progressed to business owners, as was the case with Piver. Guerlain was different again, as it was a completely new company when it was established in Paris in 1828.

GOING UP IN THE WORLD

As the industry advanced, the pioneers gave way to astute businessmen. Perfume looked like a very lucrative proposition so investors began to take an interest as early as 1860. They came from outside the industry, often from fashion, which shared the same clientele and was also an image-conscious business. One such example was Édouard Pinaud, who bought the soap company Legrand in 1830. Others had a trade background, for instance brothers-in-law Armand Roger and Charles Gallet, a provincial merchant and businessman, respectively, who took over the family business in 1862 under the Roger&Gallet name. By 1860, entering the perfume business was an industrial venture with the prospect of excellent profits. Entrepreneurial spirit and aspirations of social success, therefore, defined the perfume industry under the Second Empire.

A perfume shop at 15, rue de la Paix

In 1841, Guerlain opened a retail store at the prestigious address of 15, rue de la Paix, Paris. The inside was later fitted out in the luxurious style of the Second Empire of Napoleon III, with tall ebony or mahogany display cabinets, fringed drapes and heavy, complex gas chandeliers. Shop assistants at a corner counter welcomed customers and the focus was on advising and selling.

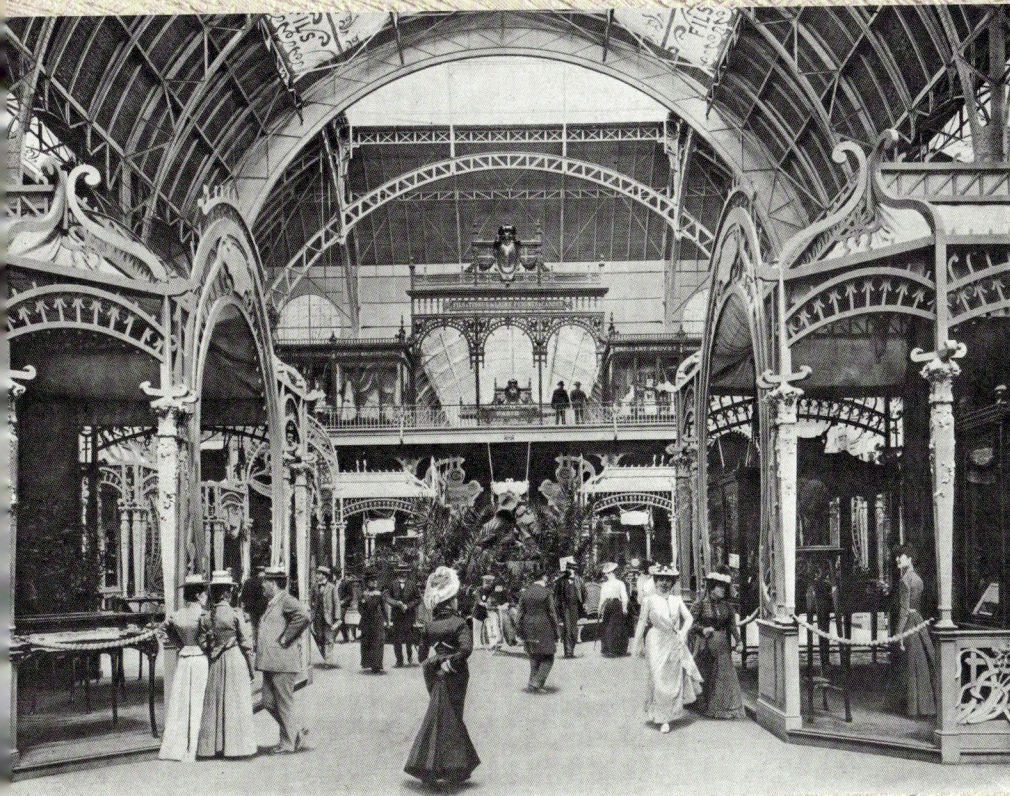

THE IMPORTANCE OF THE SALESROOM

Elegant stores were opened to attract a Parisian clientele and to sell off the ever-greater volumes produced by industrial methods. A perfume shop became a prestigious, sumptuous salesroom for receiving customers. From the 1860s, the exteriors were given a facelift with more vibrant colours, and each display was more creative than the next. Parisian high society of the Second Empire filed past the shop fronts, which displayed the name of the founder and the brand in large letters.

La parfumerie au Champ-de-Mars (Champ-de-Mars perfume businesses), illustration for *Le Panorama*, the Paris Exhibition, 1900.

PERFUMES IN THE CITIES AND BEYOND

To sell their goods across France, perfumers very quickly established a nationwide network of sales representatives to work with merchants or agents who bought the goods in cash for resale. Some perfume companies set up branches outside the cities and sent catalogues to local residents who were likely to be good customers. The exquisite, illustrated catalogues showcased the brands and mentioned the medals won at international exhibitions, the steam-powered factories and the boutiques. Around 1880, some large perfume brands such as Roger&Gallet, Pinaud and Piver made their appearance in department stores.

Roger&Gallet at 8, rue de la Paix in Paris, lithograph, 1914.

By setting up shop in the 'new products' section, they reached new, middle-class customers who would never have dared set foot in a luxury boutique. The elegant, eclectic, upmarket clientele, often royalty, continued to buy from the luxury brands such as Guerlain, the self-proclaimed 'aristocrat of the perfume world'. The lower middle class went to Gellé Frères or Bourjois and the working class shopped for their personal care products in the general perfume stores that sprang up on the large boulevards of Paris.

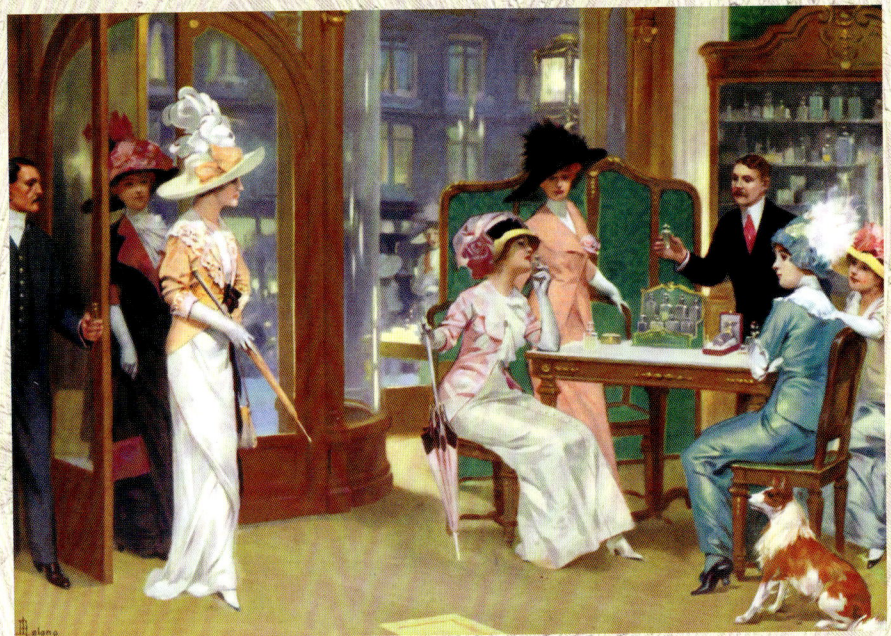

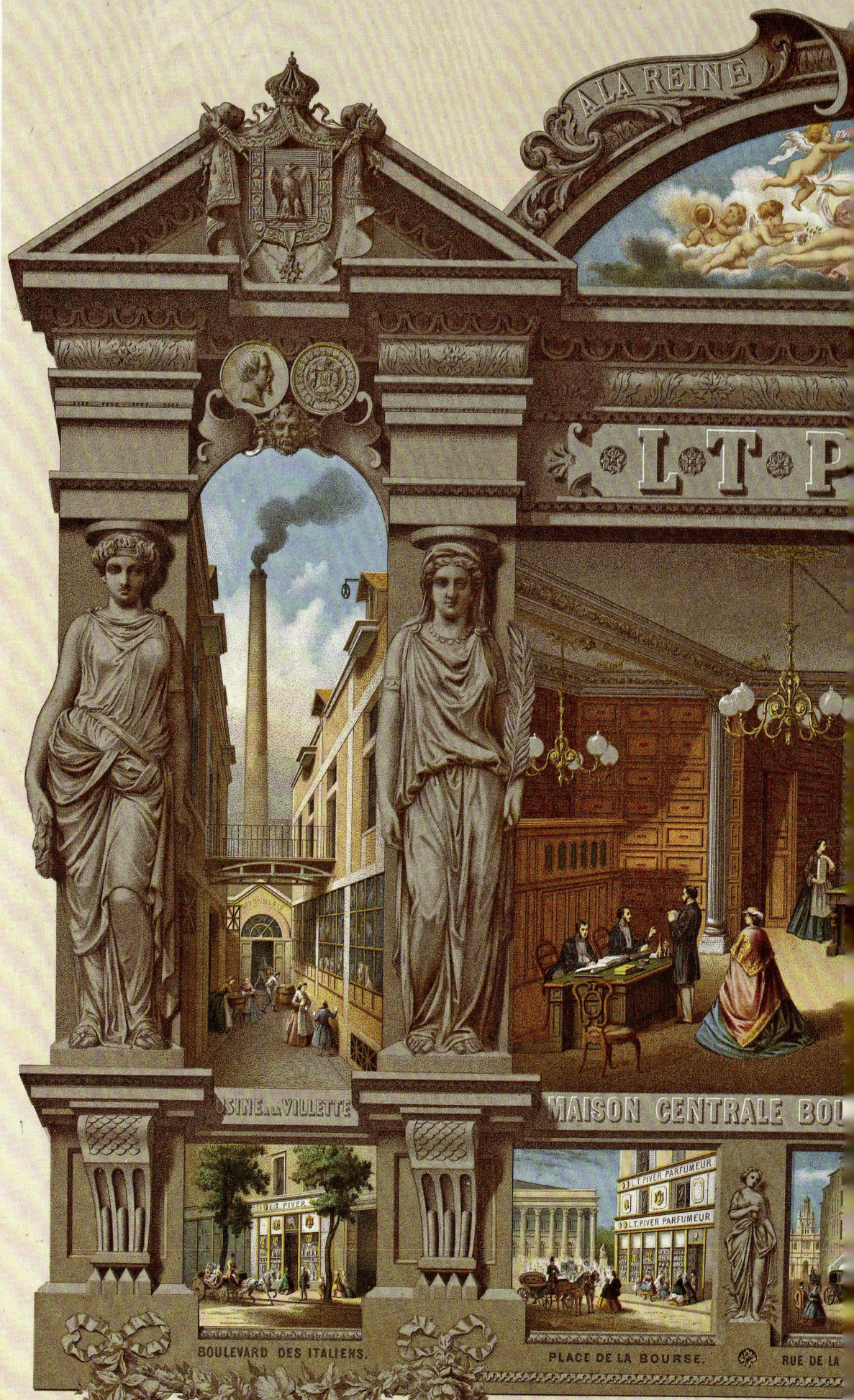

À LA REINE

L·T·P

PARFUMEUR DE

PA

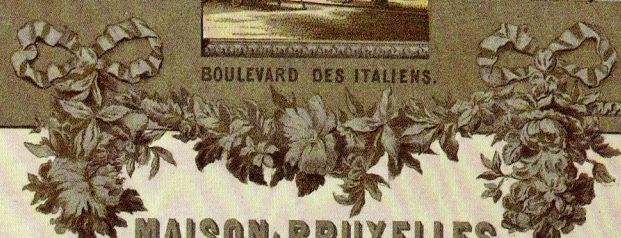

MAISON À BRUXELLES

USINE DE LA VILLETTE

MAISON CENTRALE BOU

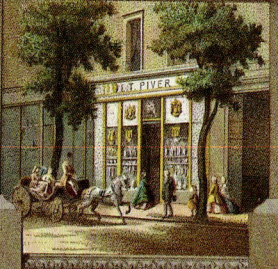

BOULEVARD DES ITALIENS.

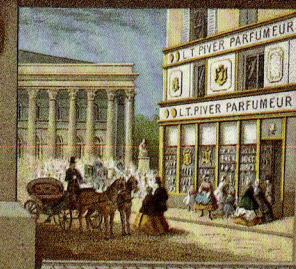

PLACE DE LA BOURSE.

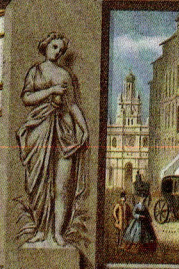

RUE DE LA

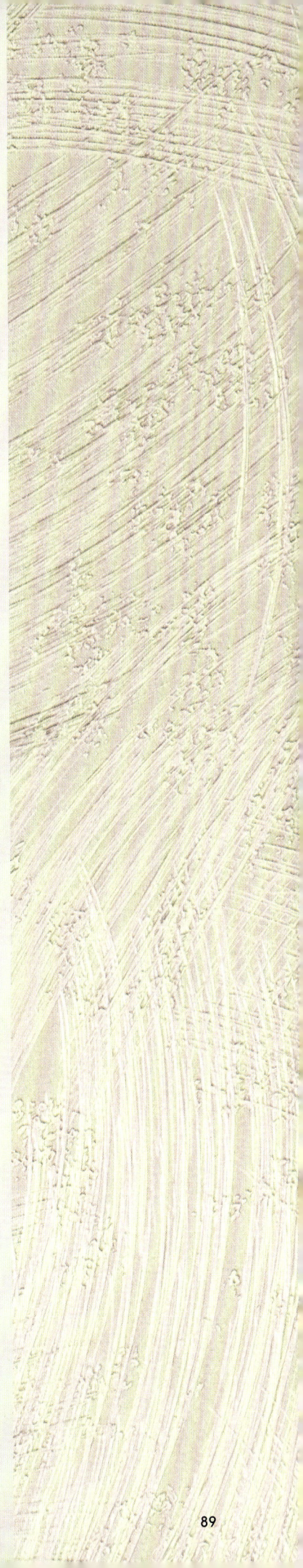

DES FLEURS

...VER

...RD DE STRASBOURG 10.   ...USINE A GRASSE

...D'ANTIN.   PLACE VENDÔME.   BOULEVARD POISSONNIÈRE.

M. L'EMPEREUR
...IS

MAISON A LONDRES

Success at home and abroad

Although France had some competition from abroad, it was not significant until the 1960s. Thanks to clever sales and marketing, French perfume exports soared from 1850 onwards. With brands vying for royal favour, foreign courts became clients and perfumers opened branches throughout the world. By the end of the nineteenth century, Guerlain was exporting to every country in Europe and even the United States. The brand's price lists at the time stated that it adapted the manufacture of its export products to suit every type of climate. Perfumers subsequently established subsidiaries in Europe and further afield and the smaller concerns, unable to keep up with the new demands of the industry, gradually disappeared.

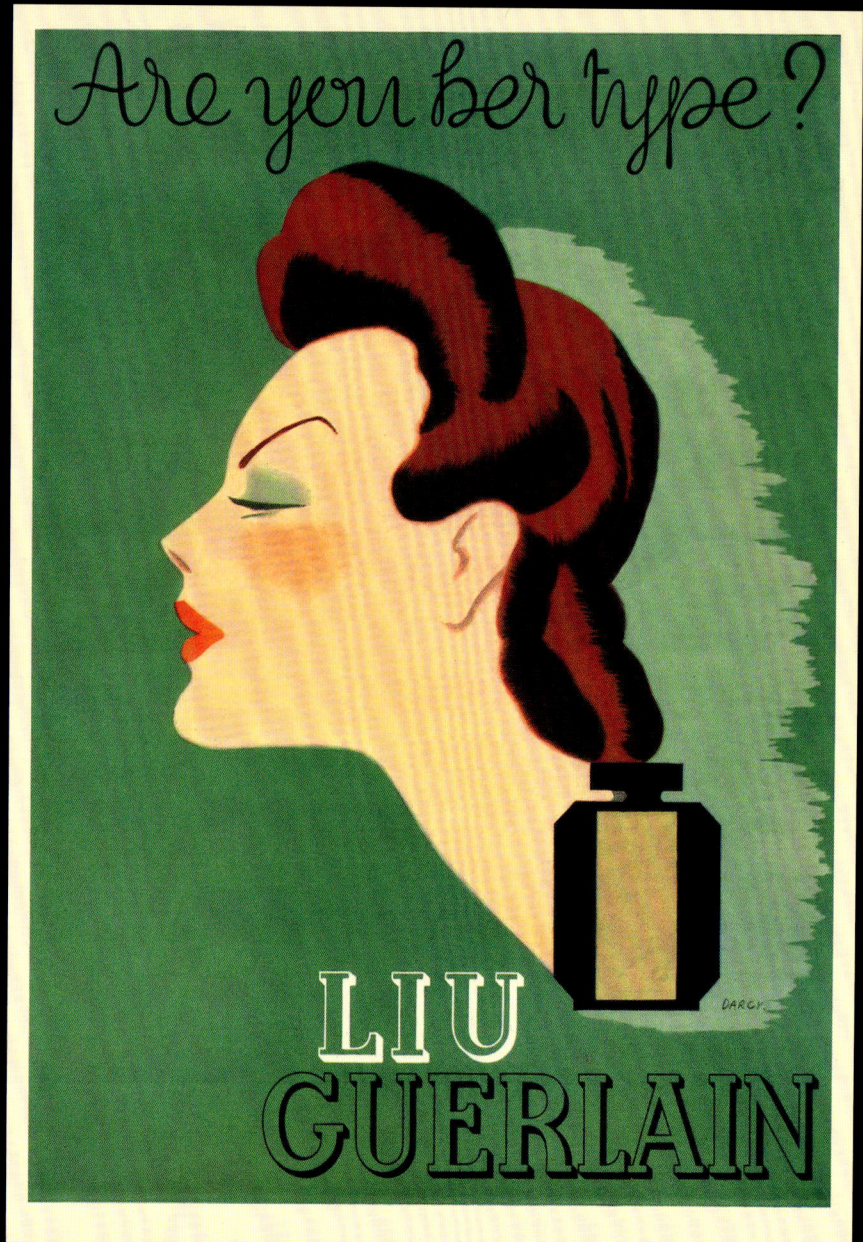

Are you her type?

LIU
GUERLAIN

Guerlain poster for Liu perfume, 1950s.

ENTER THE MULTINATIONALS

From the 1970s and 1980s, the perfume profession became a tighter-knit community as it faced growing rivalry from detergent manufacturers. The perfume business was at the height of its growth and had attracted large multinationals looking to diversify. They invested heavily to establish themselves as serious market players and achieved rapid results. Having gained greater international recognition and a broader customer base, perfume found itself in the paradoxical position of being both a luxury and a mass-market product. And because its future lay in a globalized world, it had to adapt to a wide range of cultures. From the 1980s, no perfume could find a place on the market without international visibility. Prestige remained its unique selling point and selective distribution was key to the promotion of French products. However, while France retained its position as market leader, there was increasing competition from other countries; together, American and Japanese groups accounted for a large proportion of international production.

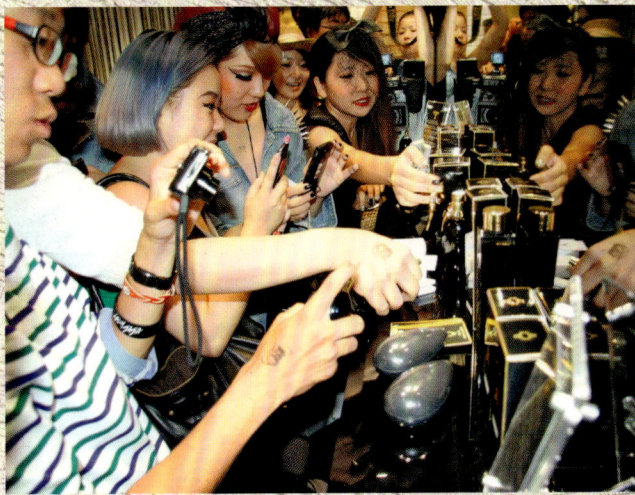

The Lady Gaga perfume store in Tokyo, 2012.

THE ADVENT OF MARKETING

Marketing as a set of techniques to devise, design and update and sell products came on the scene in the 1970s. Its aim was to create new demand with a view to meeting customer expectations and adapting production, sales and distribution accordingly. The first heavily marketed, lifestyle perfume was Charlie, launched in 1973 by the US brand Revlon. Perfume became a significant consumer product and brands' marketing strategies kept in step with the increasingly varied demands of customers who wore perfume every day. It was no longer a status symbol but remained a reflection of the wearer's personality and played a role in seduction. For customers to invest emotionally in a perfume, it had to be a quality product that was not readily available and had a genuine backstory. Yet, in today's fast-moving industry, brands and perfumes appear and disappear at lightning speed. Since the 2000s, there have been some 450 launches each year. The financial stakes are ever greater, supply outstrips demand and the market is expanding worldwide, at the risk of trying to please everybody and pleasing nobody.

NICHE PERFUME BRANDS

The concept of niche perfume brands came about in the late 1980s and referred to the small operations outside the mainstream industry which were creating experimental, highly unusual fragrances. Some were independent, others part of large groups, but they were all sceptical about marketing methods and, above all, wanted to bring meaning back to perfume, with the product being given priority over promotion. These brands had a strong identity and a significant olfactive slant because much of their production budget was spent on quality raw materials. And confidentiality was key to its success. In the bird world, a niche is a habitat in a protected area. The niche stores were hidden sanctuaries where well-trained staff offered a highly personalized service. In 1992, Serge Lutens designed the upmarket Salons du Palais-Royal as 'a symbol, a dream', the perfect symbiosis of Parisian chic and Japanese refinement.

Niche brands are innovative and often foreshadow future trends. For example, when in 2000 Lyn Harris created Miller Harris, an English perfume house offering subtle

A selection of Miller Harris perfumes, 2020 .

perfumes with touches of poetry and nostalgia, she used only high-quality natural ingredients, reflecting a return to nature. Harris had grown up in the Yorkshire countryside and spent her holidays in Scotland on her grandparents' farm, immersed in the scent of her grandfather's carpentry workshop and her grandmother's jam cooking.

Such brands are at the luxury end of the market. They champion the values of singularity and expertise, create value and generate margin. In short, they take the industry back to its roots. These are collections with integrity and a story to tell.

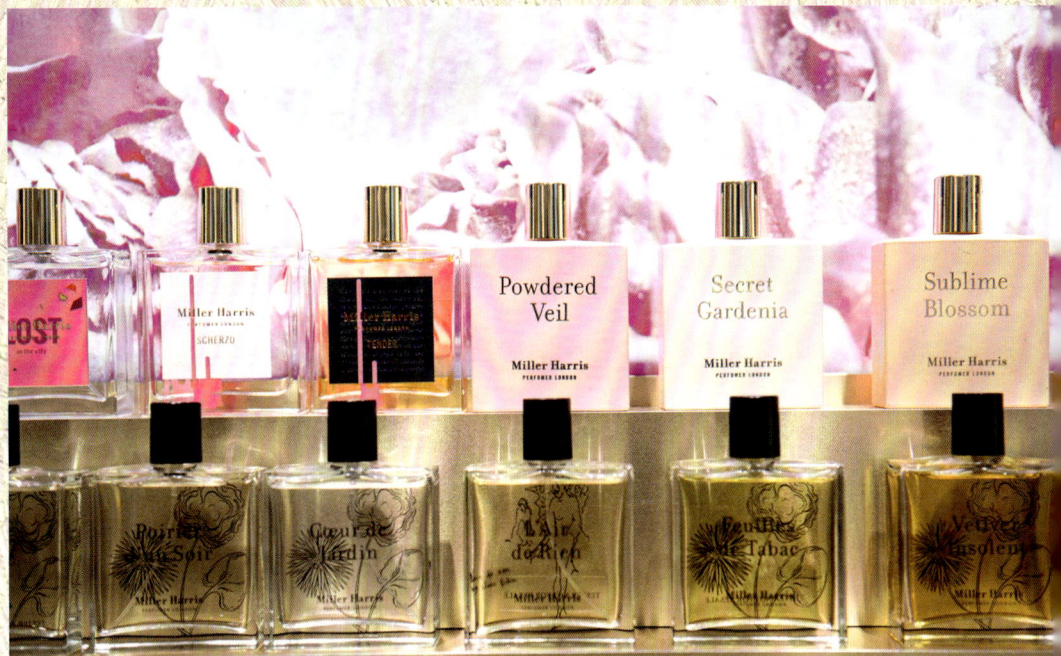

A MASS-PRODUCED INDUSTRIAL PRODUCT

NEW PEOPLE ENTERED THE INDUSTRY AND TECHNIQUES WERE DEVELOPED IN A CONSTANT QUEST FOR PERFECTION; ARTISTRY AND SALES AND MARKETING CAME TOGETHER TO BETTER MEET DEMAND AND CREATE THE DREAM. PERFUMERS TURNED PERFUME FROM WHAT WAS ESSENTIALLY A PERSONAL BODY-CARE PRODUCT INTO THE ULTIMATE GIFT. ONE STEP TOWARDS LUXURY BUT PRODUCED BY THE THOUSAND:

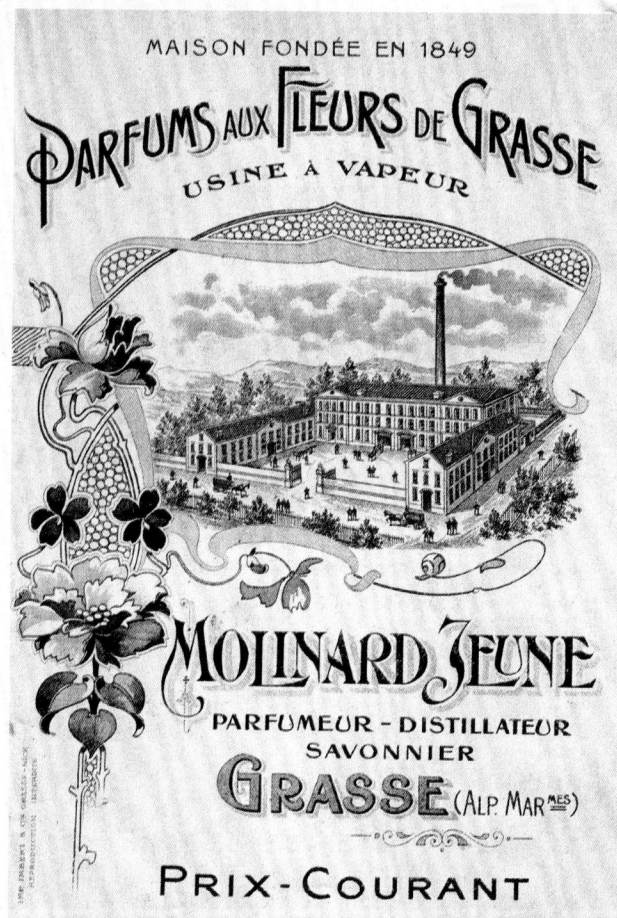

Advertising card depicting the steam-powered factory of Molinard Jeune, a company founded in 1849.

FRENCH PERFUME, THE BEST IN THE WORLD

Having inherited the products and mindset of the Ancien Régime perfumers, their nineteenth-century counterparts evolved from craftsmen and merchants to become industrialists. They attempted to reconcile the two trends to establish a luxury perfume industry, a subtle blend of craftsmanship and elegance driven by industrial machinery. At World's Fairs and International Exhibitions, French perfumery made its name and earned a reputation of being the best in the world. The 1900 Paris Exhibition, in particular, marked a turning point and left no doubt as to French supremacy in the field. The few industry statistics available paint a picture of prodigious growth. Perfume was a particularly attractive business proposition at the time.

A PERIOD OF TRANSITION AND GREAT CHANGE

Between 1890 and World War I, the perfume industry underwent a period of transition, capitalizing on its knowledge of botany, physiology, chemistry and applied mechanics to introduce steam-powered machinery, mechanize operations and improve the distillation process. Other groundbreaking innovations included extraction using volatile solvents, solid perfumes, organic chemistry, the creation of what was known as the 'model' factory and the industrial research laboratory. Reporting on the 1889 International Exhibition, Louis-Désiré L'Hôte correctly observed that perfume making had become a veritable industry that had taken inspiration from advances in mechanics, physics and chemistry. Following the example of chemical manufacturers, many industrialists had brought young chemists into their factories. These scientists would play an important role in the perfume industry. After 1889, the number of artificial fragrances increased. The most important products were patented. As for the others that had entered the public domain, such as vanillin, heliotropin, coumarin and hawthorn, stiff competition drove down the selling price.

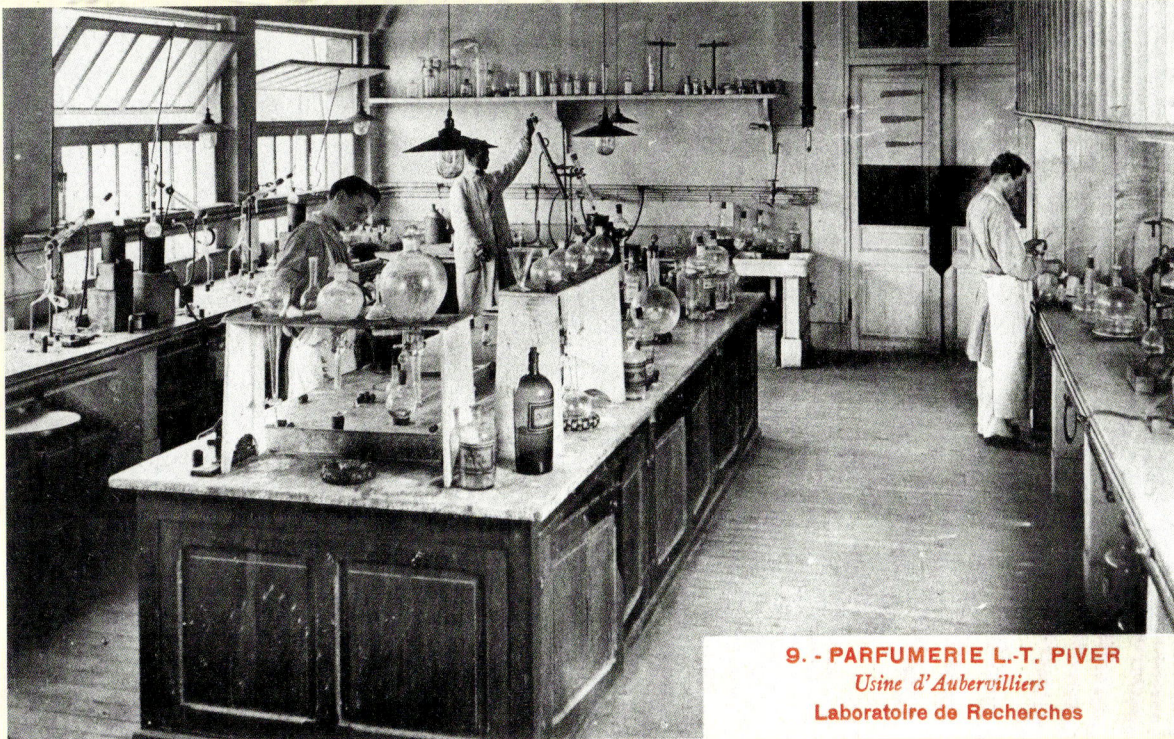

9. - PARFUMERIE L.-T. PIVER
Usine d'Aubervilliers
Laboratoire de Recherches

The L.T. Piver perfumery: the factory at Aubervilliers and its research lab. Postcard, circa 1910.

PERFUME BECOMES AN INDUSTRIAL PRODUCT

Gradually, the processes for making synthetic products moved out of the laboratory and into the factory. Catalogues listed 100% synthetics alongside many variations of products that were blends of various known fragrant compounds, sold under fancy names or the name of the corresponding essence. Before the outbreak of World War I, scientists and engineers had become perfume-chemistry experts. And yet, perfumers were reluctant to use synthetic products in their compositions because they felt they were not in keeping with the art and were harmful to health (see page 84). Some even believed their use showed a distinct lack of taste. However, immediately after the war, perfumers began to investigate these substances, which offered a number of advantages. Because of their ability to stabilize and intensify the scent, and their potential for mass production, they could add to the available range of fragrances on offer and be useful as bases and fixatives. These 'artificial' notes took the art of perfume out of the every-day world and into the realm of dreams.

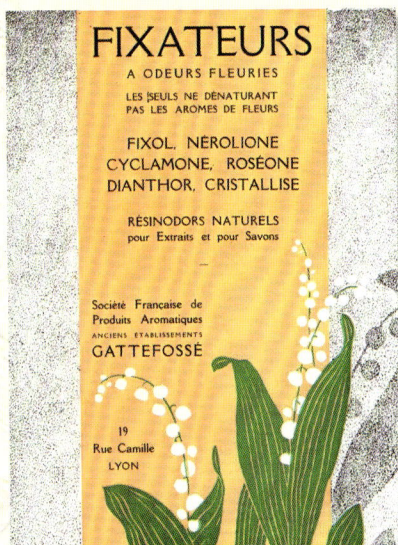

FIXATEURS
A ODEURS FLEURIES
LES SEULS NE DÉNATURANT
PAS LES AROMES DE FLEURS

FIXOL, NEROLIONE
CYCLAMONE, ROSÉONE
DIANTHOR, CRISTALLISE

RÉSINODORS NATURELS
pour Extraits et pour Savons

Société Française de
Produits Aromatiques
ANCIENS ÉTABLISSEMENTS
GATTEFOSSÉ

19
Rue Camille
LYON

Fixatives, from 'La Parfumerie moderne: revue scientifique et de la défense professionnelle' (Modern Perfumery: A Scientific and Professional Journal), 1921.

François Coty: revolutionary

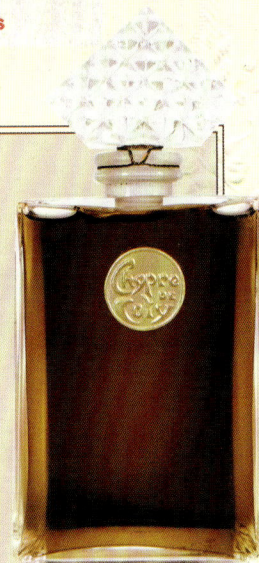

François Coty turned the rules of perfume design and creation on their head, enabling industrialization on a larger scale. His intuition and strategic thinking took perfume into a new era. He firmly believed that the market could be expanded to include the middle classes, and even some of the lower classes. He was a man of vision who wanted to make high-quality natural fragrances. To achieve this, he experimented to find the perfect balance of fine natural ingredients (absolutes) and mass-produced synthetic products to obtain the strength and clarity that were missing from existing perfumes. In doing so, he established the modern perfume families, particularly the florals, ambers (orientals) and chypres, based on traditional perfume accords.

Chypre by François Coty, 1917.

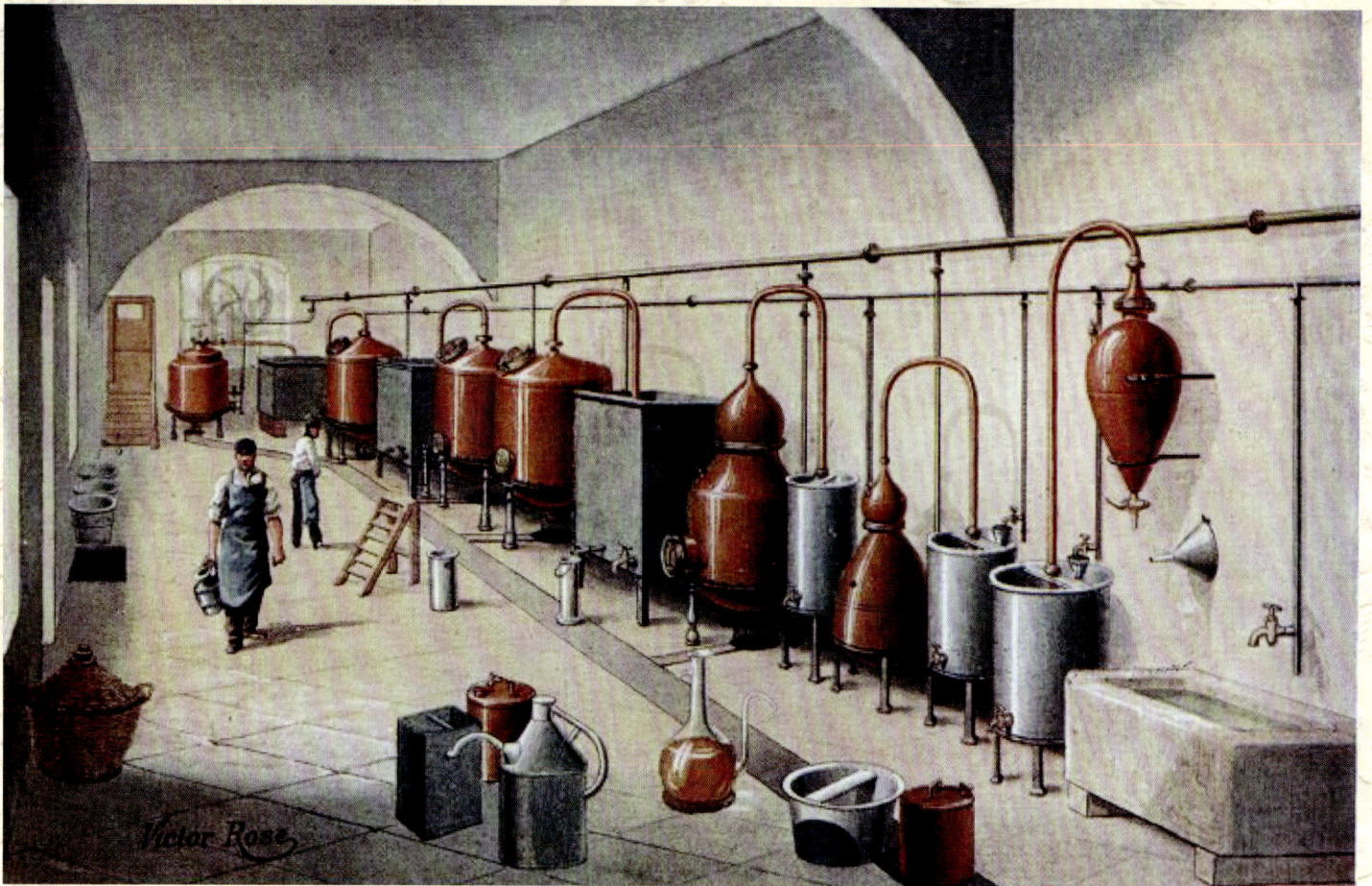

Distilling room at the former Robertet factory in Grasse, in *La Parfumerie Française et l'art dans la présentation* (French Perfumery and the Art of Presentation), published by *La Revue des marques de la parfumerie et de la savonnerie* (Review of Perfume and Soap Makers), 1925.

MECHANIZATION AFTER WORLD WAR I

At the end of World War I, a flurry of creations and styles positioned modern perfumery at the frontier of art and industry. Factories grew in size and wealth but the structure did not change. Mechanization made it possible to meet growing demand while adhering to the eight-hour day for factory workers brought in by a 1919 Act of Parliament. French manufacturers had to find ways to stay competitive in the face of foreign competition, which meant increasing output to keep costs down. This they achieved by standardizing working methods and introducing widespread mechanization, training workforces to operate the machines efficiently in order to deliver optimal quality.

MAN AND MACHINE

The Grasse companies combined manual operations (such as flower harvesting and sorting) with processes that had now been mechanized, such as pomade preparation. Having embraced industrialization, the perfumers made what were known as *communelles*, judicious blends of natural essences with similar properties. By blending the raw materials, they were able to obtain a large volume of essences of consistent quality. New products were created which could not have been made by hand. Because nothing less than perfection would do, in 1927 François Coty introduced vertical integration, bringing different aspects of the manufacturing process in-house at Cité des Parfums (Perfume City), a vast industrial complex he had established at Suresnes. Each stage, from administration to crystal production, engraving, printing, production of metal boxes and lipstick cases, powder-box filling and manufacture of the perfume itself, was seamlessly integrated on site. The packing departments preparing the finished goods for shipment and the lorries delivering them to France and beyond completed the picture. In the 1920s, synthetic floral notes were developed and produced in industrial quantities. Natural flower essences were hugely expensive to produce because of the massive volume of flowers required, so it was clearly beneficial to use synthetic notes.

Acceptance of synthetic bases

The merits of artificial products were finally acknowledged at the 1925 Paris Exhibition. The creation process now had one foot in the garden and the other in the lab; the perfumer's art was now to blend natural and synthetic products to create distinctive bases for the brands, and gain fame for the perfume houses. Guerlain's bases were known as 'Guerlinade'. A Coty perfume could not be confused with another perfumer's creation. From then on, each perfume house derived its own unique style from its bases, the elementary structures perfumers built from preconfigured components from their own fragrance palette. Production now depended on each perfumer's skill and the chemical knowledge gained during training.

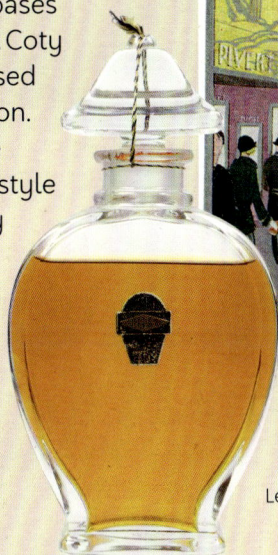

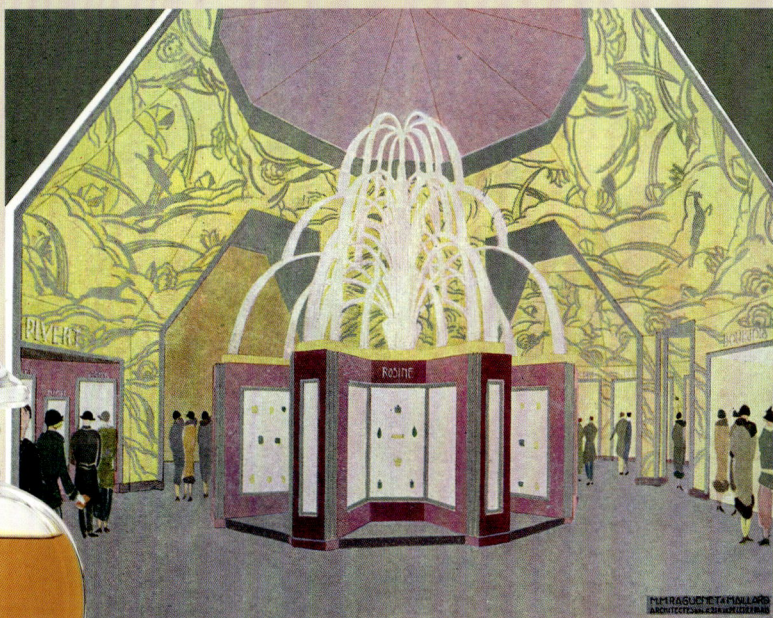

Above: Perfume section at the International Exhibition of Modern Decorative and Industrial Arts, *La parfumerie française et l'art dans la présentation* (French Perfumery and the Art of Presentation), in *La revue des marques de la parfumerie et de la savonnerie* (Review of Perfume and Soap Makers), 1925.

Left: Guerlain's Guerlinade, Baccarat bottle, 1922.

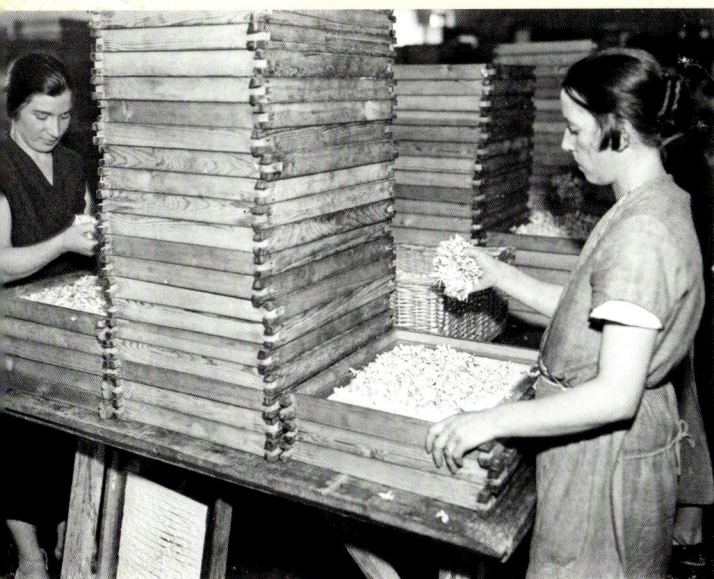

Enfleurage, at the company Roure-Bertrand Fils et Justin Dupont, in Grasse, 1931–4.

PERFUMES IN THE INTERWAR PERIOD

Synthetic components gave floral bouquets more staying power, for example in Joy, launched by Patou in 1935, which was made from ultra-precious Bulgarian rose and jasmine essences from Grasse. Émeraude (Coty, 1921), Shalimar (Guerlain, 1925), Bois des Îles (Chanel, 1928) and Tabu (Dana, 1931) were ambers, florals, woods or sweet ambers, with oriental notes. The chypres were also in demand and fell into the categories of floral, fruity, aromatic and leather. Examples included Chypre (Coty, 1917), Mitsouko (Guerlain, 1919) and Crêpe de Chine (Millot, 1925). In the 1930s, leather notes for women were in vogue after the release of perfumes such as Tabac Blond (Caron, 1919), Cuir de Russie (Chanel, 1927), Scandal (Lanvin, 1932) and Kobako (Bourjois, 1936). The various families were combined in many ways to create some truly exquisite fragrances. The perfume industry's heyday continued after World War II, thanks to the changes and new developments made possible by product innovation and the invention of new processes. Little by little, perfume became a mass-market item and entered every level of the social sphere. It was no longer the preserve of the elite.

ADVERTISING GETS IN ON THE ACT

THE RISE OF MODERN PERFUME MIRRORED THAT OF ADVERTISING. POSTERS AND SLOGANS HAD TO BE EYE-CATCHING AND MEMORABLE. IN THE MIDDLE OF THE 1937 RECESSION, JOY WAS ADVERTISED AS 'THE WORLD'S MOST EXPENSIVE PERFUME'. GABRIELLE CHANEL POSED FOR HER NO. 5, AND GUERLAIN'S 'ARE YOU HER TYPE?' POSTERS ADVERTISED PERFUMES FOR BLONDES, BRUNETTES AND REDHEADS (SEE PAGE 90). THE FIRST ADVERTISING CAMPAIGNS HAD ARRIVED!

EARLY BUCOLIC-STYLE ADVERTISING

At the end of the nineteenth century, the country scenes so popular in eighteenth-century advertising were still proving to be a good way for brands to assert their identity, appeal to women and promote a certain lifestyle. It was common to look back to the time of the great perfumers to the royal family and to capitalize on a legacy of gallantry and aristocracy. Beribboned women radiated a reassuring purity, like a scene from an old-fashioned romantic comedy. The illustrations were in soft colours and, like a painting, often contained in a rococo-style frame. Rural scenes depicted women playing gentle games and dancing joyful farandoles, as in the time of Marie-Antoinette. They could have been paintings by Watteau or Boucher of happier times gone by – which could be found again through perfume. This representation of fragrance as synonymous with happiness and refinement was used in adverts in the 1900s for product lines such as Manon Lescaut (Bourjois), Parfumerie Louis XV (Rigaud) and Souvenir de la Cour (Roger&Gallet, 1908). Perfumers wanted to portray the real and recognizable. However, this tendency to seek inspiration in the past was gradually replaced by the fantastical, ethereal personas of the Art Nouveau movement, which were more evocative of carnal and sensual olfactive profiles.

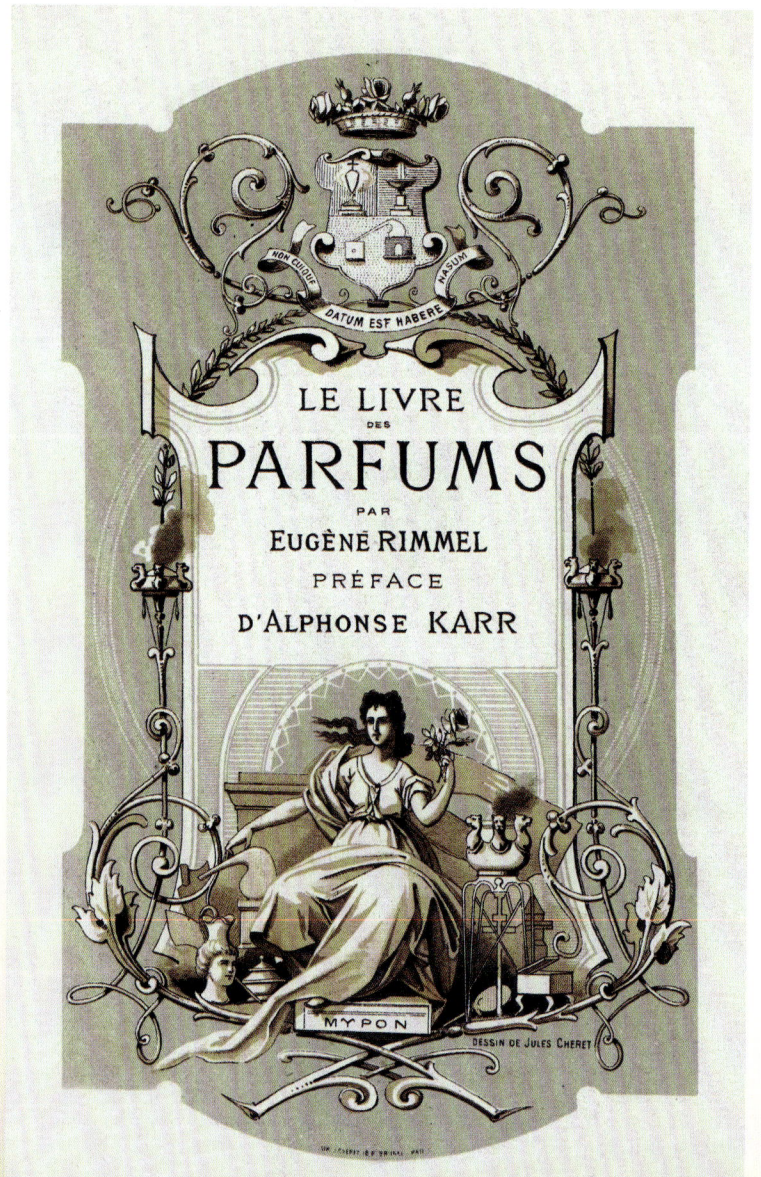

Illustration by Jules Chéret for the cover of *The Book of Perfumes* by Eugène Rimmel, 1870.

JULES CHÉRET: FAMOUS BELLE ÉPOQUE ILLUSTRATOR

Jules Chéret (1836-1932), the man behind the modern poster, was considered something of a pioneer in the world of advertising. He had initially set his sights on training as a lithographer before he became a regular visitor to the Louvre and attended evening drawing classes at the École des Beaux-Arts in Paris. After a first trip to London in 1854, where he discovered Turner and Constable's landscapes, he created a much-acclaimed poster for the Offenbach operetta *Orpheus in the Underworld* in 1858. He was again in London from 1859 to 1866, where he worked for the perfumer Eugène Rimmel. He illustrated Rimmel's work *The Book of Perfumes* and created floral labels and decorations for him. His colourful ads promoted events, places and brands, including Roger&Gallet. Jules Chéret's signature style made use of bold colours and always featured his 'Chérettes' – happy, free-spirited women in motion. He was awarded a gold medal at the 1889 International Exhibition in Paris and his work inspired famous painters such as Henri de Toulouse-Lautrec and Pierre Bonnard.

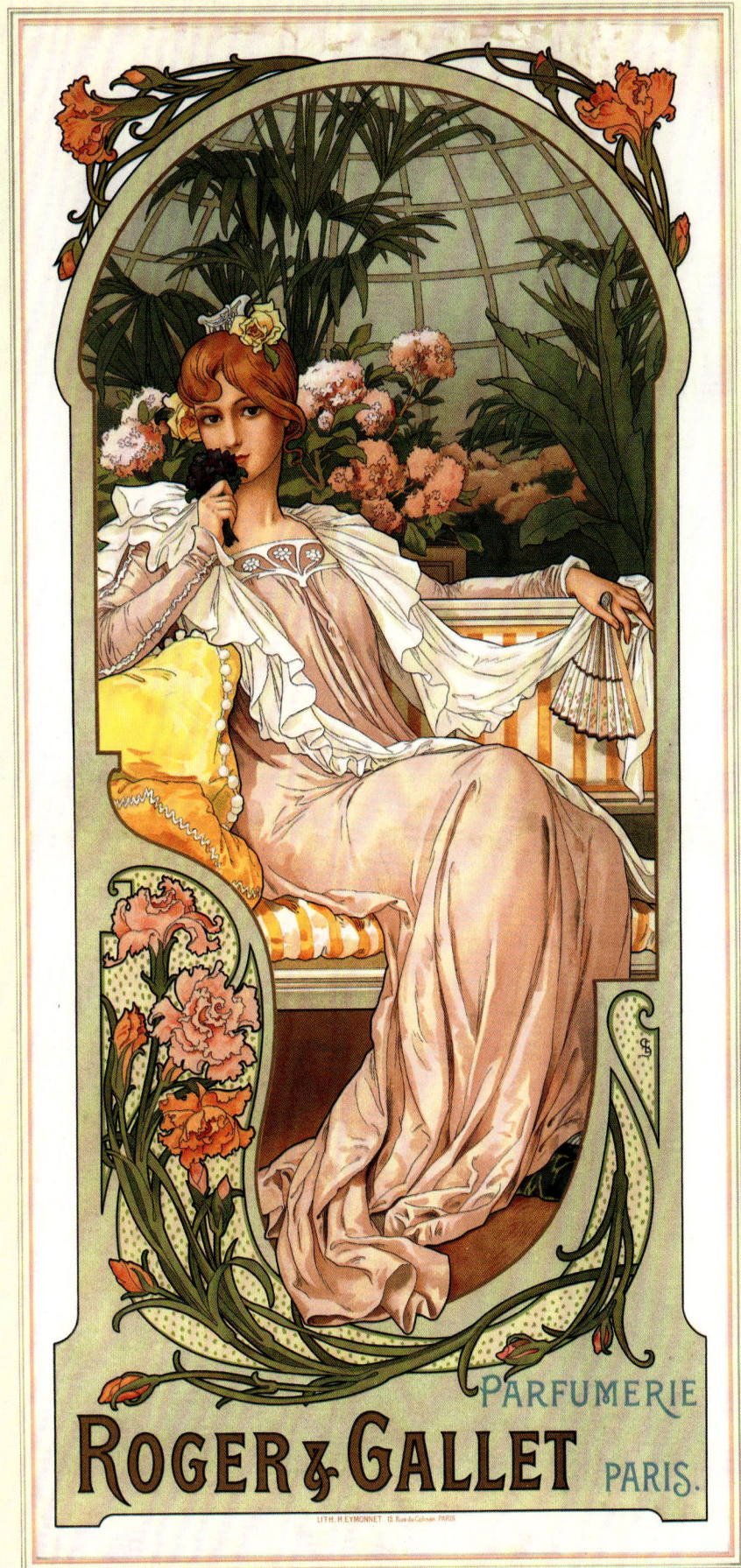

Roger&Gallet advertising poster by Elisabeth Sonrel (1874–1953). Roger&Gallet archives.

ALFONS MUCHA AND HIS 'FLOWER WOMEN'

Alfons Mucha, a Czech artist born in 1860, was an Art Nouveau decorative painter and poster illustrator. He designed posters advertising new industrially made products such as bicycles, cigarettes and, of course, perfumes. A decorative female figure always took centre stage in his mystical, magical, ethereal posters. A talented illustrator, he was known as the 'father of advertising' and was influenced by the burgeoning concept of the mythical Parisian woman.

In 1896, Rodo asked him to design a poster for his newly released perfume spray (the poster was printed by Ferdinand Champenois). Mucha was then commissioned by Houbigant to design their stand at the 1900 Paris Exhibition. In the space of a few years, this type of decorative advertising would be adopted by almost all the perfume brands and, in 1910, Roger&Gallet created an advert that was a perfect replica of one of Mucha's. Showing the influence of the Art Nouveau movement, golden-haired, wasp-waisted 'flower women' with their open bodices and seductive smiles became the iconic images of perfume advertising. Playful and sensual, they stretched and arched their backs provocatively, ruffling lightweight fabrics to reveal a glimpse of their slender legs. And so was born the dream of the Art Nouveau woman as a goddess displaying a fleeting hint of sensuality, very much in keeping with the biomorphic arabesque shapes of Mother Nature. Advertising was becoming increasingly allegorical and it reproduced literary themes that took perfume into the realms of the sensual and emotional.

Opposite: Poster advertising the launch of 'Rodo' perfume. Alfons Mucha, colour print, 1896.

Guerlain's L'Heure Bleue, 1912

On a beautiful late summer's afternoon in 1911, Jacques Guerlain was walking with his son along the banks of the Seine. Daylight was fading and dusk was on the horizon. They witnessed a twilight sky turning a deeper blue than the usual sky blue, caused by a phenomenon known in physics as Rayleigh scattering. In this blue hour, Jacques Guerlain felt that everything was in perfect harmony. He is said to have experienced something so intense that the only way he could express it was in a perfume. And yet, the Belle Époque had run its course and was coming to an end. The world was going mad and there were rumblings of war. Jacques Guerlain himself talked about having a sensation of impending doom. During World War I, handkerchiefs sprayed with L'Heure Bleue, the perfume inspired by that moment and worn by his wife Lily, were handed out to soldiers in the trenches. It became something of a talisman, one of the most beautiful perfume metaphors to this day, intended to provide an invisible, but comforting, female presence to cheer up the soldiers.

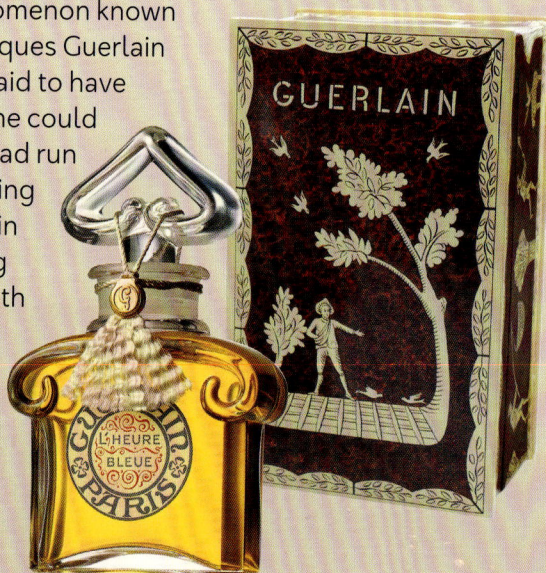

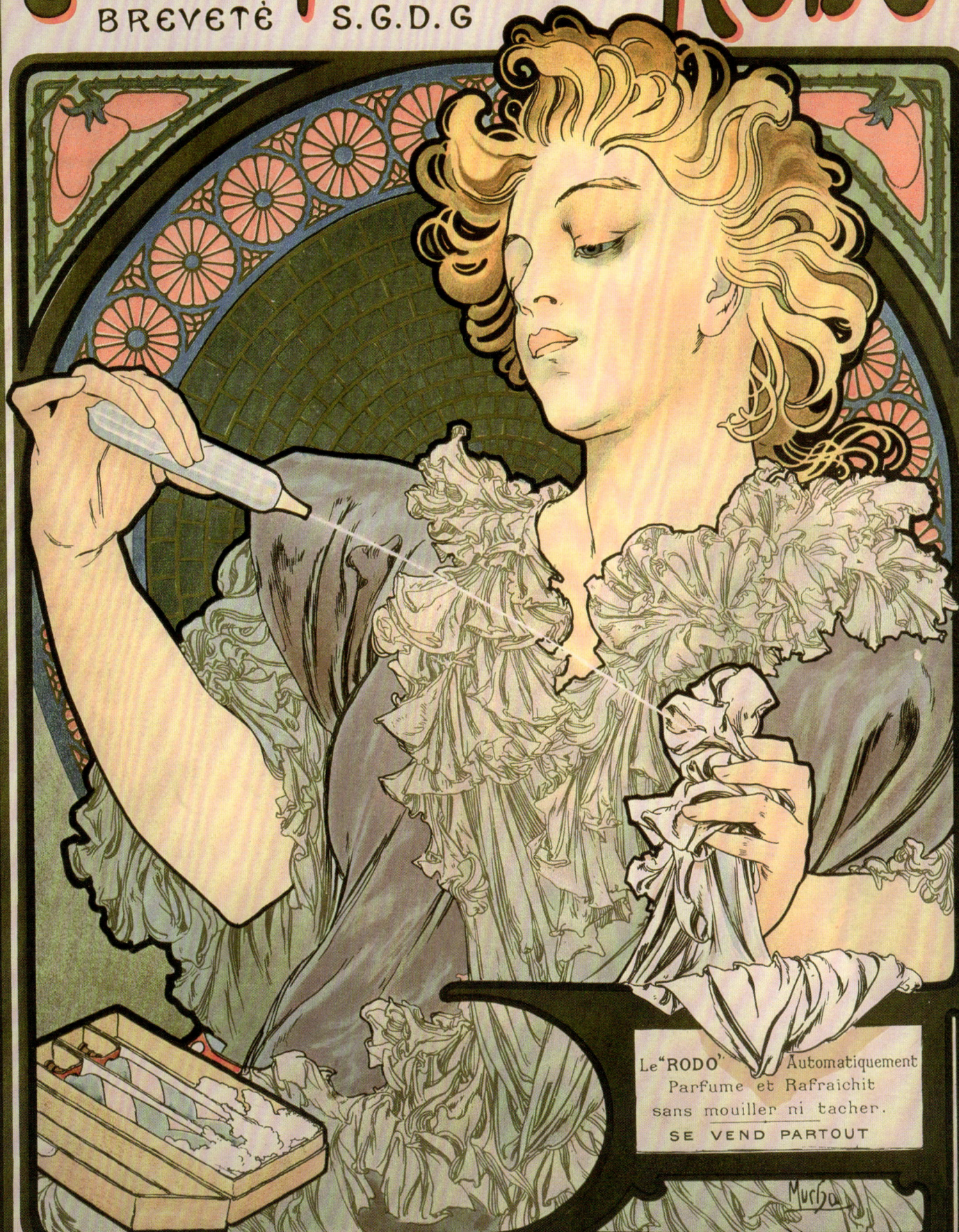

WOMEN'S EMANCIPATION AND ADVERTISING

In the 1920s, women embraced shorter hair and shorter hemlines and began to smoke openly in public. A flawless, even tan with no visible lines marked out the social elite, who could afford to spend their free time in the sun. Perfumers brought out suntan oils. Makeup became the working woman's best friend because it could hide signs of fatigue and was the perfect way to add an elegant, seductive touch. Sports and cars would be the new passions of women, who asserted their social identity in an interwar period that resonated to the stirring tunes of the Charleston, foxtrot, tango and other dances of the time. Women enjoyed nightlife, flirted, earned their own living and dressed the part.

Adverts depicted active women on the move and the corresponding images were often car- or cigarette-related. Sport prompted the concept of a unisex fragrance. Thus, the copy for Patou's 1929 perfume Le Sien proclaimed that men and women were equal on the playing field, that sports fashion was classic and practical, and so a perfume that was too feminine would not strike the right note. It referred to a scent that was straightforward and wholesome, with an 'outdoors' feel, so it was suitable for men but also chimed with the personality of the modern woman who played golf, smoked and was a demon behind the wheel.

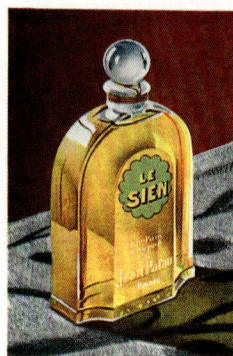

"A FEMME SPORTIVE PARFUM MASCULIN"

"Le Sport est un terrain où la femme et l'homme sont égaux. Avec la Mode de Sport, sobre et pratique, un parfum trop efféminé est une fausse note.,

"Le Sien" est un parfum d'inspiration plutôt masculine., Je l'ai composé dans cette note franche, saine, très "en dehors" qui convient à l'homme, mais qui s'allie bien aussi avec la personnalité de la femme moderne qui joue au golf, fume, et conduit sa voiture à 120 à l'heure.,"

JEAN PATOU

"le sien"

Advert for Le Sien by Jean Patou, 1929.

The first 'faces' of perfume

In 1853, Pierre François Pascal Guerlain created Eau de Cologne Impériale in honour of the wife of Napoleon III, the Empress Eugenie, his one-time muse who had become his patron and benefactor. However, the first 'face' hired officially by a perfume house was the sublime actress Sarah Bernhardt, in 1890, who appeared in a large number of perfume and makeup adverts. Until around 1860, actresses in the theatre were the only women to wear makeup, or greasepaint as it was known, on stage and in their everyday lives, and to spray themselves liberally with perfume. Bourgeois norms did not permit virtuous society women to do likewise. When, in the late nineteenth century, morals changed and makeup was permitted, some actresses became ambassadors for the art of self-adornment and shared their beauty secrets with other women. It was their faces that appeared in the first adverts painted on the walls of major capital cities.

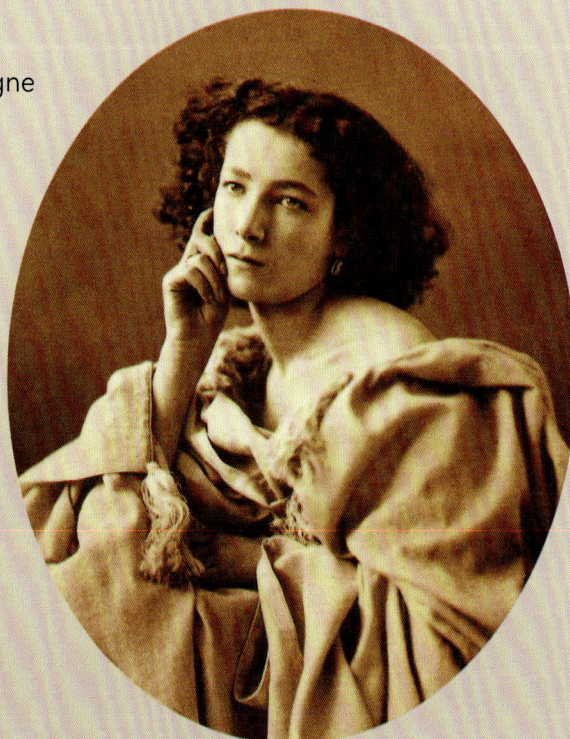

Sarah Bernhardt photographed by the French photographer Nadar, 1859.

GABRIELLE CHANEL AND THE BRAND'S MUSES

Muses played a very important role in advertising's psychological hold on women. The oldest image of Chanel No. 5 is from 1921. It is a lithograph by Sem, the illustrator and famous caricaturist and friend of Gabrielle Chanel, depicting a flapper raising her face and arms towards the magical bottle – an image truly representative of the importance of the launch. It shows the new woman in all her femininity reaching out towards No. 5 which, for her, epitomizes promises and dreams. Next, Gabrielle Chanel put herself in front of the camera in a 1937 photo by François Kollar. In it, she is leaning against the fireplace of the Ritz suite she called home, overlooking place Vendôme. There followed a series of stunning muses selected by the expert eye of artistic director Jacques Helleu, whose sole desire was to have Chanel No. 5 represented by the most beautiful women in the world. He also called upon the biggest names in photography and cinema to bring together in one advert the image of the bottle set off to perfection by a face. He was always inspired by his love of cinema and a desire to tell true stories in which there was a woman, a perfume and a man – or at least the promise of love.

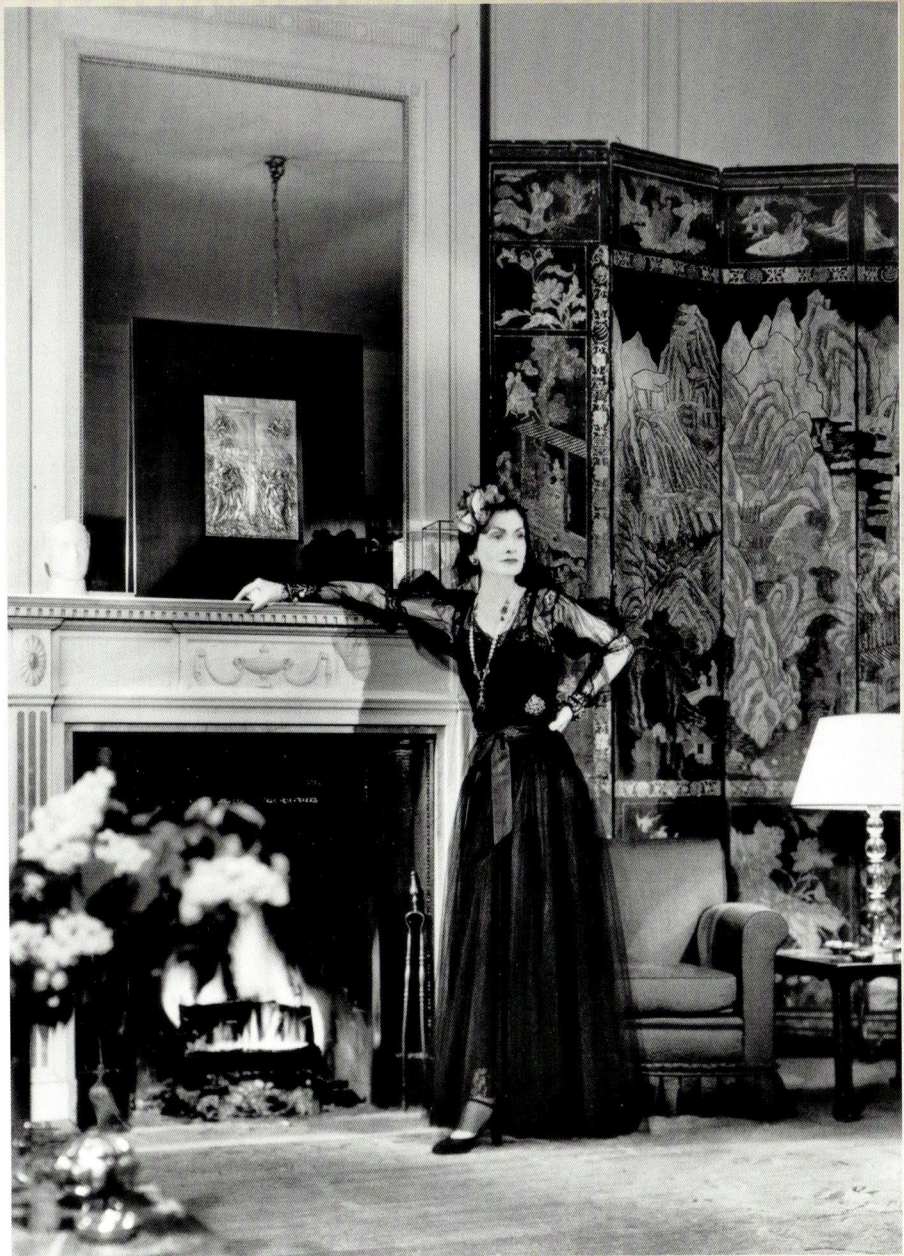

Gabrielle Chanel in her suite at the Paris Ritz in 1937. This François Kollar photo was selected for the Chanel No. 5 advertising campaign.

HOLLYWOOD ICONS

The concept of muses and icons with whom women could identify rose with the popularity of Hollywood cinema in the 1920s and 1930s. Women copied the hairstyles, dress and mannerisms of its glamorous stars. Perfume was femininity in a bottle, a golden liquid that could turn them into goddesses in their own right. Joy (1930) was dedicated to American women and film stars such as Louise Brooks, as was *Coty's Muse* (1947). In Billy Wilder's film *Sunset Boulevard* (1950), Gloria Swanson's character, Norma Desmond, sprayed herself liberally with Narcisse Noir by Caron (1911). Fracas by Piguet (1948), made for actress Edwige Feuillère, had and continues to have devoted fans, among them Marlene Dietrich, Madonna, Kim Basinger, Naomi Campbell and Princess Caroline of Monaco. Youth Dew, launched in 1953 as the sexiest perfume of all time, was the signature scent of the 1950s femme fatale. In her book *My Way of Life*, Joan Crawford confessed that she could never live without it.

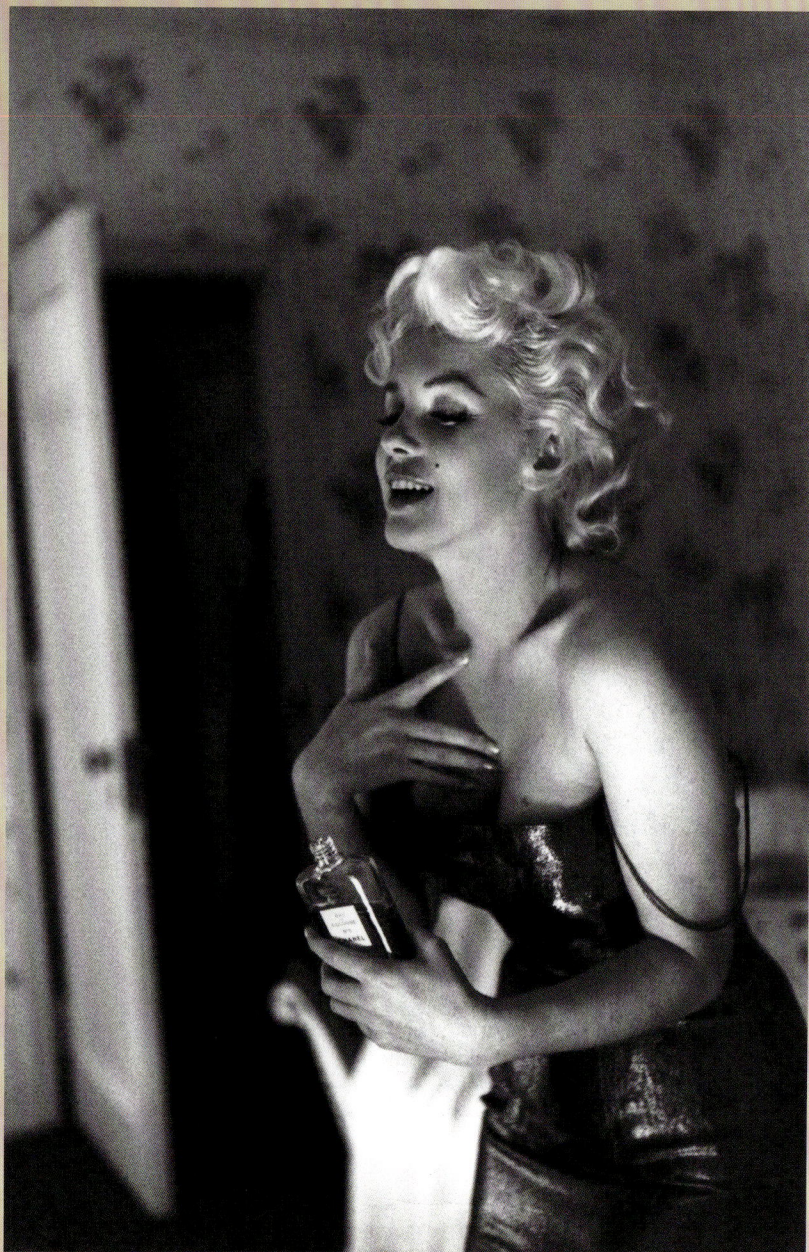

Marilyn Monroe and Chanel No. 5

In 1952, Chanel No. 5 aficionado Marilyn Monroe said, 'I lose my sense of smell without it.' The whole world, hanging on to every word that left her fabulous lips, was charmed by a famous anecdote. When asked what she wore in the morning, she replied a skirt and blouse. When she was then asked what she wore in bed her response was, 'Just a few drops of No. 5.' This free publicity worked its magic and Gabrielle Chanel must have been delighted, and possibly amused, by it. Both women had perfected the art of seduction, so Marilyn Monroe's spontaneous comment tied in nicely with this image, as did the photos of her clasping a bottle of No. 5 — a marvel of grace and sensuality, just like the soul-enhancing properties of the perfume itself.

POST-WAR DELUSIONS OF GRANDEUR

After World War II, research and sales and marketing in the perfume world were dominated by a quest for quality and continuous innovation. Marketing teams focused their efforts on advertising to a particularly receptive, and increasingly demanding, 1950s market. Socio-cultural change had affected lifestyles, which were now observed and analysed.

It was almost always women who appeared in 1950s perfume adverts and most of the houses signed exclusivity contracts with models who would become the face of the brand. The famous Chanel No. 5 (1921) has had many ambassadors over the years, including Ali McGraw, Lauren Hutton, Catherine Deneuve, Carole Bouquet, Nicole Kidman and Audrey Tautou. Their beauty has been immortalized by the most talented photographers, such as Richard Avedon, Helmut Newton and Patrick Demarchelier. In 1957, Hubert de Givenchy gifted Audrey Hepburn her own personal perfume. When his company admitted they wanted to put it on the market the same year, she jokingly refused and so the name of the perfume became L'Interdit, which means 'forbidden' in French. The first publicity launch that broke the mould was for Poison by Dior in 1985, and it was a huge success. In 1989, Guerlain invested a record-breaking $50 million into its Samsara advertising campaign.

Marilyn Monroe applying Chanel No. 5, 1955.
Photograph by Ed Feingersh.

SUPERMODELS AND FILM STARS

The 1990s witnessed the advent of a new phenomenon: the super-model. These women were the elite, the most in demand and the highest paid, of the modelling world. They graced international magazine covers and walked the haute couture runways. Naomi, Cindy, Linda, Christy, Claudia, Kate … they became muses for designers and friends and very quickly claimed the limelight. Kate Moss, who shot to fame when she was photographed for Calvin Klein's iconic Obsession campaign, became the face of a certain social style, the icon of a whole generation. Linda Evangelista famously declared in 1990, the same year she posed for Fidji by Guy Laroche, that she wouldn't get out of bed for less than $10,000 a day.

Some adverts shot at the end of the twentieth century and beginning of the twenty-first century were filmed by movie directors, the longest of them by Baz Luhrmann for No. 5 in 2004. It lasted for 180 seconds and starred Nicole Kidman. Other Hollywood actresses who have represented perfumes in major campaigns include Charlize Theron, Natalie Portman, Jennifer Lawrence, Scarlett Johansson and Cate Blanchett.

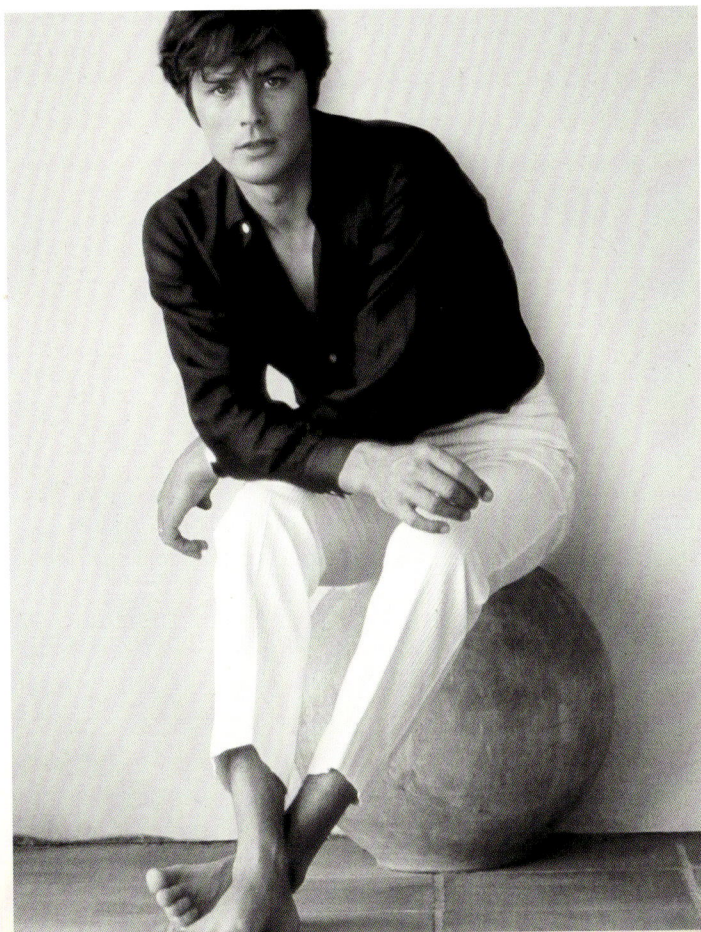

Nicole Kidman, photographed by Patrick Demarchelier for the Chanel No. 5 campaign in 2006.

This iconic 1966 photo of actor Alain Delon, taken by Jean-Marie Périer, was used again in 2009 for Dior's Eau Sauvage campaign.

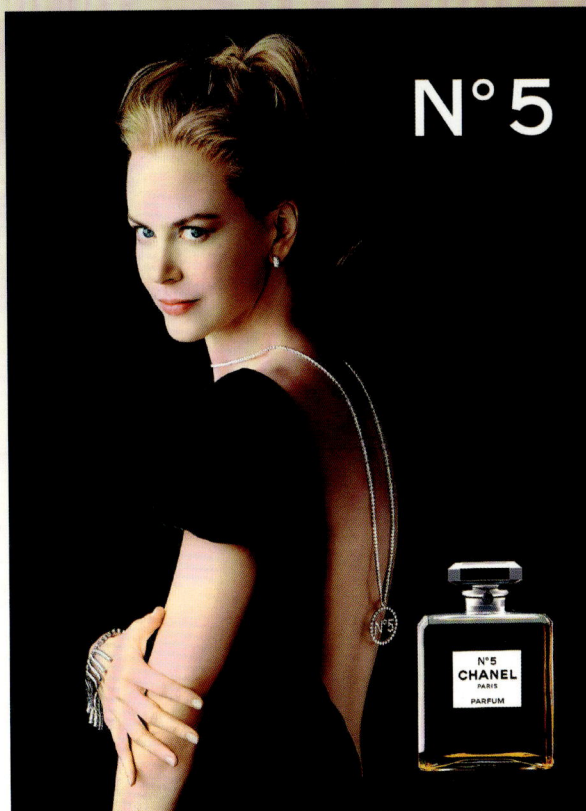

MALE PERFUME AMBASSADORS

Today, male fragrances also have their ambassadors. They can be male or female, as long as they do not overshadow the product. Dior's first perfume for men, Eau Sauvage, created by Edmond Roudnitska in 1966, also appealed to women because of its light fragrance. It was the world's best-selling male perfume in the last 25 years of the twentieth century. The fragrance was sporty, classic and elegant, as was the bottle with its rounded corners and silver-grey 'belt'. The accompanying, rather risqué, advertising by René Gruau featured a naked man applying perfume in his bathroom. There followed a series of adverts with male celebrities, including footballer Zinédine Zidane, wearing a black turtleneck sweater pulled up to under their eyes to emphasize their 'wild' look (Eau Sauvage means 'wild water'). Alain Delon proved to be a worthy successor in 2009, this time with images from the 1960s. The iconic photos, taken by Jean-Marie Périer in 1968 while Delon was filming Jacques Deray's *La Piscine* (The Swimming Pool), speak louder than words.

In 2015, Johnny Depp was made the face of Dior's Sauvage, a move that was so successful for the brand, they renewed his contract in 2023.

MASTER GLASSMAKERS: GLASS AND CRYSTAL

ACCORDING TO THE HEAVY-DRINKING FRENCH POET ALFRED DE MUSSET, THE BOTTLE WAS IRRELEVANT PROVIDED THE CONTENTS GOT YOU DRUNK. FOLLOWING THIS LOGIC, IT IS A MERE ACCESSORY WHOSE MAIN PURPOSE IS TO PRESERVE PERFUME AND ONLY THE CONTENTS HAVE THE POWER TO AWAKEN THE SENSES. YET BOTTLES HAVE ALWAYS HAD A VERY IMPORTANT ROLE IN PERFUMERY. SINCE ANCIENT TIMES, THEY HAVE BEEN NEEDED TO PRESERVE FRAGRANCE AND, WITHOUT A BOTTLE MADE BY A MASTER GLASSMAKER, THERE IS NO PERFUME !

BACCARAT: FROM CARAFES TO PERFUME BOTTLES

The Baccarat glassworks was founded by royal decree in 1765, during the reign of Louis XV. The factory, located on the banks of the River Meurthe in Lorraine, produced all sorts of glassware, mainly drinking vessels and windowpanes. Bought in 1816 by Aimé-Gabriel d'Artigues, a former director of the Saint-Louis glass factory, it began to make crystal and was rewarded with a gold medal at the 1855 International Exhibition. In 1860, by popular demand, Baccarat added 'bottles for perfumers' to its catalogue, fashioning them on the model of small wine and liqueur carafes.

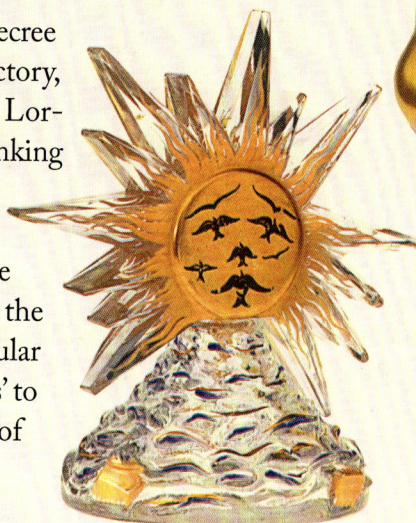

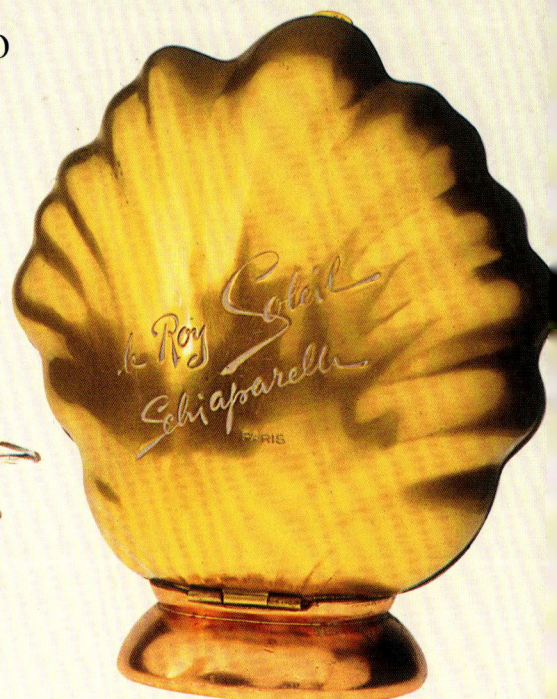

Le Roy Soleil perfume bottle with a special case by Salvador Dalí for Elsa Schiaparelli. Mould-blown clear crystal painted with gold and enamel, Baccarat ,1945.

Guerlain, Elizabeth Arden, Dior ... they all loved Baccarat!

Baccarat featured prominently at the 1925 Paris Exhibition, with a pavilion on the Esplanade des Invalides; its artistic director, Georges Chevalier, who ran the Baccarat workshops in the 1920s, created some extraordinary products for the occasion. The company joined forces with major brands to design exceptional bottles for famous fragrances, such as the black crystal one for Liu by Guerlain. In 1939, Baccarat designed a hand holding a golden bottle for Elizabeth Arden's It's You. In 1947, Ferdinand Guéry-Colas created the overlay crystal amphora bottle for Baccarat, of which only 200 were made, and in 1956, a bottle in the shape of an upside-down amphora topped with a gilded bronze bouquet of flowers was perfect for the floral fragrance of Diorissimo. In 1997, Baccarat launched Une Nuit Étoilée au Bengale, the first in a series of three of its own perfumes, which was followed by Les Larmes Sacrées de Thèbes and Un Certain Été à Livadia. However, the company was also forced to succumb to industrialization and include moulded crystal in its production, creating new decorative elements such as 'Torsade' (twist), 'Laurier' (laurel leaves), 'Serpent' (snake), 'Russe' (Russian) and 'Rosaces Multiples' (a repeat rosette pattern), all of which became fairly popular.

SAINT-LOUIS AND CRYSTAL: THE MIDAS TOUCH

◆

The Saint-Louis crystal works were founded in 1767 in Saint-Louis-lès-Bitche (Lorraine), which had been home to a thriving glass industry since the sixteenth century. In 1781, François de Beaufort oversaw experiments in crystal manufacturing, which were a huge success. The raw materials (silica, lead and potash) were combined and melted at a high temperature to produce a mass that was worked in an almost liquid state. The French Revolution was not conducive to the growth of luxury industries, so the crystal factory did not go into full production until 1800.

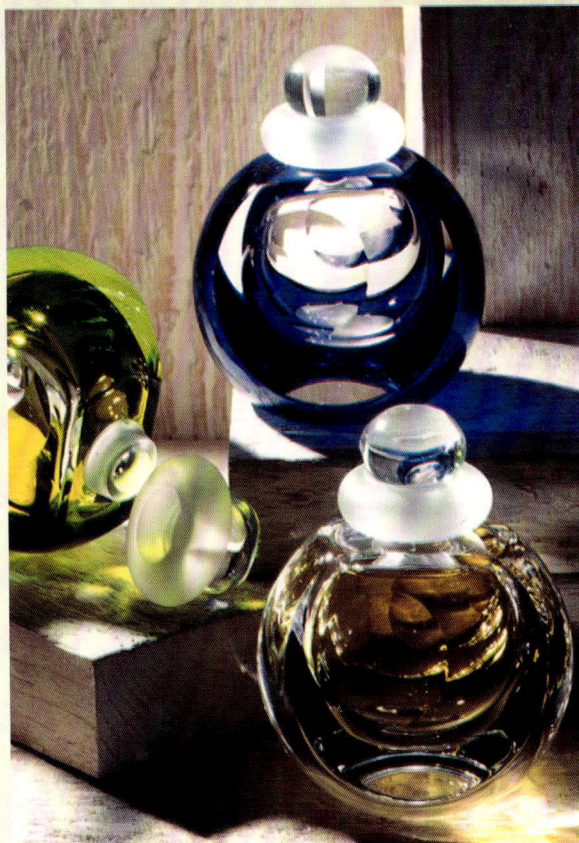

Eau de Saint-Louis, 1992.

The first bottles

The first real perfume bottles saw the light of day in the 1830s. New casting techniques were used to achieve a 'diamond-cut' look. Glass overlays were developed in 1837 and coloured glass in 1844, then along came opaline crystal under the reign of King Louis-Philippe. Between 1848 and 1850, more colours became available to glassmakers, who created wonderful opaline bottles with pigeon blue and multicoloured overlays. Flat rib pieces appeared in the Second Empire.

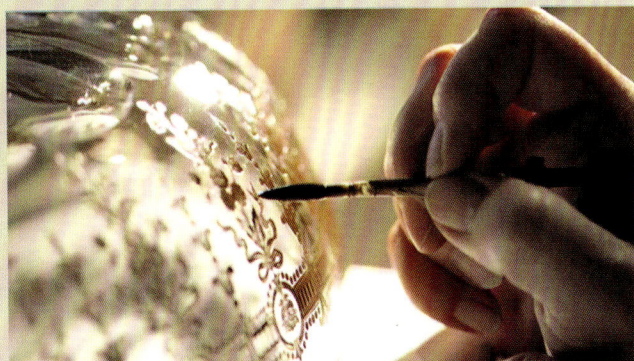

Fine gold decor.

The trademark Saint-Louis fine gold decor

Around 1870, acid etching enabled the Saint-Louis glassworks to develop what would become their trademark fine gold decor. There were figurative bottles in the shape of monuments or everyday objects, such as barrels, used for Eau de Cologne. Saint-Louis made bottles for Piver, Coty, Chanel and Bourjois.

The Jean Sala years

In 1938, Saint-Louis began a collaboration with Jean Sala, a master glassmaker known for the finesse of his animal figures and vases. He also made a diverse range of wash sets in faceted crystal. Business boomed during this period where the company counted the likes of Christian Dior, Coty, Chanel and Balmain among its clients.

In 1992, after making bottles for many perfumers, the Saint-Louis company launched its own perfume, Eau de Saint-Louis. The perfume itself might evaporate but you still have the bottle, which never loses its charm. Perfume bottles have become collectors' items and some fragrances are still sold in exquisite crystal versions today.

DÉPINOIX GLASSWORKS: SERVING THE PERFUME INDUSTRY

◆

In 1846, Théophile Coenon founded a company that specialized in the manufacture of exclusive perfume bottles. In 1888, it passed into the hands of his son-in-law, Constant Dépinoix, who expanded the business and took it to an international market. When he was joined by his son Maurice, the company became C. Dépinoix et Fils, located at rue de la Perle in Paris's 3rd arrondissement, and went on to become one of the most specialized glass manufacturers, making over 10,000 different types of perfume bottles. It was then that Maurice Dépinoix began his career as an artist and workshop owner. He managed and modernized the company by buying the Société Parisienne de Verreries, which had a factory in the 13th arrondissement, making Verreries Dépinoix (Dépinoix Glassworks) one of the largest glass producers in the interwar years. He had a particular fascination with black glass, which gave the bottle volume and strength.

Brosse

Caut-Thirion, which traded in small glass items for the perfume industry, became Verreries Brosse (Brosse Glassworks) when the company's heiress married Luc-Léon Brosse in 1880. In 1919, it was bought by Émile Barré, a company that was buying up factories in the Bresle Valley and, through this acquisition, came to focus on mainly decorative glass bottles and atomizers. In 1933, Georges Schwander joined Verreries Brosse and was awarded a gold medal at the 1925 Paris Exhibition.

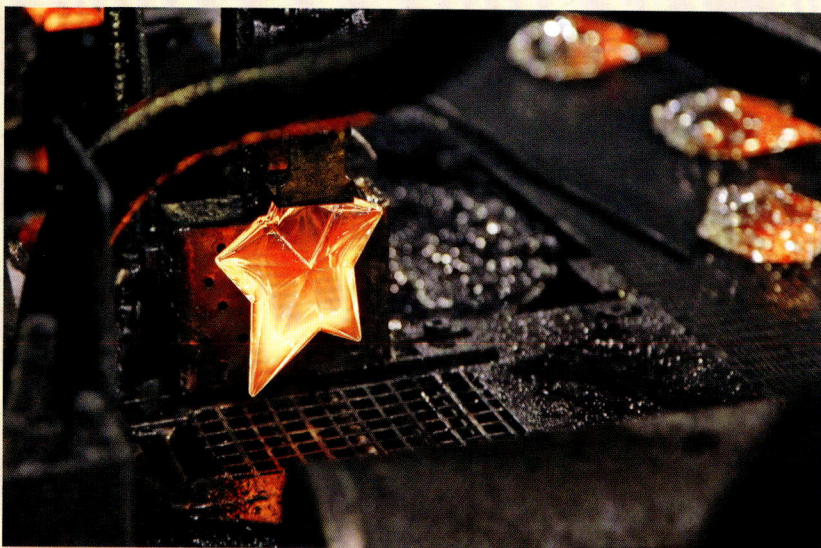

Thierry Mugler's Angel, bottle by Verreries Brosse, 1992. Photograph by Kai Jünemann.

Iconic creations of the Roaring Twenties

In the 1920s, Verreries Brosse created many Art Deco bottles with oriental style and decoration, mainly for Grenoville and Mury. Brosse also made a large quantity of spray bottles for DeVilbiss, Marcel Franck and Kitzinger Frères. In contrast, they also created a series named Golliwogg for Vigny Parfums; these were in the form of the black caricature, now considered offensive.

Creations for the big names in perfume

The Verreries Brosse name is linked to some of the most famous perfumes. There is the round black Arpège bottle, which was created in 1927 for the fashion designer Jeanne Lanvin and is still in production today, and the bottle for Chanel No. 5 (1921) with its clean lines, unfussy design and simple yet sophisticated black and white lettering on the label. Brosse also worked for some of the big names in fashion and perfume, among them Coty, Guerlain, D'Orsay, Roger&Gallet, Elizabeth Arden, Lucien Lelong, Patou, Nina Ricci, Worth and Revillon. Their greatest technical achievement, however, was the semi-artisanal star-shaped bottle they designed for Mugler's Angel perfume (1992). Thierry Mugler's brief was for a bottle that opened doors to the marvellous and ethereal. It is by staying at the forefront of progress that Verreries Brosse have retained their leading position in the perfume-bottle market.

LALIQUE: FROM JEWELLERY TO BOTTLES

◆

René Lalique arrived in Paris with his parents in 1862. He began work as an apprentice with Louis Auroc in 1876 and in 1878 he went to London to study art. On his return to Paris in 1880, he designed his first fine jewellery pieces in stones and precious metals. Fast forward ten years and he had his own workshop in rue Thérèse, where he already employed a staff of 30. Before he was commissioned by François Coty in 1909 to design the famous glass label for the L'Effleurt bottle, Lalique had been better known for the incredible jewellery he created in glass, enamel, horn, ivory and semi-precious stones for Sarah Bernhardt and many other women of the nobility, bourgeoisie and stage.

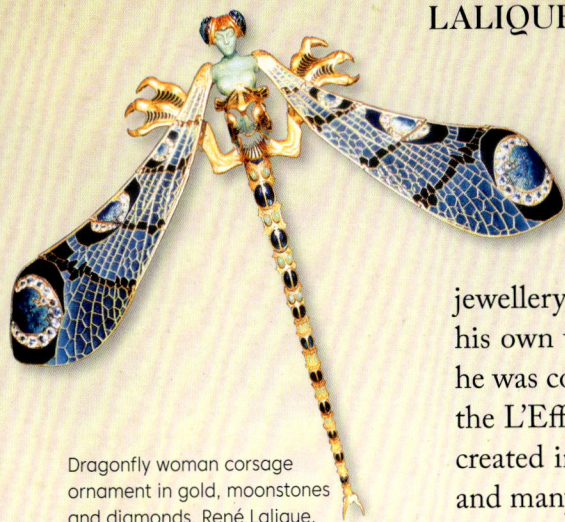

Dragonfly woman corsage ornament in gold, moonstones and diamonds, René Lalique, 1897–8.

Perfume bottles: adventures in glass

For François Coty's commission in 1909, René Lalique created a press-moulded panel from which an Art Nouveau-style woman seems to be emerging like a flower exhaling its scent. Coty was so happy with the experiment that he ordered the bottles and encouraged Lalique to open his own glass workshop. Like his jewellery, Lalique's bottles featured women and flowers, two of his favourite Art Nouveau themes. Arys, Corday, D'Orsay, Guerlain, Houbigant, Piver, Molinard, Roger&Gallet, Volnay, Worth and many other famous perfumers vied with each other to work with him. He was responsible for the two most beautiful creations of the Worth fashion house, Dans la Nuit in 1924 and Requête in 1944. Le Jade (Roger&Gallet, 1925), Cœur-Joie (Nina Ricci, 1946), Je Reviens (Worth, 1932), Imprudences (Worth, 1938), Leurs Âmes (D'Orsay, 1912) and Poésie (D'Orsay, 1914) were also presented in Lalique bottles.

With more than 400 perfume bottles to his name, René Lalique would be often imitated (but never equalled), especially in the 1920s and 1930s. He also sold empty bottles to be filled with the customer's favourite perfume. When he died in 1945, his son Marc took over and created the exquisite dove bottle for Nina Ricci's L'Air du Temps (1948) and the Femme bottle for Marcel Rochas (1944).

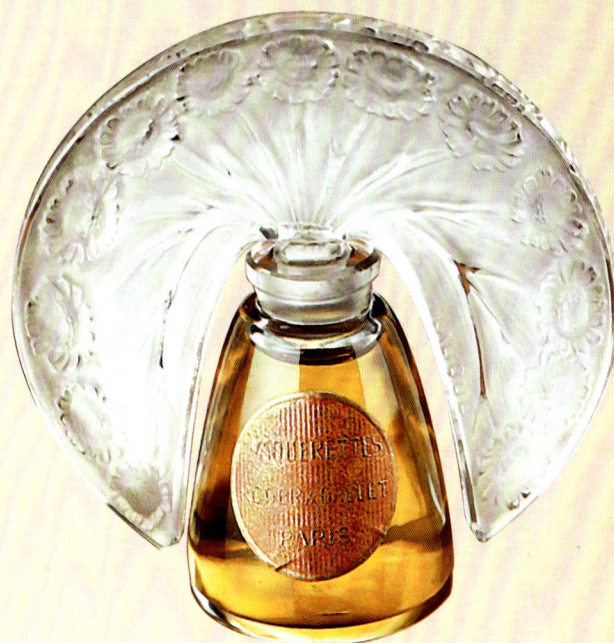

René Lalique bottle for Pâquerettes by Roger&Gallet in 1908. Roger&Gallet archives.

A man of many talents and international renown

René Lalique was awarded a top prize at the 1897 Brussels International Exhibition and then the National Order of the Legion of Honour the same year. By the 1900 Paris International Exhibition, his name was known throughout the world. Lalique also turned his hand to architecture, and his glasswork adorned the Coty building in New York (1911), the interior of the ocean liners Île-de-France and Normandie and the prestigious Orient Express trains.

POCHET & DU COURVAL:
FOUR CENTURIES OF EXCELLENCE

◆

On 9 January 1623, the Countess of Eu, in Normandy, granted François Vaillant of Courval permission to set up a glassworks, part of which was located on her land. Normandy had many forests, which were a good source of the firewood needed to melt the glass. A second furnace was built in 1662 to make crystal glass, the then owner, the Marquis of Senarpont, having obtained permission to work with both glass and crystal. Pochet, the company selling the Du Courval glassware, was founded in 1780 in rue Jean-Jacques Rousseau in Paris. Its owner, Jean-Baptiste Prosper Pochet, ran three shops. In the early nineteenth century, the company began to produce bottles, which became its main, and then sole, business.

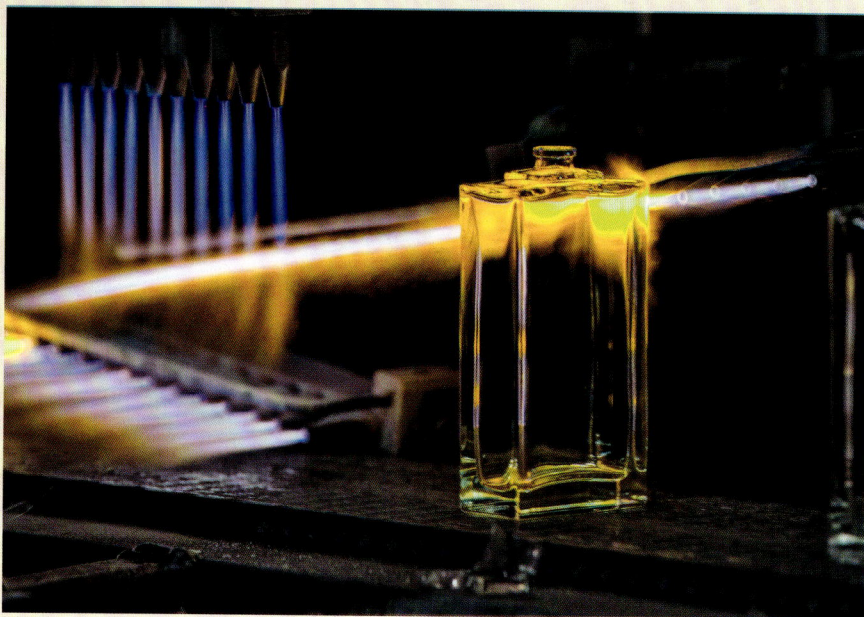

Fire polishing a bottle.

The story continues

The construction of warehouses and a factory began at quai de Valmy, by one of Paris's canals, in 1869. Verreries Pochet & Du Courval was registered as a company on 11 November 1934 and produced on average 1.2 million bottles and stoppers each day. With their cutting-edge technology, they combined tradition and innovation, industrial capacity and an eye for aesthetics to make the designer's dream a reality. The biggest names in the design world, including Serge Mansau and Pierre Dinand, have found in Pochet an outlet for their creativity. Drawing on 400 years of experience, Pochet's glass-making and firing experts still design their own moulds.

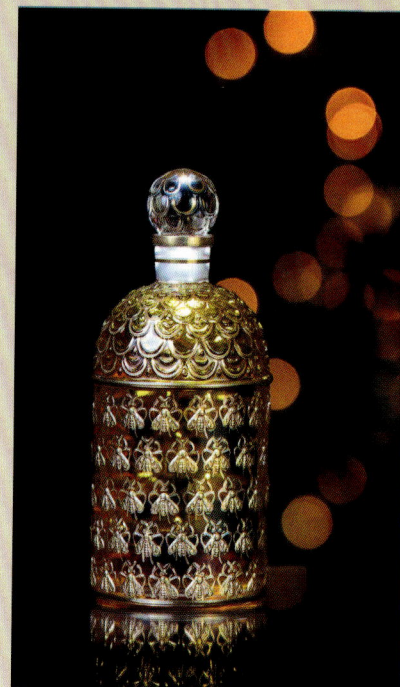

Guerlain's iconic bees

In 1853, Pochet created Guerlain's famous bee bottle for its Eau de Cologne Impériale, which took its inspiration from the Vendôme column, erected to commemorate the Great Army of Napoleon I. The iconic gold bees of the semi-manufactured bottle marked it out as one of the great innovations of its time. Each bee and each of the tiles was hand painted in fine gold and the bottle carried the Imperial coat of arms. It was the first of many fruitful collaborations between Guerlain and Pochet. This famous bottle is still available today with white or fine gilt bees.

In the 1970s, there was a need to resort to a wider variety of shapes and materials to meet the demands of a fast-growing market. With the advent of the consumer society, the attitudes of both men and women changed rapidly, which in turn fired a desire for ever-different fashions and products. Thus was born the 'one perfume, one bottle and one packaging' strategy to streamline both manufacturing needs and aesthetic requirements. Designers translated trends and the creator's brief into bottle designs, and manufacturing processes were pushed to the limit to bring these ideas to fruition.

Serge Mansau and Pierre Dinand: two great designers

Serge Mansau (1930–2019) had been producing bottle sculptures and working as an illustrator and stage designer since 1960. He was able to take his work further by collaborating with glass manufacturers because he also liked to use blown glass, carved wood and a variety of colours. At ease with modern materials, he worked with the biggest names in perfume. In 1974, he treated the creation of the bottle for Dior's Diorella as a work of art, setting the glass into a metal base. The man with 650 bottles to his name, among them some of the best known in the world, died on 17 February 2019, having shaped the perfume industry for over 50 years.

In 1977, twenty years after creating the Madame Rochas bottle, and ten years after founding Ateliers Pierre Dinand, the man himself (1931-) translated the creative genius of fashion designer Yves Saint Laurent into a bottle for his Opium perfume. He based his design on the ancient, lacquered wood *inrô*, or small case, of the samurai, which he recreated in a magnificent nylon material (see page 53). His bottle for Paco Rabanne's Calandre was inspired by a radiator grille. It was wrapped in galvanized plastic, a first in the history of perfume. Other French design greats who created beautiful perfume bottles include Frederico Restrepo, Joël Desgrippes, the Dragon Rouge agency, Véronique Monod, Thierry de Baschmakoff and Raison Pure.

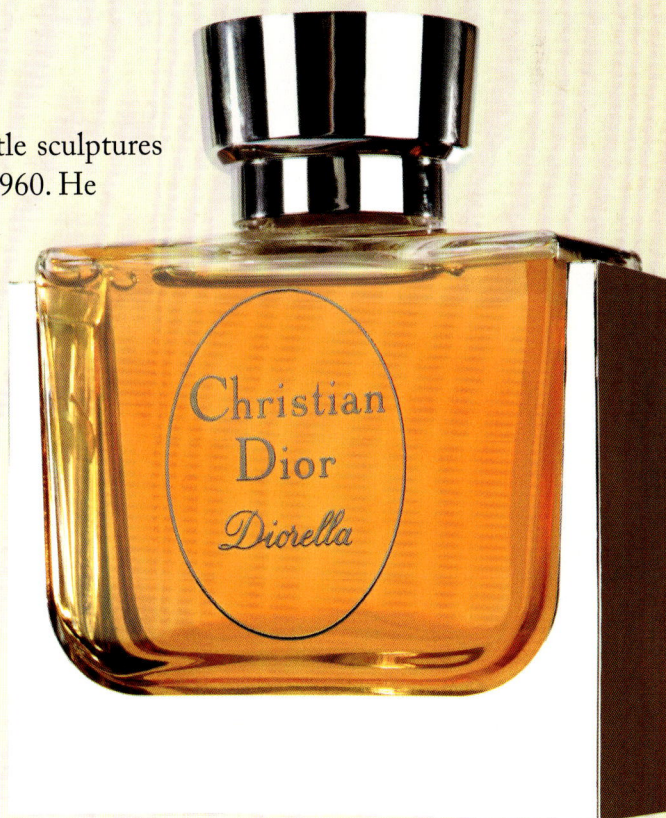

Special edition Diorella by Dior, created by Serge Mansau in 1974.

THE FIRST FRAGRANCES FOR MEN

IN THE NINETEENTH CENTURY, AFTER THE FRAGRANT FOLLIES OF THE LIBERTINES AND VARIOUS DANDY SUBCULTURES, PERFUME FOR MEN WAS A TABOO SUBJECT. VAUNTING ITS MERITS RISKED CASTING DOUBT ON THE MALE IDENTITY. AS A RESULT, THE FIRST FRAGRANCES FOR MEN DID NOT APPEAR ON THE SCENE UNTIL THE EARLY TWENTIETH CENTURY.

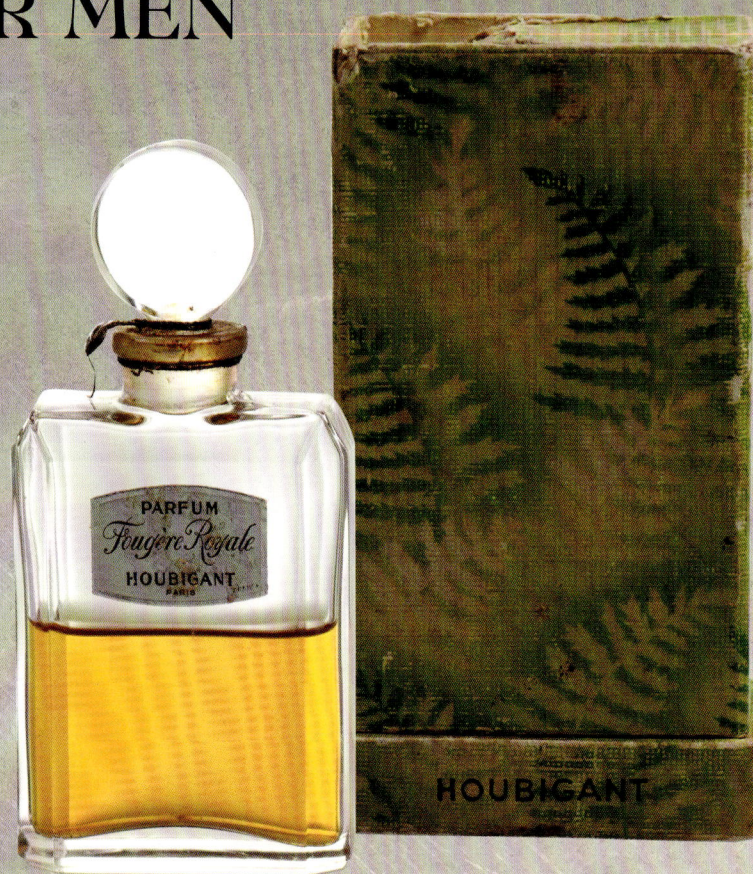

Fougère Royale by Houbigant, 1882.

FROM NO SMELL TO PERFUME JUST FOR MEN

After France became a republic again in 1848, a whiff of cleanliness was the only smell you were likely to get from elegant gentlemen who had been won over by the capitalism that was making them wealthy. Or, at the very most, a smell of tobacco, which was a mark of success. This was the start of the era of cleanliness that would prevail until the 1960s. In other words, if men smelled nice it was because they were well-groomed rather than the result of any deliberate attempt to use perfume as part of their attire or to attract a partner. They were of little interest to the perfume industry in the nineteenth century, although there were some cosmetic products available, such as Hungarian pomade, for styling and adding a shine to sideburns or moustache, and dyes to darken them. There were also balms, oils and *philocomes* ('hair-friendly' pomades) available to style the hair and promote its growth. Guerlain's Eau de Chypre took the burn out of shaving and toned the skin, and Eau de Cologne was widely used for ablutions or rubbed on the body. These became available in different fragrances, such as Russian leather and oriental amber.

FOUGÈRE … JUST FOR MEN?

In 1882, organic chemistry entered the world of perfume and Paul Parquet at Houbigant capitalized on this new development to create Fougère Royale, with a forest-floor accord of citrus, lavender, wood and coumarin. Like most perfumes of its time, it was initially made for women, but the hay-like aroma of the coumarin mixed with lavender and geranium made it very popular with dandies, because it reminded them of the lavender and wood fragrances of a barber's shop. As a result, the fougère (fern) family became almost exclusively used for male fragrances, raising the question as to whether men and women were naturally drawn to certain scents. When Aimé Guerlain released Jicky in 1889, it confirmed this hypothesis. The perfume caused confusion because women didn't understand it but men, the dandies at least, adopted it because they had not been able to find a male fragrance they liked. They loved Jicky for its fresh scent (bergamot, lemon and rosewood) fused with lavender and an assortment of herbs (basil, rosemary), and amber (coumarin, opoponax and vanillin) and animal (civet) notes.

FRAGRANCE FOR MEN BECOMES FASHIONABLE

Dunhill for Men by Dunhill was launched in 1936. Two years later, in 1938, Schiaparelli brought out Snuff, which came in a bottle shaped like a pipe, the quintessential male accessory. In 1947, fashion designer Jacques Fath launched Green Water, an aromatic citrus scent for men. The perfume industry in the 1950s and 60s benefited from the strong American culture that influenced Europe. US perfumers sold shaving and skincare products alongside their eaux de toilette. Green Water was also very popular with Americans. In 1948, Rochas launched Moustache in France. This fougère laced with rare fruit, moss and woody essences was the first luxury fragrance for men and its fresh, elegant scent was the perfect fit for the 1950s masculine ideal.

Advert for Moustache by Marcel Rochas, 1950.

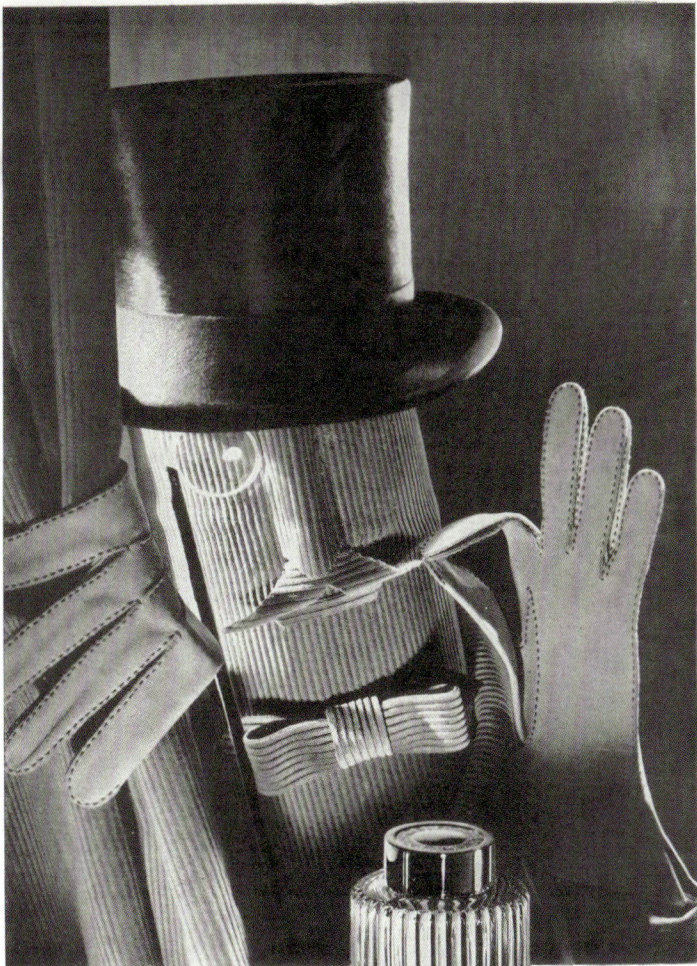

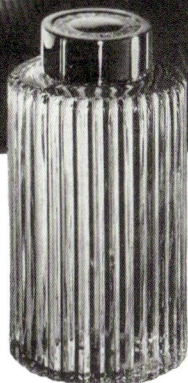

MOUSTACHE
parfum piquant
création
MARCEL ROCHAS

PARFUM
EAU de TOILETTE
EAU de COLOGNE

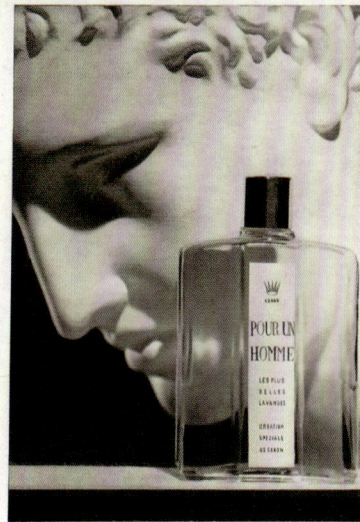

PARFUM DE JEUNESSE ET BEAUTÉ
POUR un HOMME
LES PLUS BELLES LAVANDES
de CARON

Pour un Homme by Caron, the first fragrance specifically targeted at men

Caron launched a series of successful perfumes that were aimed at women but had some masculine qualities (including Tabac Blond in 1919 and En Avion in 1930), but they did not decide to tackle the male market until 1934. When a bottle of Pour un Homme was opened, the immediate scent had to be one men recognized and associated with shaving, so lavender, but different and slightly edgy, closely followed by vanilla and amber. The bottle was smooth and classic with a black cap. It was an overnight success. For the first time ever, cleanliness was linked to attractiveness. A clever way to get men to think about fragrance differently without frightening them off.

Advert for Pour un Homme by Caron, 1954.

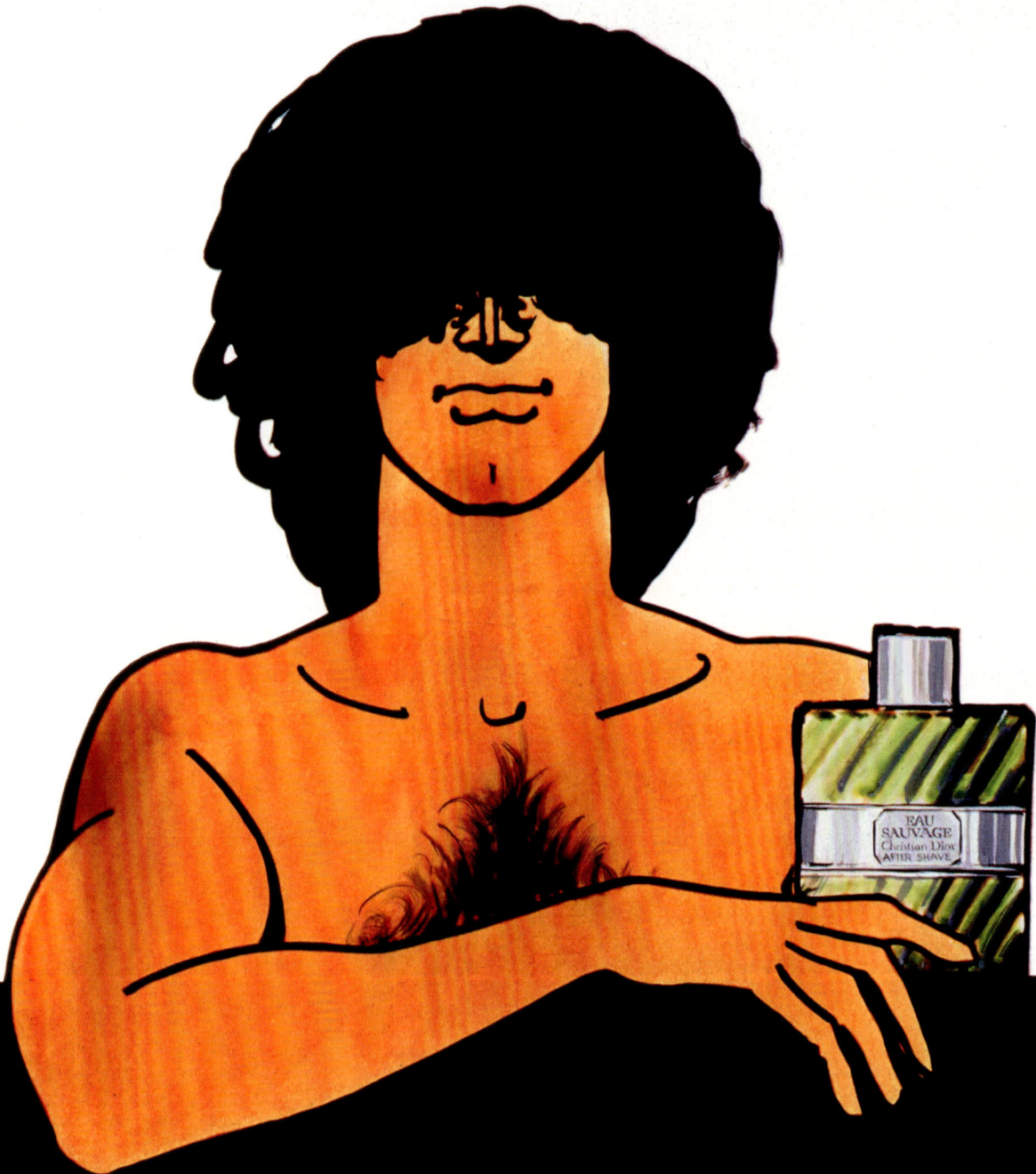

Ink and gouache illustration by René Gruau for Dior's *Eau Sauvage*, 1972. © Société René Gruau.

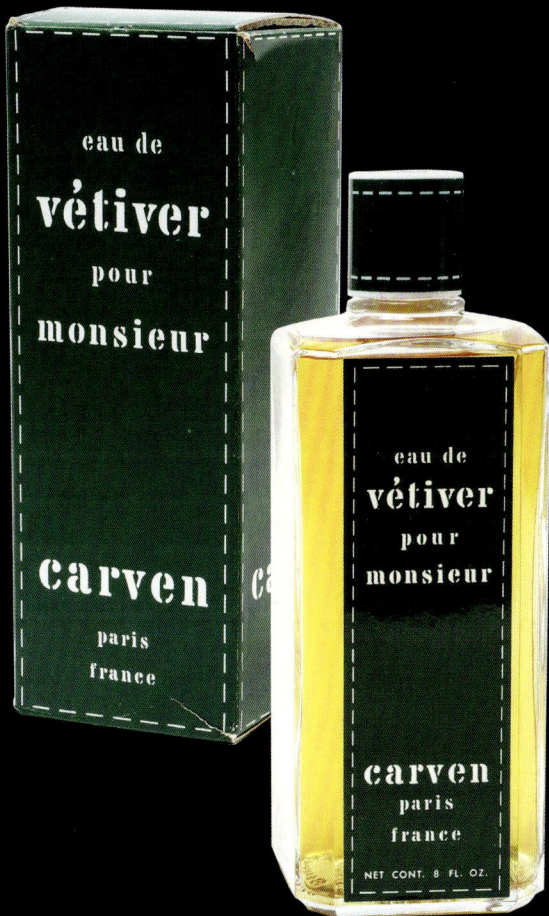

Wood for men

The late 1950s saw the advent of the wood family, the embodiment of male strength. Indeed, if we go back to the origins of perfume, early man burned wood mixed with resins to honour the gods, but also as a symbol of strength and immortality. The wood family includes scents that range from warm and opulent (sandalwood and patchouli) to drier, elegant notes (cedar and vetiver). In fragrances for men, these woody aromas are reminiscent of roots, earth and conquest. In 1957, Carven was the first to release a perfume in this genre named Vétiver, followed by Givenchy in 1958 and Guerlain in 1959.

FOR MONSIEUR

In the 1950s, particularly in France, the male stereotype was elegant, conventional and protective rather than seductive. It was against this backdrop that the perfume industry launched a vast number of products with 'Monsieur' (Mister) in their name. Chanel's Pour Monsieur (1955) was an elegant, refined eau de toilette from the chypre family, a successful fusion of freshness from citrus, depth from wood and warmth from dried spice. Class, elegance and allure was what the male fragrance market was all about. Memorable 1960s names included Monsieur Balmain and Monsieur by Givenchy, Monsieur Lanvin, Monsieur Worth, Monsieur Rochas … There was absolutely no doubt as to who the target market was!

Davidoff's advertising campaign for Cool Water with model Christian Hogue from the Elite agency, Paris, 2019.

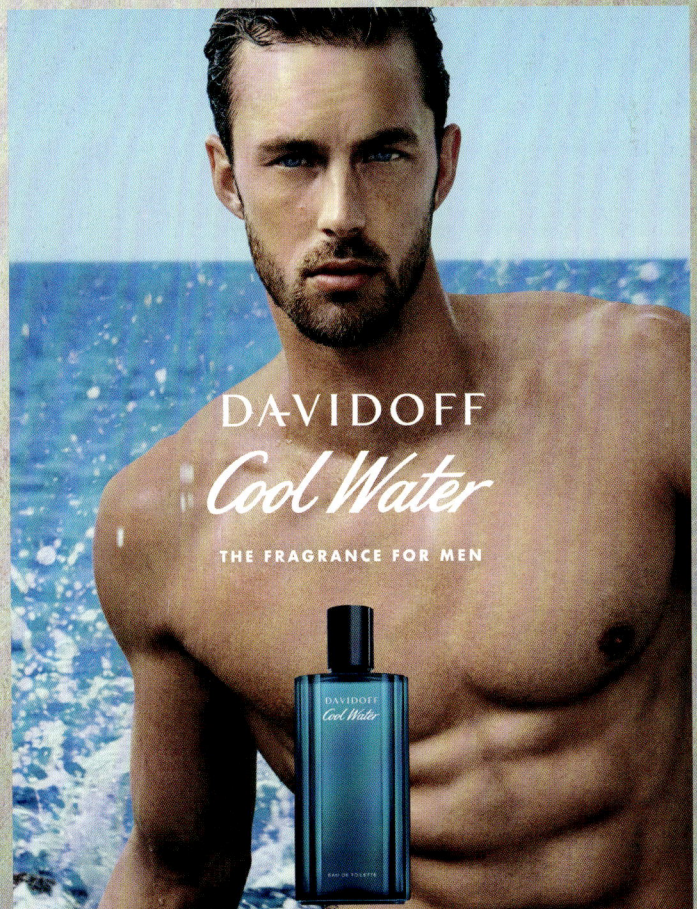

GETTING ALL MEN ON BOARD!

Subsequently, the twentieth century saw a growth in the male fragrance market, which only really took off in the late 1960s. The names were masculine, and fragrances such as Balafre (scar) by Lancôme, Guerlain's Habit Rouge (red hunting jacket) and Équipage (crew) by Hermès brought the worlds of hunting and exploration into the bathroom. There was still a massive gap in the market for products for men who secretly wanted perfume but could not access it. It was several decades before certain taboos were broken and a new era dawned in which new generations were comfortable with fragrance for men. In 1964, Fabergé made a quest to conquer the male market with Brut. Its black opaque bottle mirrored its rugged image in an attempt to convince men that wearing perfume did not make them any less virile. The first attempts at diversification involved making more masculine versions of existing women's perfumes, for instance Aramis was the male version of Cabochard by Grès, and Fabergé's Brut that of Canoë by Dana.

This changed in the 1980s and 1990s with the introduction of bona fide male fragrances. One of the first, R by Paco Rabanne, was from the fougère/tobacco family. Azzaro pour Homme in 1978, then Drakkar Noir by Guy Laroche in the early 1980s, introduced strength, freshness and tenacity to reinforce the virility factor. Freshness was still key. It had been achieved to some extent by Dior's Eau Sauvage in 1966 but it was now pushed to the extreme. This 'new freshness', harking back to an original purity, was introduced by Davidoff with Cool Water in 1988, and it was a revelation.

AN END TO GENDER STEREOTYPES

Gradually, as perfume became associated with image, its masculine attributes were reinforced. It capitalized on traditional male stereotypes and the different elements – name, colour codes and the design of the bottle – reflected the scent of the perfume itself. The male expression became more refined, more feminine, and the 1989 release of Joop Homme, an amber fougère, started a trend for florientals which led Jean Paul Gaultier to bring Le Mâle to the market in 1996. As the popularity of male perfumes grew, their concentration increased and they became available as extracts and elixirs, which had previously only existed in women's fragrance. These new, exclusive products required more precise application, a far cry from the usual morning splash. As the perfume worlds of both genders merged, a third category arose that in some way questioned the traditional codes. Echoing the words of Jean Paul Gaultier, it was felt that men should have the same choice and freedom as women.

Advert for Le Mâle by Jean Paul Gaultier, 1990s. Photograph by Jean-Baptiste Mondino.

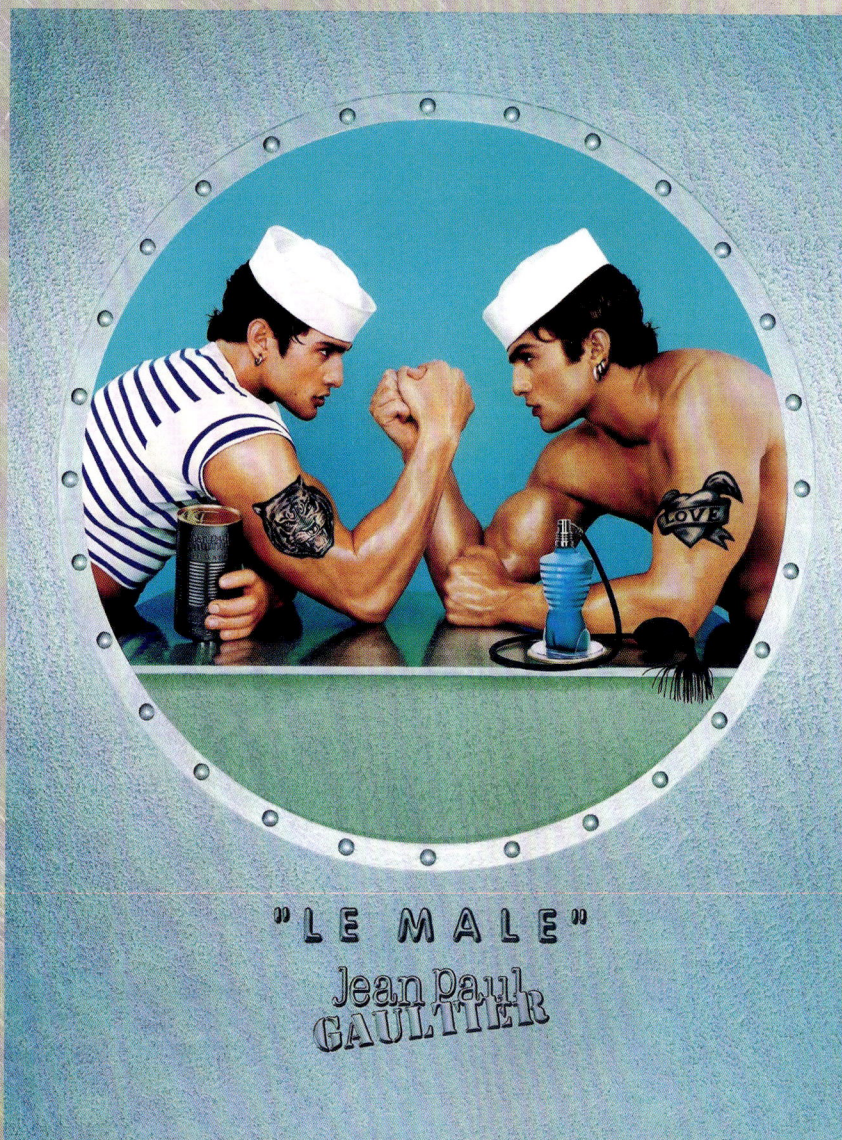

"LE MÂLE"

Jean Paul GAULTIER

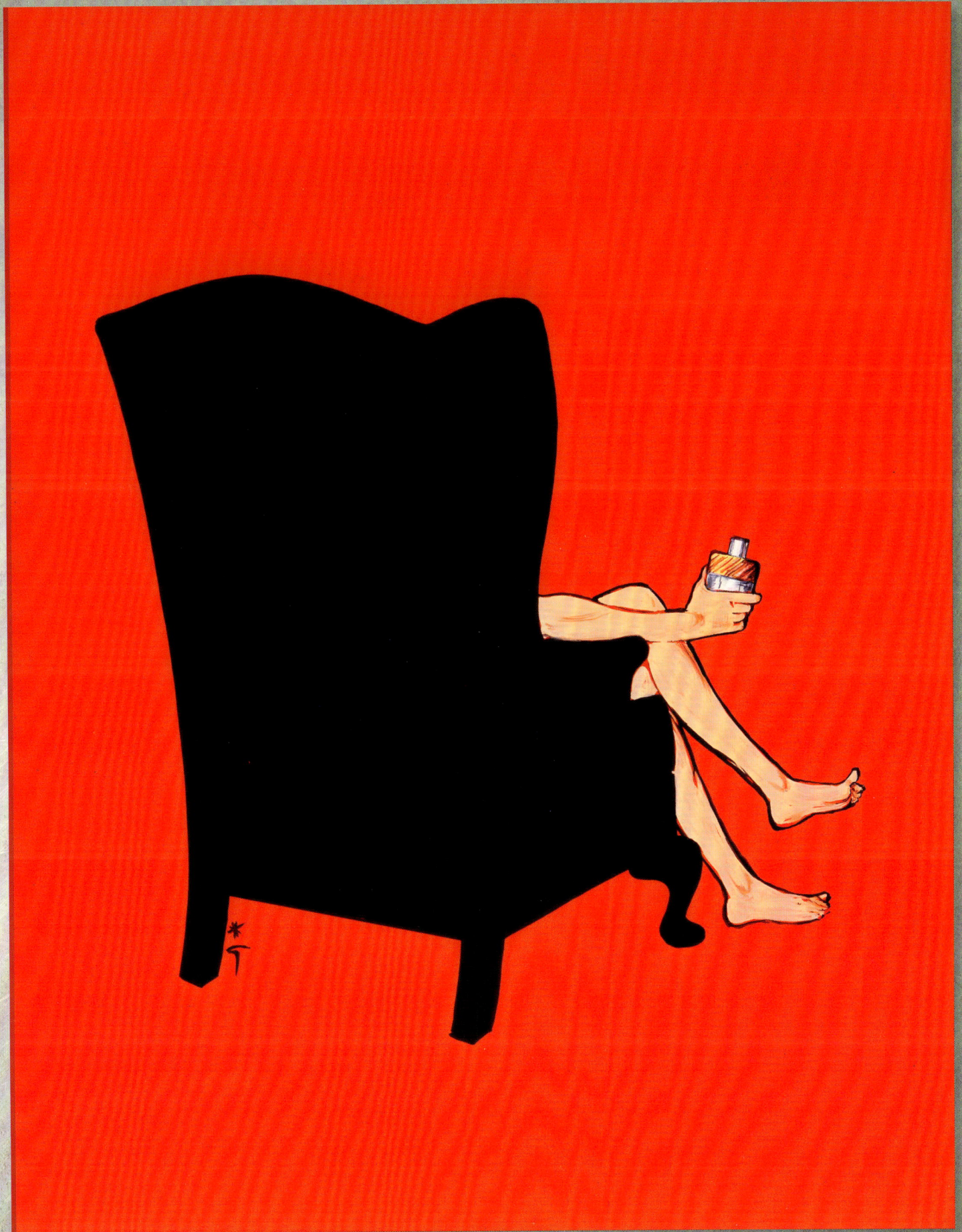

Ink and gouache illustration by René Gruau for Dior's *Eau Sauvage*, 1972. © Société René Gruau.

Couturier-Perfumers: Fashion Meets Perfume

In the first half of the twentieth century, perfume and couture combined to create a particular style which was so successful that it led to the demise of the traditional Paris perfumers. Only a few big names survived.

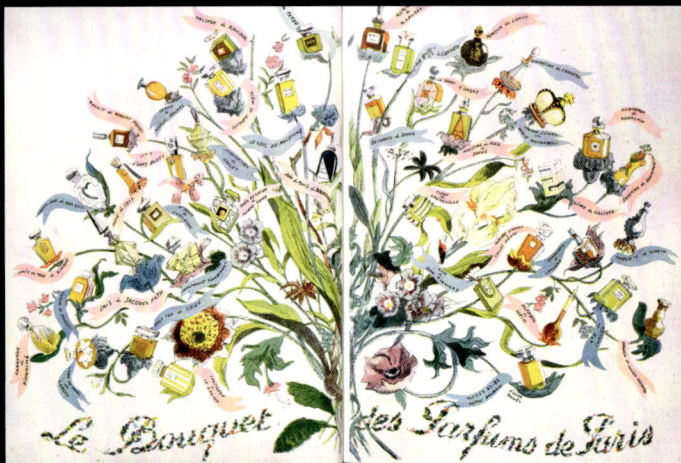

Le bouquet des parfums de Paris, illustration for *Vogue* magazine, 1 February 1947.

Perfume and fashion go back a long way

In the second half of the eighteenth century, Marie-Antoinette's stylist Rose Bertin was already working with her perfumer, Jean-Louis Fargeon, to create perfumed gauze flowers. This link with the fashion industry had been established by the Guild of Glover–Perfumers when it was set up in 1190, and perfume became a secondary trade for artisans in the leather industry and, more broadly, those in fashion. In the nineteenth century, the perfume industry encompassed lingerie makers, corset makers and even shoemakers. Scented leather, perfumed gloves, a tiny drop of perfume on the hem of a dress – all ensured the wearer left a fragrance in their wake, which became known in French fashion as a *sillage*. The perfume given off by the swish of a skirt could be extremely evocative. This association was of great interest to fashion designers, who could create a complete style with a dress, hat and a fragrance, and also worked in perfumers' favour – the Parisian fashion clientele made a great outlet for luxury perfume. In addition, perfume was extremely lucrative and profitable, so it could finance the much higher outlay of couture.

Perfumer-designers

In the early twentieth century, haute couture expanded to incorporate perfumery. This could happen in a number of ways. Couturiers might buy manufacturing formulas from a perfume house or employ their own perfumer–designer. With the merging of the two worlds, perfumers began to work for couturiers and became known as 'noses'. Famous noses included Henri Alméras at Patou, Ernest Beaux at Chanel, Maurice Blanchet at Worth, André Fraysse at Lanvin and Maurice Shaller at Poiret and Revillon. Fashion and perfume became intrinsically linked as two creative industries. The concept was extended to leather (Hermès) in 1951 and then jewellery in 1976, with First by Van Cleef & Arpels. For customers who could not afford a designer dress or high-end bag or piece of jewellery, couture perfume was an achievable first step towards the luxury end of the market. Next on the scene were more affordable perfumes from ready-to-wear brands, such as Chloé by Lagerfeld (1976) and Anaïs Anaïs by Cacharel (1978), and designer perfumes, often the figure-heads of a new fragrance trend, such as Parfum de Peau by Montana (1986) or Angel by Mugler (1992).

Draper Emmanuel Boulet and Paul Poiret, French fashion designer and decorator, at the Rosine perfume factory in Courbevoie, circa 1925.

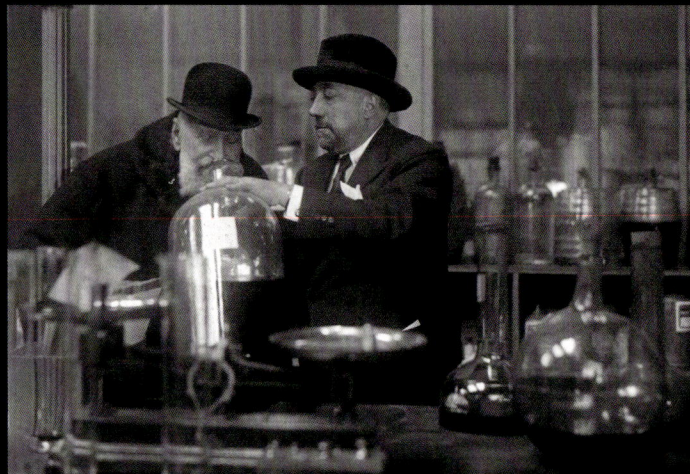

CHARLES FREDERICK WORTH,
inventor of haute couture
✦ 1825–1895 ✦

The couture house was established by Charles Frederick Worth, who arrived in Paris in 1845. He was initially employed as a salesman for a Paris textile company, Gagelin et Opigez, and one of his clients, Marie Vernet, later became his wife. Her outfits were much admired, so the company opened a couture department, which was run by the married couple before they set up their own company on rue de la Paix in 1858.

Worth laid the foundations for haute couture by showing ready-made garments which customers could try on and then have adjusted to their requirements. He broke new ground by using living models, known as 'sosies' or stand-ins, one of whom was his wife, Marie. The shows were held on a set date in luxury salons. Worth was introduced to the famous Princess Metternich of Austria and later became the couturier of Empress Eugenie and other European royals. When he died, his son Jean-Philippe Worth, also a couturier, took over the business with his brother Gaston. In his hands, the company grew considerably, dressing elegant Belle Époque women. Gaston's sons Jean-Charles and Jacques, Jean-Philippe's nephews, later ran the company.

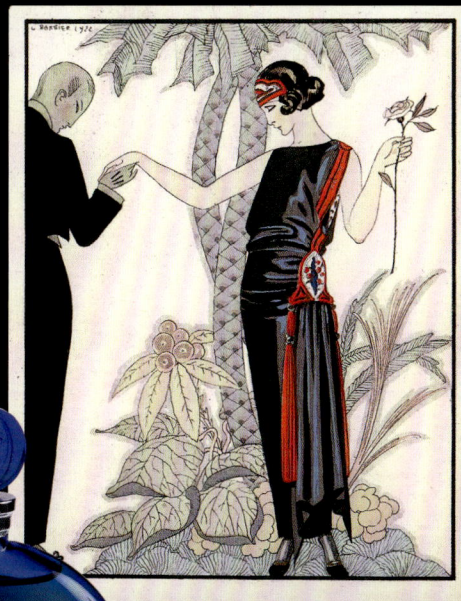

Above: Espérez, an evening dress designed by Charles Frederick Worth, reproduced in a drawing by Georges Barbier which appeared in the fashion magazine, the *Gazette du bon ton* (Journal of Good Taste), 1922.

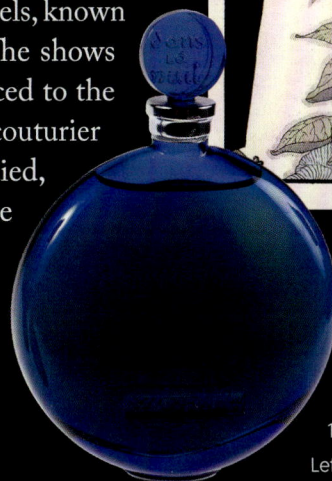

Left: Dans la Nuit, bottle by René Lalique for Parfums Worth, 1924.

R.B. Sibia poster for Les Parfums Worth, 1947.

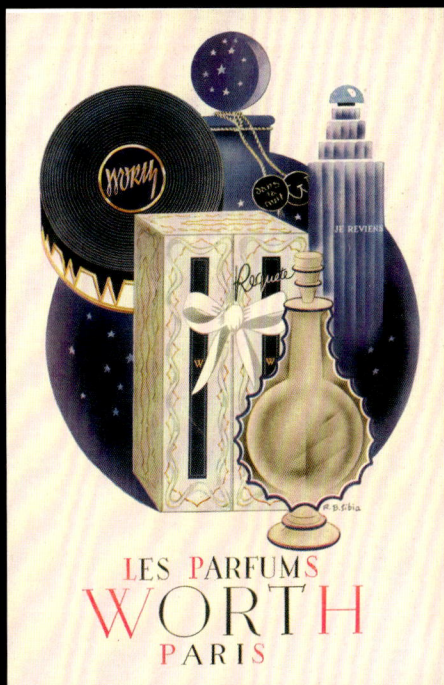

JE REVIENS OWED ITS SUCCESS TO … THE WAR
The Parfums Worth branch of the company was probably the brainchild of Jacques Worth, who enlisted the services of the perfumer Maurice Blanchet, the founder of Coryse Salomé perfumery. Notable creations included Dans la Nuit in 1924 and Je Reviens in 1932. The latter, with its slightly dusky scent of narcissus combined with jasmine, tuberose and ylang-ylang, owed its success to the war because American soldiers who had been sent to fight in Europe took it home to their wives and girlfriends. By 1947, Je Reviens was enjoying the same international success as Chanel's No. 5 and Soir de Paris by Bourjois. René Lalique created a round blue crystal bottle, as voluptuous as a hot summer's night, decorated with a moon and stars. Inspired by the recent construction in New York of the Chrysler Building and Empire State Building, a second version of the bottle was shaped like a skyscraper. Very few Europeans had crossed the Atlantic at the time so they dreamed of these buildings, symbols of the modern world. Roger Worth ran the company from 1941. It was later bought by Paquin and a British branch continued to operate until the 1970s.

Jeanne Lanvin, a mother's passion
⟻ 1867-1946 ⟼

Jeanne Lanvin went to work with a milliner to learn the trade at the age of 16. She proved to have a true talent for hat making and set up her own business on rue du Marché-Saint-Honoré. As orders flooded in she had to move to rue du Faubourg-Saint-Honoré. With Count Emilio di Pietro, whom she married in 1896, she had a daughter, Marguerite, who was the centre of her life. Lanvin's garments were simple, elegant and refined. She launched a mother-and-daughter collection, dressed her own daughter and launched a childrenswear line in 1908.

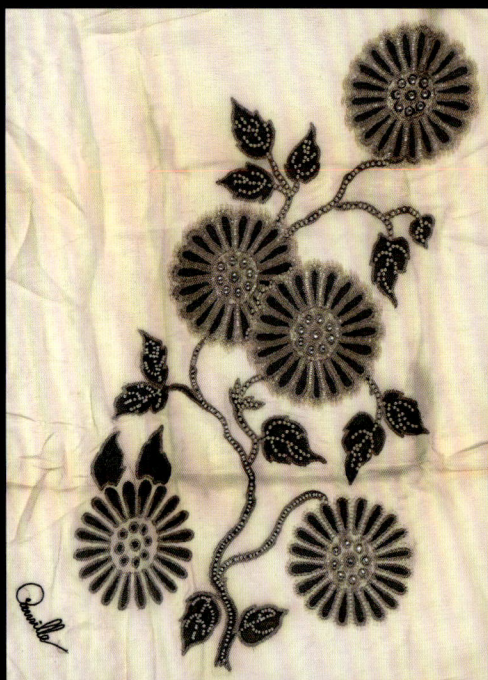

Daisy (common marguerite) embroidery, circa 1925.

Moving in artistic circles in the Roaring Twenties

Lanvin's business took off again when its exquisitely cut garments, eveningwear and sportswear line proved popular with the women of the Roaring Twenties. At the time it had 1,200 employees and Lanvin branches opened outside Paris and in Madrid, London and Rio de Janeiro. Jeanne was a great art lover and collected paintings by the great masters, including Renoir. She was bowled over by a Fra Angelico Madonna and the mauve-blue colour used by the artist became 'Lanvin blue'. She also surrounded herself with young artists such as Paul Iribe and Eugène Printz and was friends with the photographer Nadar. Jeanne Lanvin was a businesswoman, fashion designer and trailblazer. She also chased publicity, flooding fashion magazines and theatre programmes with adverts. Actresses, in particular, endorsed the brand by wearing her clothes on and off stage.

Lanvin after Jeanne Lanvin

In 1938, Jeanne Lanvin was presented with the rosette of the National Order of the Legion of Honour by actor and director Sacha Guitry. She died in 1946 and her daughter took up the reins until her death in 1958, when Yves Lanvin, a nephew of Jeanne, took over the business. The brand was bought by the Midland Bank in 1989 and then L'Oréal in 1990. In 2001, the company became independent again under the ownership of the investor group Harmonie S.A. A women's fragrance, Rumeur, which remained true to the Lanvin roots, was launched in 2006, and Jeanne Lanvin in 2008.

Parfums Lanvin: 'I'm talking perfection'

Between 1923 and 1924, the perfumer Maria Zede (known as Madame Z) created a diverse range of fragrances – Le Sillon, La Dogaresse, Où Fleurit l'Oranger and My Sin – for Jeanne Lanvin. Established in 1924, Parfums Lanvin, launched 14 perfumes in the space of two years. Lanvin hired Paul Vacher and André Fraysse and in 1927, for the 30th birthday of her daughter Marguerite, who was now a musician, they created Arpège. 'I'm not talking fashion or budget, I'm talking perfection' were Lanvin's words in commissioning it. When Marguerite inhaled the perfect accord of the finest and rarest raw materials that made up this perfume, with its exquisite black and gold ball-shaped Armand Rateau bottle, she exclaimed, 'It's just like an arpeggio!' (*arpège* in French). Arpège was followed by other subtle, elegant creations: Scandal (1932), Eau de Lanvin (1933), Rumeur (1934) and Prétexte (1937).

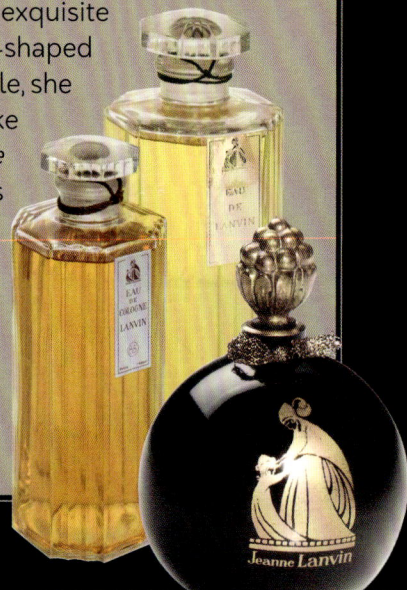

Eau de Lanvin, Eau de Cologne Lanvin and Arpège (1927).

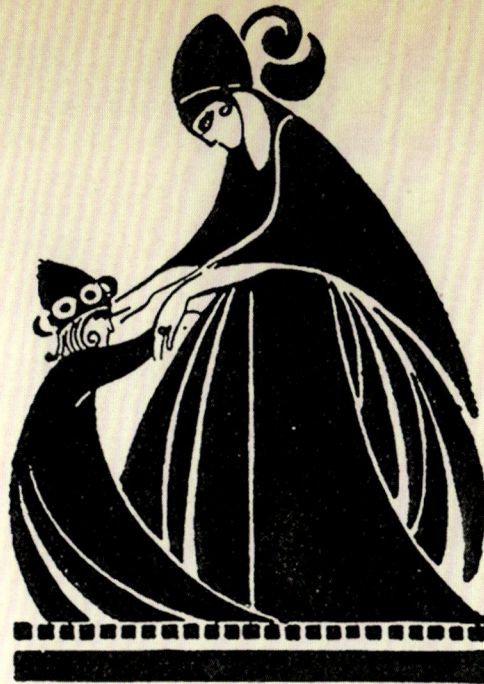

Advert for Lanvin perfumes in the *Gazette du Bon Ton* (Journal of Good Taste) , 1925.

PAUL POIRET,
the first couturier-perfumer
1879–1944

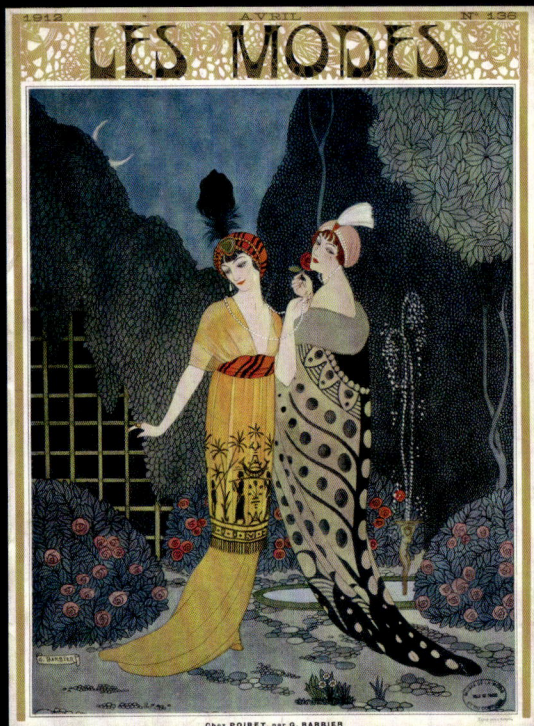

When Paul Poiret founded Les Parfums de Rosine in 1911, he reconnected with the Ancien Régime tradition of marrying fashion with perfume. Poiret was born into a family of cloth merchants in 1879. He had started his career as a fashion designer with Doucet in 1898, and then worked at Worth from 1901 to 1903 before opening his own couture house. He had a vision of a new, more liberated woman in softer, lighter fabrics, roomy coats and, most importantly, high-waisted dresses that would free her from the straitjacket that was the corset. Inspired by the Ballets Russes, a dance company much in vogue at the time, his brightly coloured, oriental-style creations were all the rage. Poiret's wife, Denise, was his ambassador to ladies in Parisian high society and Poiret dazzled them with magnificent soirées hosted in his private mansion on avenue d'Antin. He dressed all the actresses of the time, including Gabrielle Réjane and Sarah Bernhardt, and started a trend for Oriental-style fashion.

Poiret's daughters, Rosine and Martine

Poiret's Les Parfums de Rosine and L'Atelier de Martine were named after his daughters, born in 1906 and 1911 respectively. He engaged the services of great creatives such as his father-in-law, the draper Emmanuel Boulet, illustrator Fabiano and perfumer Henri Alméras, who created a series of perfumes for the brand: Nuit de Chine, Le Fruit Défendu, Aladin, Borgia, Arlequinade, Sakya, Monni and Le Parfum de ma Marraine, the latter a tribute to the wartime penfriends of soldiers. Poiret also wrote the book *En habillant l'époque* (Dressing the Era), published in 1930 and translated in 1931 with the title *King of Fashion: The Autobiography of Paul Poiret*. He is credited with the concept of fashion shows. Prior to this, couturiers unveiled their creations at court balls or on theatre stages. An extravagant visionary, Poiret died penniless in 1944, just before the opening of an exhibition organized in his honour. Jean Cocteau had a few years earlier produced an illustration of a woman dressed in Poiret slipping away into the background behind the silhouette of Gabrielle Chanel with the caption: 'Poiret s'éloigne, Chanel arrive' (Poiret is out, Chanel is in).

Just for fun!

Poiret took the idea of marrying fashion with perfume from Viennese workshops, which combined activities such as fabrics, clothing and jewellery. Why not add perfume to the mix? He would tell clients how wonderful they looked in his dresses, then add that they would be absolutely ravishing with a tiny drop of his perfume. He claimed he made perfumes 'just for fun' but would research the blends himself, and his vision was to introduce a range of new scents.

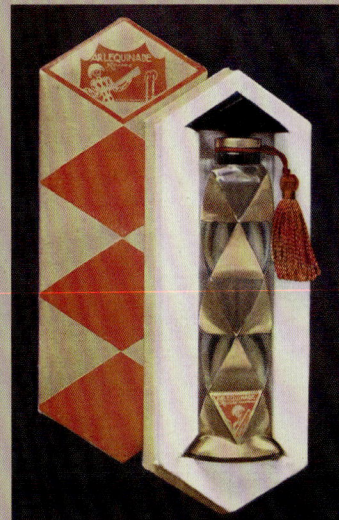

Arlequinade, circa 1924. The moulded column has a Harlequinesque diamond motif and the stopper has a decorative tassel.

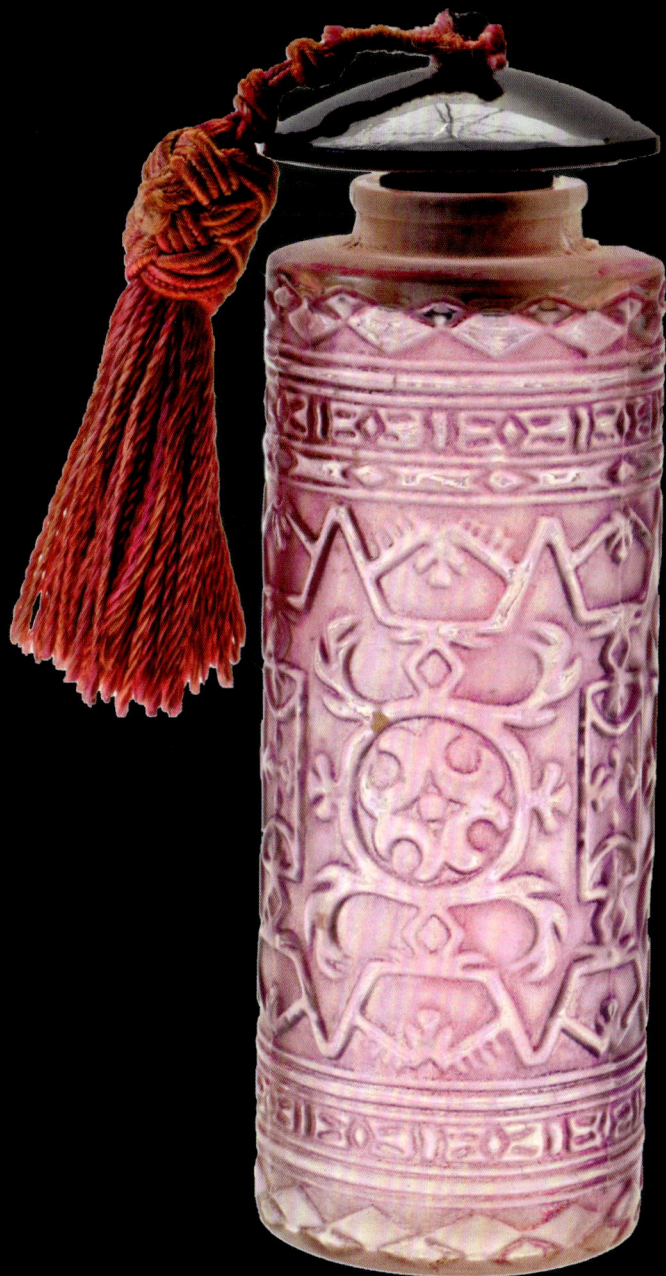

Bottle for Les Parfums de Rosine by Paul Poiret, 1925.

GABRIELLE CHANEL,
the irresistible Mademoiselle

1883-1971

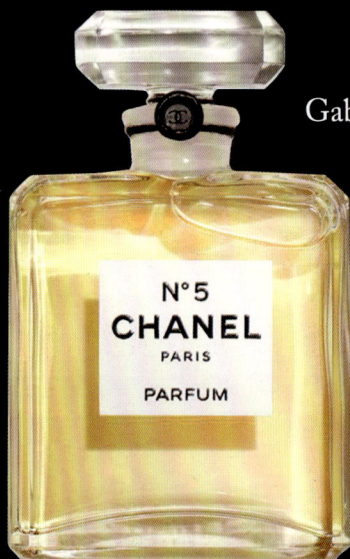

Gabrielle Chanel, described by novelist André Malraux as one of the three most important French figures of the twentieth century alongside de Gaulle and Picasso, was born on 19 August 1883, but there was no newspaper announcement of her birth. The daughter of an impoverished couple from Cevennes who sold haberdashery door to door, she was born in the workhouse in Saumur. Her mother died when Gabrielle was very young and her father placed her in the care of a convent. In 1903, while working for a company that made wedding trousseaux and baby clothes, she was known as Coco, a nickname her father gave her when she auditioned as a singer at La Rotonde in Moulins (central France). She would later become Mademoiselle Chanel and rule the world in her own unique manner. But how did she get there? What were the breakthroughs that led to this success?

Early successes

In 1907, the young Gabrielle met Étienne Balsan, a young, upper-middleclass cavalry officer, who invited her to live with him at his estate near Compiègne. There she discovered indulgent, high society life and was initiated into the joys of horse riding. She was a different breed of woman and decided she wanted to work. Encouraged by her new lover Boy Capel, a British polo player and brilliant businessman, she set herself up as a milliner in Paris in 1910. She bought straw hats from the Galeries Lafayette department store, decorated them tastefully and, thanks to her friends who wore them, this became her first successful venture.

She opened her first boutique in Deauville in 1912 and, using a stock of jersey material she had purchased from Rodier, made her first clothes during World War I. Her vision was to rid the world of outdated fashion so she took the bold move of using a soft knit fabric, until then primarily used for men's underwear, to create flowing garments, shirt dresses, sailor tops and cardigans. The style was simple and the emphasis was on cut, comfort and freedom of movement. Gabrielle Chanel's success was gaining momentum.

Coco: an ambassador for women's emancipation

Attitudes changed at the end of the war. With men at the front, women had taken on responsibilities and discovered independence, an ideal championed by Gabrielle Chanel. As early as 1917, she cut her hair, exposed her skin to the sun and was photographed in her white silk unisex beach pyjamas. When, in December 1919, Boy Capel died in a tragic car accident, she threw herself headlong into her work. In 1920 in Biarritz, she fell in love with Grand Duke Dimitri Pavlovitch and pinched his tunics and fur-lined cloaks to have them embroidered and give them a feminine touch.

Homage to Chanel No. 5 by the illustrator Sem, 1921.

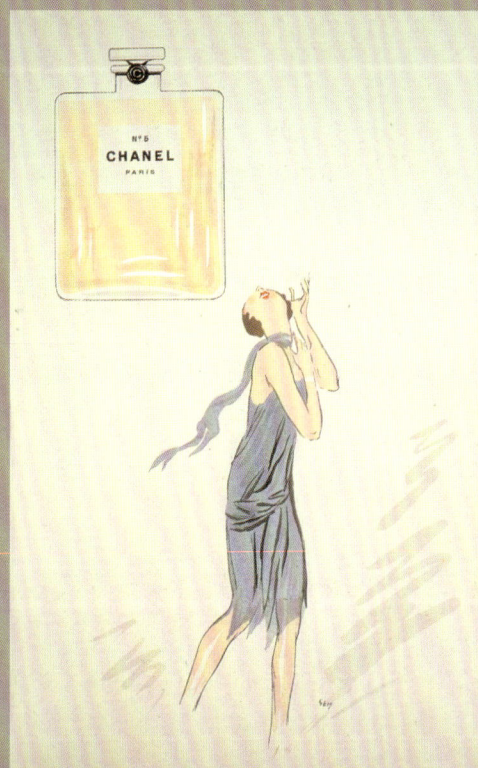

Chanel No. 5, a winning formula: 'A perfume for women that smells like a woman'

Gabrielle Chanel had a highly developed sense of smell. On a trip with the Grand Duke in 1920, she met Ernest Beaux, who was the nose for Laboratoires Chiris & Rallet at the time. She told him she was looking to create a very expensive, one-of-a-kind, perfume that would be the envy of other perfumers. She added that she would put everything into the perfume rather than the presentation, which would be a simple, straightforward design: 'No name, just a number.' And so the famous, ultra-modern No. 5, the first floral abstract in the history of perfumery, was born in 1921. It was so successful that the small-scale production could not meet demand. In 1924, Chanel signed an agreement with Pierre and Paul Wertheimer, the owners of Bourjois, and established Parfums Chanel to distribute her perfumes worldwide. Ernest Beaux became technical director of the laboratory and created other perfumes for Chanel.

Suzy Parker in 1957 posing for the Chanel No. 5 advert. Photograph by Richard Avedon, courtesy of the Richard Avedon Foundation.

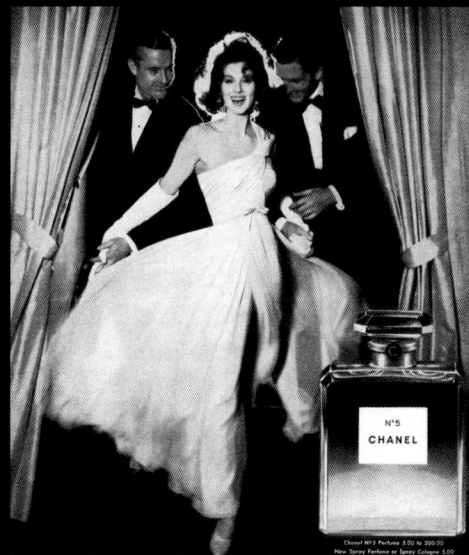

every woman _alive_ loves Chanel N° 5

CHANEL

The image of the modern woman: 'Chanel is above all a style'

Having launched her own unique style, Gabrielle Chanel was the epitome of the modern woman with her suntan, short hair, tiny waist and charisma. She rubbed shoulders with most of the artists, poets and musicians of the time, including Sergei Diaghilev, founder of the Ballets Russes, Igor Stravinsky, Pablo Picasso, Erik Satie and Jean Cocteau, all of whom would provide her with inspiration. Between 1924 and 1930, during a six-year relationship with the Duke of Westminster, Chanel adopted a more English style. She embraced striped tops, sailor knits, gold buttons, berets, white collars and cuffs, tweed jackets, sports jackets and comfortable cashmere knits with the sole purpose, it seemed, of turning the simple into something remarkable. In November 1932, she exhibited her unique 'Bijoux de Diamants' fine jewellery collection in the magnificent setting of her private mansion at 29, rue du Faubourg-Saint-Honoré in Paris. In 1954, 15 years after it closed on the outbreak of World War II, the Chanel couture house reopened for business. Her collection was not well received in France but her creative force made an impact in the United States, where her suits were extremely popular. In 1957, she received a fashion Oscar in Dallas and styled the world's biggest stars, including Elizabeth Taylor, Romy Schneider and Marlene Dietrich. A workaholic until her dying day, she forever maintained that 'Chanel is above all a style. Fashion passes, style remains.'

After the launch of No. 5 in 1921, Chanel became one of the first luxury brands in history to have an extensive international presence, reaching the United States in 1924 and Japan in 1930. It was followed by a string of successes, with Antaeus, Égoïste, Coco, Allure, Chance, Coco Mademoiselle, No. 5 Eau Première and L'Eau, Gabrielle to name but a few. And of course there is the unforgettable 'Les Exclusives' collection, which was launched in 2007 to honour Chanel as one of the perfume greats and pay tribute to the history of the company and the woman herself.

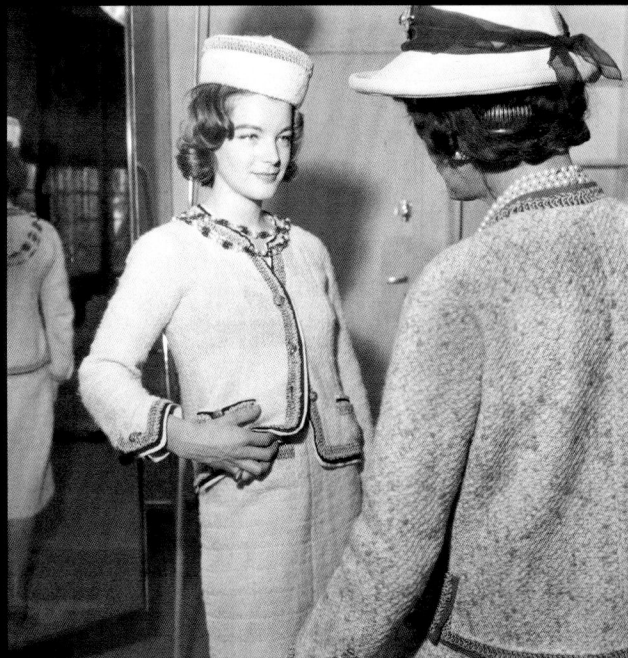

Actress Romy Schneider during a fitting with Gabrielle Chanel, 1961.

NINA RICCI,
Bringing 'dream colours' to life
✦ 1882-1970 ✦

Maria Adélaïde Nielli, known as Nina Ricci, was an Italian-born French couturier. She married Louis Ricci, a partner in the Raffin et Ricci couture house, which closed on the death of Raffin. Her son Robert was born in 1905 and, little by little, Nina achieved international fame as a fashion designer. She opened her haute couture house on rue des Capucines in Paris in 1932 and her son came on board to run the business. It was a great success, with her novel and romantic creations finding favour with the women of Paris. Although the 1930s were all about the tomboy look, trousers and short hair, Nina Ricci preferred to celebrate femininity in all its grace and beauty. Her dresses were cut from rich fabrics so the wearer not only looked truly elegant but could move with a certain decorum. On the eve of World War II, the Nina Ricci fashion house occupied three buildings on rue des Capucines and employed 450 people.

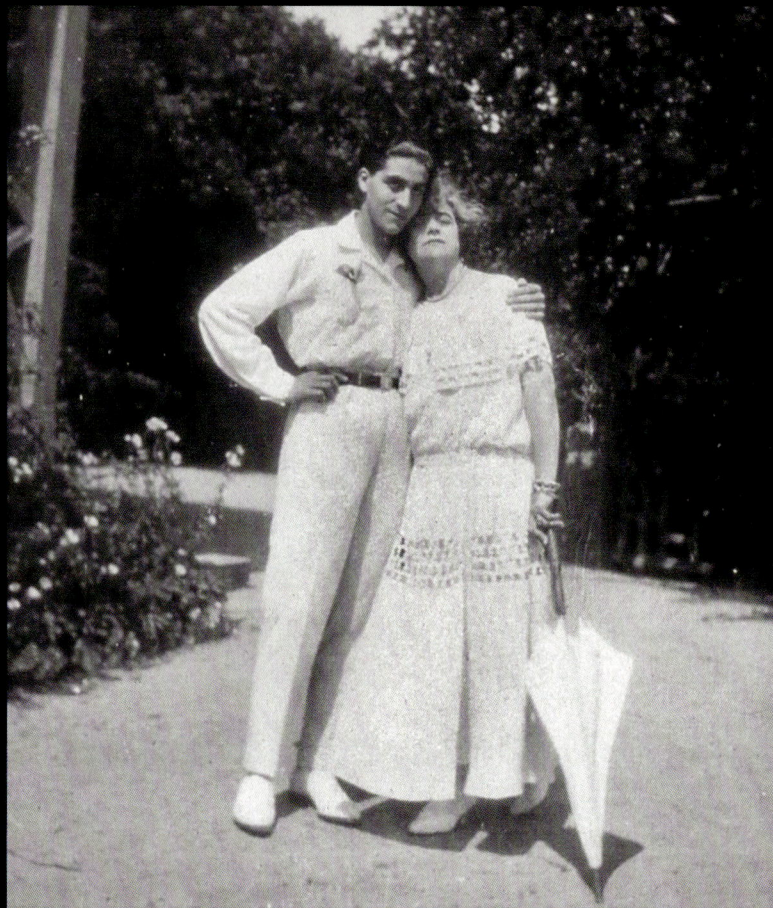

Nina Ricci and her son Robert.

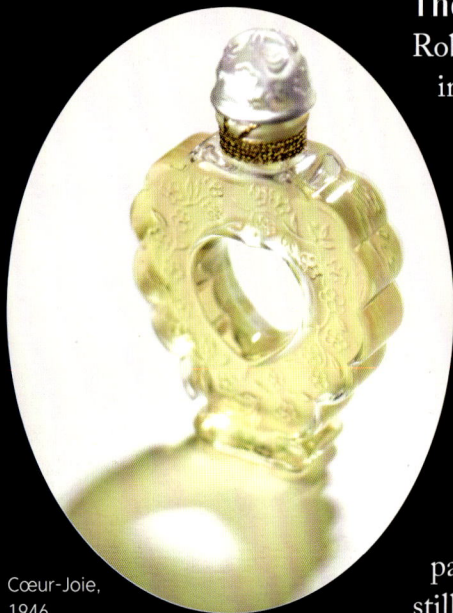

Cœur-Joie, 1946.

The first Ricci perfumes

Robert felt the company should diversify, and he had the idea of branching out into perfume. In 1946, they launched their first fragrance, Cœur-Joie, created by Germaine Cellier and presented in a bottle by Marc Lalique, a childhood friend of Robert's. Robert believed perfume elevated a woman's beauty and that this fragrance would fit the romantic, feminine Nina Ricci style. The brand's most iconic fragrance, L'Air du Temps, was created in 1948. On the subject of perfume, Robert once said that just as a dress was made to enhance the body, perfume was made to make one attractive, but in a subtler way. It was made to express a woman's personality and show her in her best light. In his words, L'Air du Temps, the first ever spicy floral fragrance, contained a little miracle that gave it a strong personality. His aim was to capture the mood of the moment, or 'l'air du temps' in French, hence the name. In 1987, Robert Ricci launched the floral Nina as a tribute to his mother. Maison Ricci is now part of the Puig group, but the diversity of its activities and quality of its creations still embody Parisian elegance and celebrate an ethereal femininity.

JEAN PATOU,
'the most expensive perfume
in the world'
━━ 1887–1936 ━━

Jean Patou was born in Normandy in 1887 and grew up in a family of tanners. Rather than taking over the family business, he decided to establish his own couture house in Paris in 1910. The bold, highly creative young man designed fashion for the upper classes, the newly emancipated sporty women and the carefree generation of the Roaring Twenties. He was an immediate success in the United States and used American models in his Paris shows. He had his own ambassador, the tennis champion Suzanne Lenglen, who created a sensation by wearing a knee-length skirt and sleeveless top on court at Wimbledon in 1921. Jean Patou's dressmaking salon, named Maison Parry, was located at 4 Rond-Point des Champs-Élysées.

Patou perfumes

The story began with Cocktail Dry, which was released in 1925, and continued with a trio of perfumes for specific hair colours, Amour-Amour for brunettes, Que Sais-Je? for blondes and Adieu Sagesse for redheads. He also launched Le Sien as a unisex fragrance that was made for men but could suit the modern, sporty woman. In 1930, to counteract the pessimism and depression after the 1929 Wall Street crash and the ensuing financial crisis, Jean Patou commissioned the company's nose, Henri Alméras, to create a perfume that would be as iconic for the brand as No. 5 was for Chanel. The result was 'Joy, the most expensive perfume in the world', according to Elsa Maxwell's tongue-in-cheek slogan. It was made from astronomical quantities of the finest and most expensive rose and jasmine essences from Grasse. Subsequent releases were Divine Folie, Normandie and Vacances. The men behind all the bottles, Louis Süe and André Mare, were interior designers whom Patou had also commissioned to decorate his rue Saint-Florentin mansion.

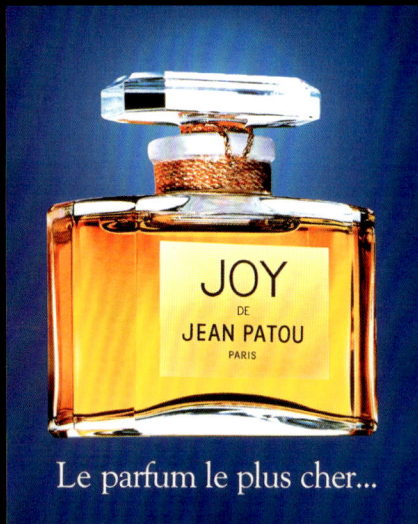

Above right: Jean Patou creation, stencil drawing by Joujou, published in 1924. Left: Joy de Jean Patou, 'The most expensive perfume...', advert, 1989.

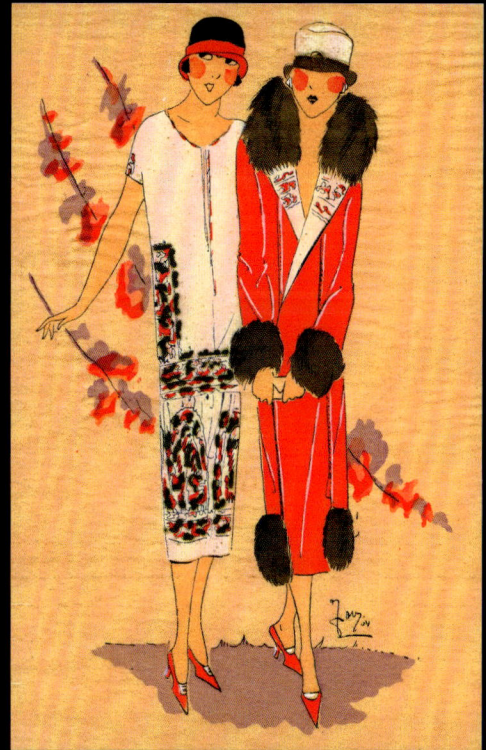

Le parfum le plus cher...

Later changes at Patou

When Jean Patou died, his brother-in-law and colleague Raymond Barbas took over and released two perfumes that perpetuated the spirit of the brand: Colony and, to celebrate the liberation of Paris, L'Heure Attendue. Jean Kerléo was the nose from 1967 to 1998 and Jean de Moüy, Jean Patou's nephew, took over the running of the company in 1980. The haute couture department closed in 1987. Jean-Michel Duriez took over from Jean Kerléo, becoming the house's fourth nose. In 2001, the brand became part of the Procter & Gamble group and the enticingly named Enjoy was launched in 2000. In 2018, LVMH took control of Jean Patou and decided to relaunch the former couture house's ready-to-wear fashion alongside its perfumes.

ELSA SCHIAPARELLI,
eclectic and extravagant
1890-1973

Elsa Schiaparelli was born into an aristocratic family and spent her childhood in Rome. She visited London and Paris in 1912 and 1914, before marrying Count Wilhelm de Wendt de Kerlor. She later divorced him and moved to Paris, where she rubbed shoulders with the leading figures of the Dada movement including the painter Francis Picabia, and also the sister of Paul Poiret, who opened doors for her in the fashion world. She established her own couture house in 1928 and her Surrealism-inspired knitwear was an overnight success. Having opened premises at 21, place Vendôme in 1935, she reigned supreme as the queen of Parisian high society and presented increasingly extravagant themed collections at her theatrical shows.

The birth of an unconventional fragrance

In August 1937, Elsa Schiaparelli founded her own perfume company and launched a perfume intended to reflect the brutal rhythm of Parisian life. She named it after her favourite expression, 'Shocking'. She opened a small manufacturing unit at Bois-Colombes and commissioned Maison Roure to create a perfume that defied all conventions. Citrus top notes developed into a surreal heart of green rose and honey nestled in patchouli and amber and ended with powdery vanilla base notes. The famous 'shocking pink' inspired by the Peruvian rose of her couture collections had become a perfume in its own right. Its packaging was the work of the artist Leonor Fini. The bottle was shaped like a dressmaker's dummy with the voluptuous proportions of Mae West, a client of Schiaparelli. The glass-paste stopper in the form of a spray of flowers referenced Elsa's dreams as a little girl when, thinking herself ugly, she 'planted' flower seeds in her throat, nose and ears to turn her face into a garden. None of them grew, but she nearly suffocated in the process. It was Elsa herself who added the V-shape, fashioned from a measuring tape, which was attached to the bottle's waist with the Schiaparelli 'S'. The bottle was mounted on a base and encased in a lace-patterned glass globe as a nod to the wedding globes of days gone by.

Hope for the war years

Marcel Vertès' sophisticated, suggestive illustration to advertise Shocking was seen as erotic at the time. Before Elsa fled to New York in 1940 she redesigned the advert, symbolically placing the Shocking bottle in a cage with a bird and the inscription 'Shocking Chante l'Espoir' ('Shocking, a song for hope'). In 1945, Salvador Dalí designed a bottle for the new Roy Soleil in the form of a rock topped by a sun-shaped stopper with a pensive face. After the war, the Elsa Schiaparelli brand lost its sparkle and both the couture business and perfume house closed in 1954.

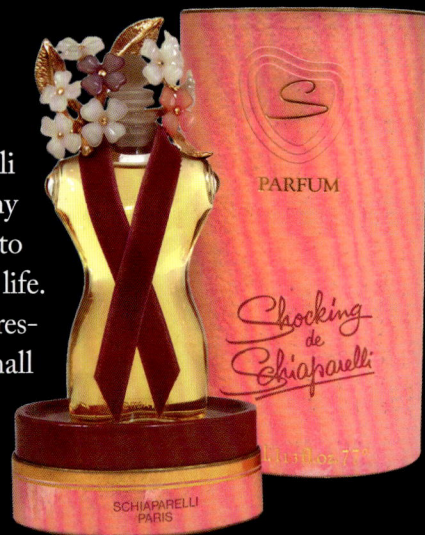

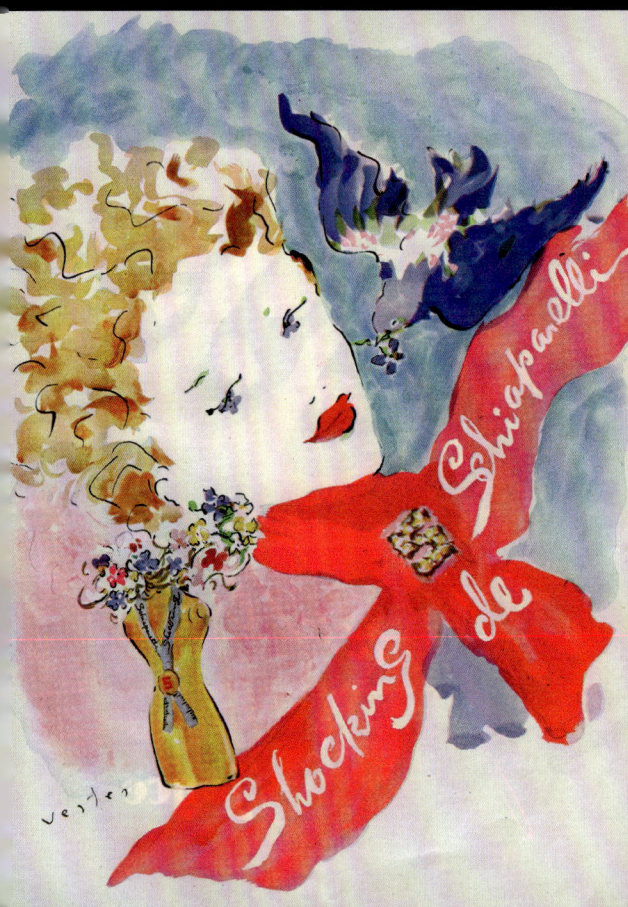

Advert for Schiaparelli's Shocking perfume, 1944.

CHRISTIAN DIOR,
'designing the wonderful'
1905–1957

'A nimble genius unique to his time whose magical name combines God [Dieu] and gold [or],' is how Jean Cocteau described his friend Christian Dior, who was born in Granville, a seaside town on the coast of Normandy, not far from the bay of Mont Saint-Michel. He was the second of five children of an archetypal bourgeois family, all well brought up and educated by governesses. From 1910 onwards, the family split its time between Granville and Paris. From a very young age, Christian stood out for his fascination with plants and flowers and his early gift for drawing. Anything shiny, ornate, floral or light-hearted could entertain him for hours. He dreamed of studying at the Beaux-Arts in Paris and becoming an architect, but his parents had a diplomatic career mapped out for him.

Creativity in his blood

From 1923 to 1926, he was a student at the Institute of Political Studies in Paris (known as Sciences Po today), but he regularly skipped classes to hang out with his friends, who loved painting and Art Nouveau in all its forms. He went with them to private viewings and parties, which opened his mind to all types of art. Failing his exams threatened to put an end to his life as an enlightened dilettante, but his father agreed to finance a painting gallery for him on the condition that their name never appeared on the front, so as not to blight the family reputation. Between 1928 and 1934, Christian Dior and his business partner Jacques Bonjean, later joined by Pierre Colle, exhibited works by Christian Bérard, Max Jacob, Picasso, Dalí, Utrillo, Braque, Léger, Dufy, Zadkine and others.

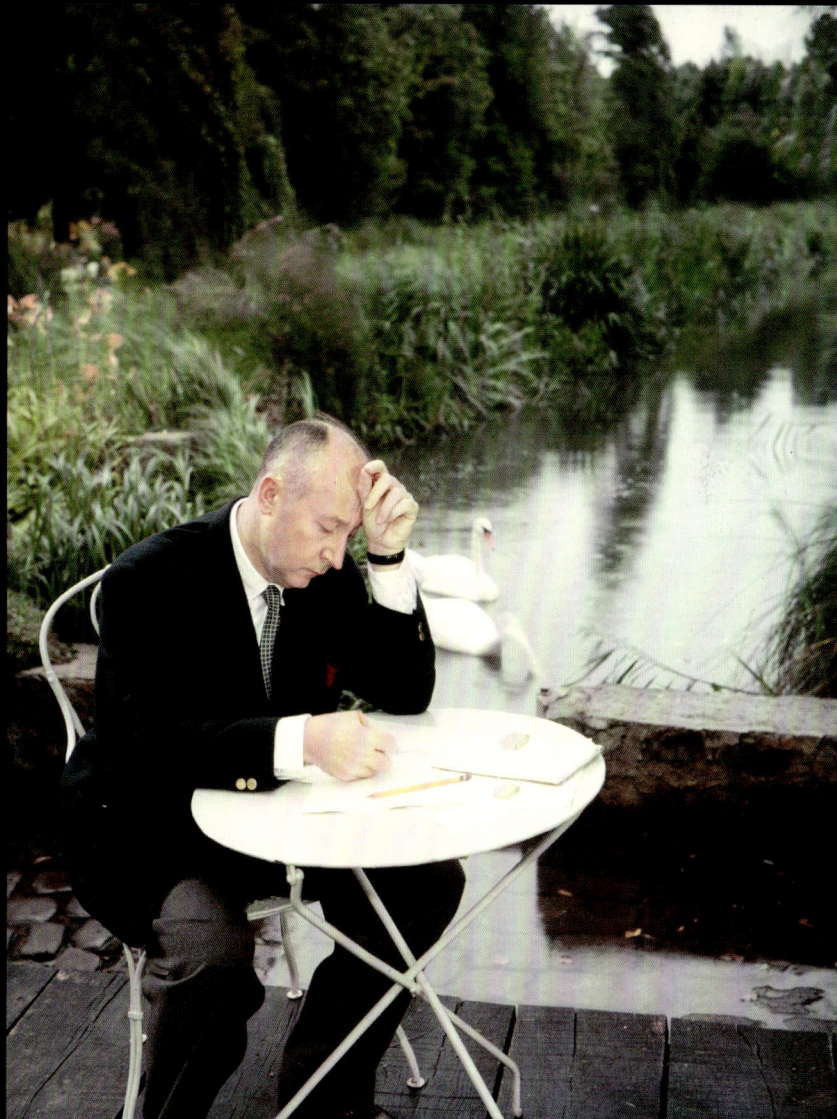

Christian Dior at work, circa 1950, France.

A difficult phase and his first sketches

Sadly, Dior's life suddenly took a painful turn. His father suffered financial ruin as a result of the 1929 economic crisis and ill-advised property dealings, and his mother died, so he had to leave the gallery. He found himself homeless with almost no income. He contracted tuberculosis, from which he recovered thanks to his friends clubbing together to send him to a clinic at Font-Romeu, and then to the Balearic Islands. He then turned his hand to drawing and used this skill to produce extraordinary, expressive sketches that enabled him to show the woman behind the outfit and so find a job as a designer.

Sudden fame

In 1941 Dior was employed by the prominent couturier Lucien Lelong, but, as his talent developed, he soon felt restricted in his supporting role. On 8 October 1946, Marcel Boussac, a textile magnate, agreed to give him the money to set up his own couture house, which opened on 16 December of the same year in a private mansion at 30, avenue Montaigne in the 8th arrondissement. Jacques Rouët was appointed managing director. On 12 February 1947, Christian Dior showed his first spring–summer collection, named Corolle, in the salons of the couture house. Those who were there could not believe their eyes. Dresses with generous bodices, slender waists and long skirts were unheard of at the time. 'It's quite a revolution, dear Christian. Your dresses have such a new look. They are wonderful, you know?' enthused Carmel Snow, editor-in-chief of *Harper's Bazaar*. The New Look, as it came to be known, crossed the Atlantic to the United States before travelling the world. In the words of the French journalist, writer and politician Françoise Giroud, one day Christian Dior was unknown and the next he had shot to stardom. Women dreamed of owning his dresses, which came to symbolize new-found happiness.

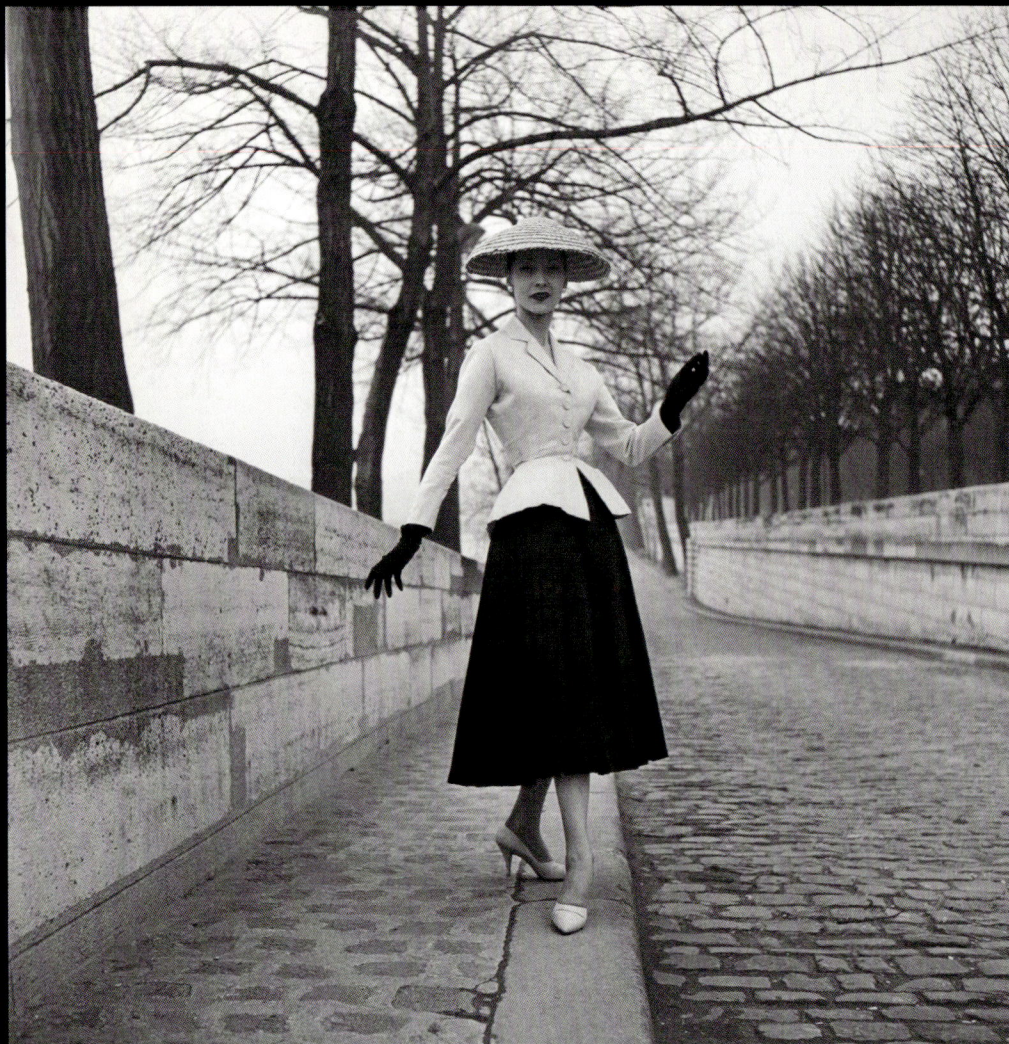

Bar suit from the Corolle collection, photographed by Willy Maywald in 1947.

From a love of botanicals to Parfums Christian Dior

As a young boy, Christian Dior adored women's perfume and flowers, having inherited a passion for botanicals and gardens from his mother. At the age of 15, he created a magnificent pergola bedecked with honeysuckle, mignonette, geraniums and roses in the clifftop garden of his childhood home. As early as 1946, he had wanted to create a perfume to 'wrap every woman in an exquisite femininity, as though each of my designs was emerging from the bottle one by one'. He saw perfume as the philosopher's stone of his world, in other words the perfect finishing touch or je ne sais quoi his dresses needed to make them truly sensational. He thought of himself as a perfume creator as well as a fashion designer. In his words, he became a perfumer so that every one of his clients could see all his dresses simply by opening a bottle, and could leave a sillage of unforgettable scent in their wake. He created the company Parfums Christian Dior in March 1947 with his childhood friend Serge Heftler-Louiche, who had lived only a few metres from his Granville house and had already made his debut in perfume working for companies such as Coty.

Four perfumes in his lifetime

In his 1951 book *Je suis couturier* (I Am a Couturier), Christian Dior remembered the women of his childhood for the scent of their perfume, which was much more persistent than present-day fragrances and lingered in the lift long after they had left. His first perfume, Miss Dior, created in honour of his sister, came on to the market on 12 February 1947. It had a distinctive couture look, with an amphora-shaped Baccarat crystal bottle designed by the painter Fernand Guéry-Colas as a nod to the harmonious curves of Dior's Corolle 'New Look' collection. As his team were putting the final touches to his first boutique on avenue Montaigne, Christian Dior is said to have told them to spray more perfume. He wanted it to fill the air so that the journalists and his customers left 30, avenue Montaigne suffused with Miss Dior. As a result, over a litre of perfume was sprayed in the store each week. Four perfumes were launched in his lifetime: Miss Dior, Diorama, Eau Fraîche and Diorissimo. The second, Diorama, was created in 1948 but due to a lack of funds was not launched until 1949. This was Edmond Roudnitska's first creation for Dior and the start of a fruitful collaboration. In 1956, Diorissimo was released and likened to a dynamic musical score driven by the warmer days and renewal of spring. Christian Dior's brief was for the fragrance of a single flower, his favourite lily of the valley, which, out of superstition, he slipped into the hem of the dresses worn by his models on fashion show days.

Left: Special edition Diorissimo bottle, designed by Christian Dior and made in clear Baccarat crystal, topped by a gold-plated floral stopper by Maison Charles, 1956.

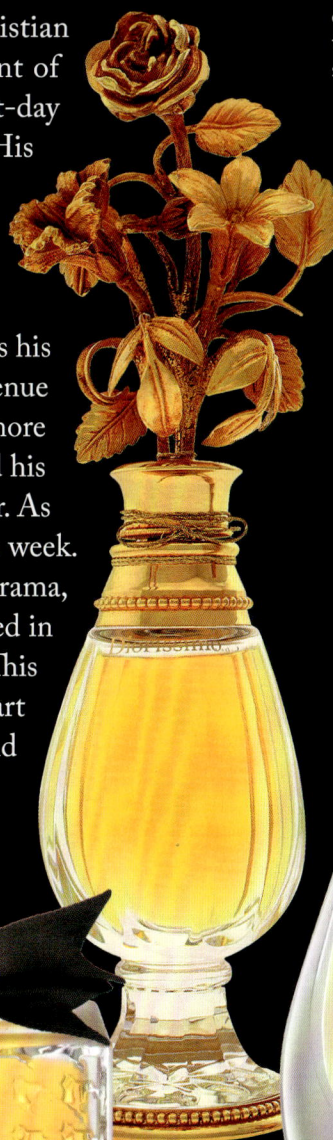

Below: Special edition of J'Adore (first released in 1999), in a Baccarat crystal bottle with a gold chain neck made in Dior's fine-jewellery workshops, 2011.

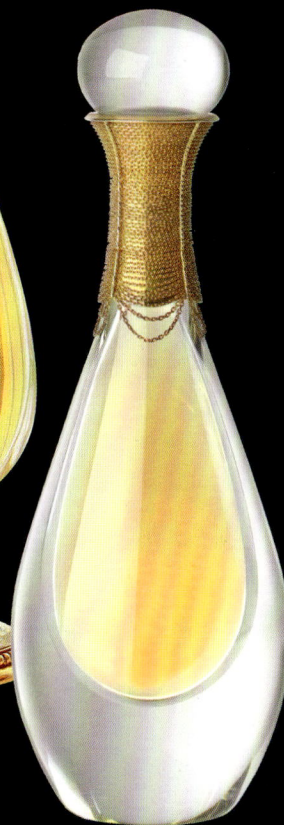

Right: Miss Dior bottle by Fernand Guéry-Colas, clear glass with a houndstooth pattern and the signature Dior swallowtail bow in black satin, 1949.

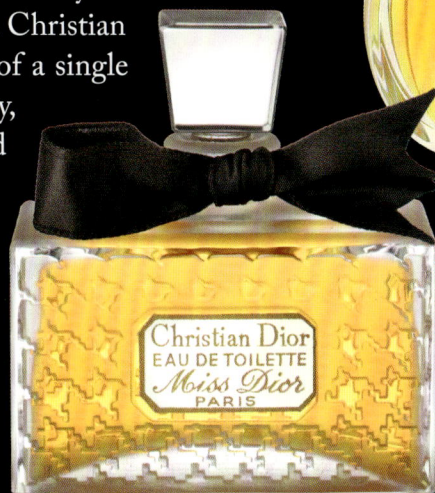

A dazzling success but fatal exhaustion

From his Zig Zag and Envol collections in 1948, it was clear he was referencing eighteenth- and nineteenth-century fashion. In 1950, Dior was made a Knight of the Legion of Honour and shortly afterwards he published his first book, *Je suis couturier*. He created relentlessly and presented six collections each year: two haute couture, two ready-to-wear, one for the stores and another for the United States. In 1957, he was the first fashion designer to be named *Time Magazine* Person of the Year. Exhausted, he suffered a fatal heart attack in October 1957.

Yves Saint Laurent, whom Christian Dior had appointed as his successor, was named artistic director.

Diorling was launched in 1963 as a posthumous tribute to the company's two founders, Christian Dior and Serge Heftler-Louiche, neither of whom lived to see Eau Sauvage take the world by storm in 1966. The first skincare range was launched in 1973 to accompany the perfumes. Since its 1999 release, J'Adore has found its natural place alongside other top perfumes in the luxury market, as has La Collection Maison Christian Dior. Each new perfume François Demachy, who was house perfumer at the time, created for this collection paid homage to the great man himself.

THE PERFUMER

THE NOSE IS NOT ONLY AN OLFACTORY ORGAN BUT ALSO THE NAME GIVEN TO A PERSON WHO MAKES PERFUME FOR A LIVING. IT THEREFORE HAS AN INEXTRICABLE LINK WITH FRAGRANCE. PERFUMERS ARE ARTISTS WORKING BEHIND THE SCENES WHO HAVE THE RARE ABILITY TO SMELL AND RECOGNIZE EVERY SINGLE SCENT. AND BECAUSE OF THE SYNERGY BETWEEN THEIR NERVE CENTRE AND MEMORY, THEIR EMOTIONAL RESPONSE TO SMELL CAN BE VERY INTENSE.

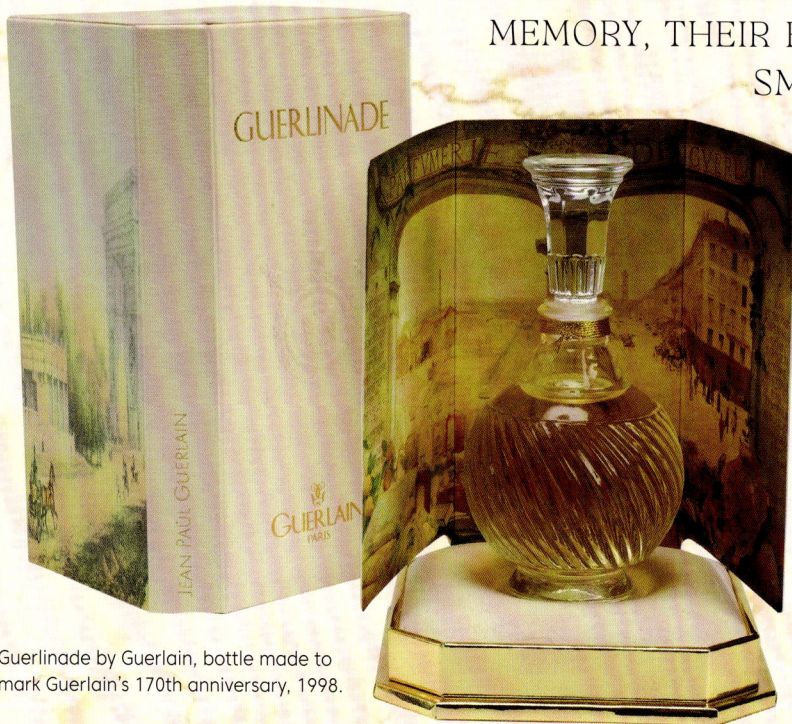

Guerlinade by Guerlain, bottle made to mark Guerlain's 170th anniversary, 1998.

THE IMPORTANCE OF THE SENSE OF SMELL

Aristophanes believed that the nose's only function was to be blown. Kant distrusted it and, for a long time, philosophers paid little regard to the sense of smell, because it was deemed too close to animal instinct. Nietzsche, on the other hand, declared 'my genius is in my nostrils', and Philippe Sollers believed that matters of desire were centred in the nose. So the sense of smell is important in life; we use it subconsciously when choosing whether to love or reject. And, for perfumers, it is fundamental to their craft and their art, because good noses find all their inspiration within. They are both artists and technicians, wizards and alchemists. Unlike apothecaries, who reproduce the same formula ad infinitum, perfumers are creative artists who touch the innermost reaches of each individual.

THE FIRST PERFUME NOSES

In the eighteenth century, Lavoisier's early scientific experiments opened up a vast terrain of knowledge which perfumers had to reflect on, learn and incorporate into their craft in order to refine it. At this time, modern perfumery was in its very early stages and perfumers' work and skill involved imitating nature as closely as possible. Change came about gradually and perfumers began to use synthetic products and their emotional memory to create scents that moved ever further away from reality, offering their clients an insight into their dreams and imagination. Paul Parquet, co-owner of Parfumerie Houbigant with Alfred de Javal, was one such creative pioneer with his exceptional Fougère Royale (1882), a bergamot and coumarin fragrance evocative of the earthy undertones of the forest floor. Aimé Guerlain conceived Jicky in 1889, establishing a new art of perfume that suggested rather than reproduced, by combining synthetic aromas and natural products. He would later tell his nephew Jacques Guerlain that a Guerlain perfume resembled what it evoked. The young perfumer created a secret formula, a unique *sillage* named Guerlinade, which would be used in all Guerlain perfumes. Noses became particularly important in the twentieth century because they had the ingenuity, skills and technical knowledge needed to make a perfume.

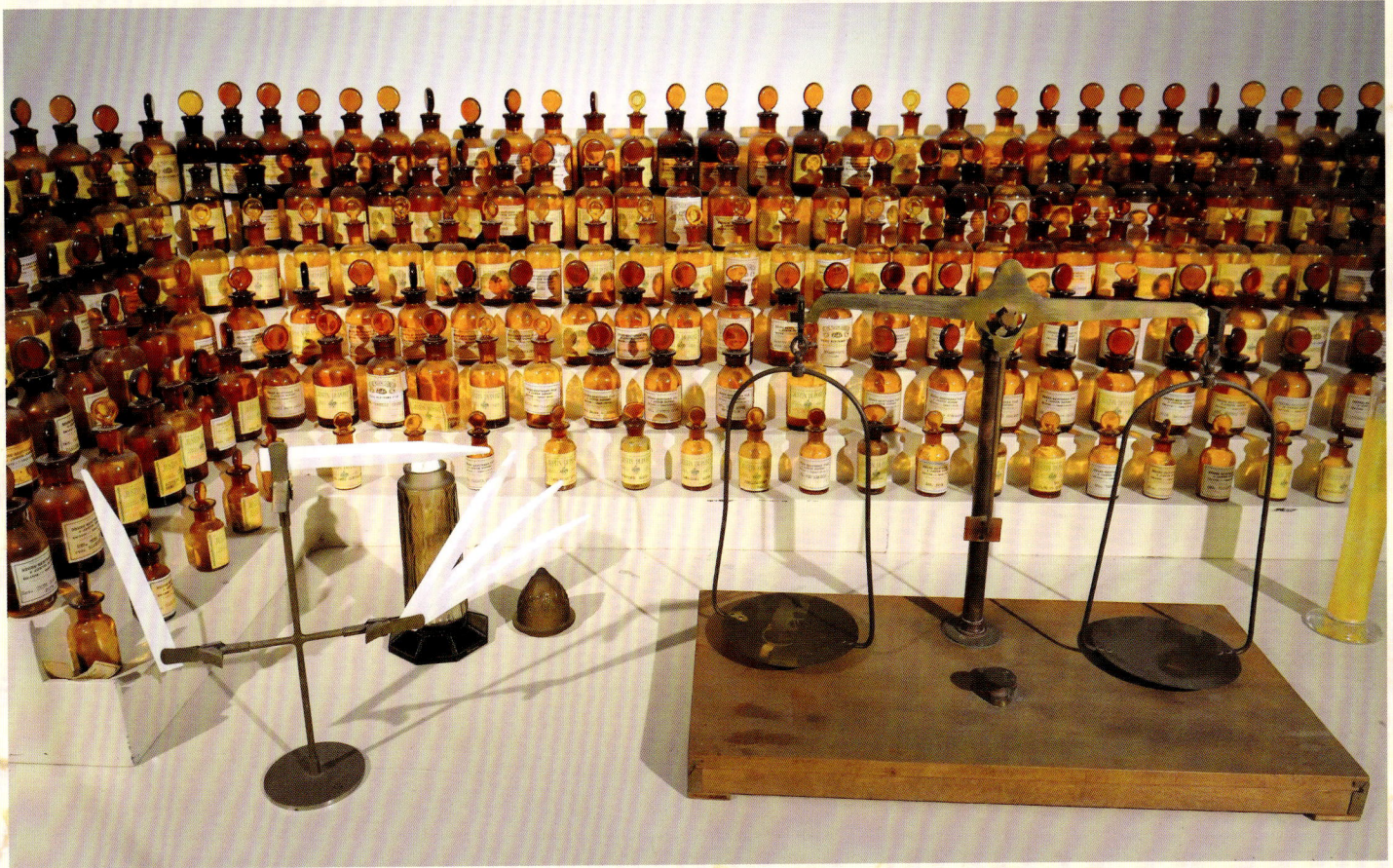

The perfume organ of the famous nose Jean Carles (1892–1966), who not only founded the first perfume school in Grasse but also created perfumes such as Miss Dior and Nina Ricci's L'Air du Temps.

A VOCABULARY BORROWED FROM ART AND LITERATURE

As perfume evolved, its vocabulary moved further away from the words used for raw materials to adopt words from other arts, including literature, embracing poetic metaphors such as departures, bodies and heart. It also borrowed from music (notes, keys, brasses, contrasts, rhythm), architecture (bases, structure, solidity) and cuisine (cold, hot, spicy, acidic). Clients used this vocabulary to describe what they wanted in a new perfume. Noses would set to work at their perfume organ, a sort of semi-circular table with several shelves containing small phials of all the essences at their disposal, and test and compose their blends. They must exercise their sense of smell every day because they have between 2,000 and 4,000 different scents to memorize, some from their palette and others from their sensory memory.

Ernest Beaux, the nose who rewrote the perfume script

According to Ernest Beaux, the famous nose behind Chanel No. 5 (1921), perfumers must first and foremost know their raw materials, and analyse and practise breaking down an aroma and commit to memory the smell of these components to create their palette. This in turn shapes the style of their personal accords, which form the basis of their work and all their compositions. The next ingredient is inspiration, which they can find in places such as literature, music or art. Ernest Beaux described the process as perfumers attempting, little by little, to translate the mental image of something lost into something concrete, the perfume. He said that the inspiration for Chanel No. 5 came to him during the Russian Civil War when he passed through a region beyond the Arctic Circle, at the time of year of the midnight sun, when the lakes and rivers exuded a particular freshness.

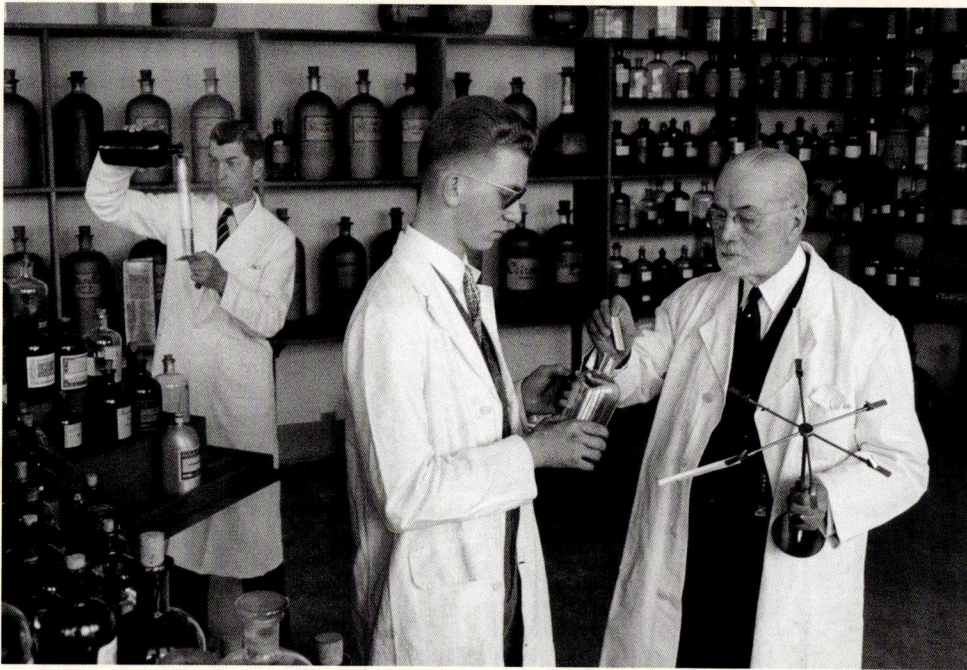

Jacques Guerlain and his son Jean-Paul in the Guerlain laboratory in Paris in 1956.

SEEKING A LOOK AND THEIR OWN PERFUMER

In the twentieth century, the look of a perfume took on a new importance and the whole creative process became an art form. In the interwar years there was a frenzy of creativity and production from the best-known designers. Until then most perfumers, such as François Coty (Coty), Ernest Daltroff (Caron) and Aimé and Jacques Guerlain (Guerlain), had owned their own house and made their own perfumes. Then, when couturiers entered the perfume world, a nose would forge links with a specific fashion house to create a perfume that reflected its style, for instance Henri Alméras (Poiret and Patou), Ernest Beaux (Chanel) and André Fraysse (Lanvin).

THE NOSE TODAY

In the early twentieth century, every major house employed its own nose, who had a good grasp of the spirit of the brand. Today, however, this tradition survives in only a few, such as Chanel, Dior, Cartier, Guerlain and Vuitton. Independent perfumers work for themselves and have significant freedom to create the perfumes they like with no constraints. Some houses outsource to companies that employ their own team of perfumers to produce the raw materials and create aromas. They follow a brief from the marketing department that describes the concept of the future perfume, which must meet the brand's criteria and market expectations. Several noses get together to produce some preliminary preparations and select the one that will be developed. However, for all perfumers, the most important thing is to create a beautiful perfume. As Edmond Roudnitska said, 'I am one with the perfume, the perfume is one with me, I am a sensory machine.'

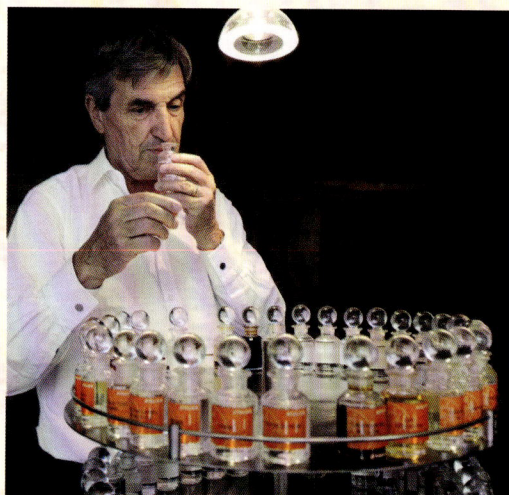

Jean-Claude Ellena, Hermès nose from 2004 to 2016.

LEARNING THE TRADE

After the Guild of Glover–Perfumers was disbanded in 1791, there were several routes into perfumery in France. Some perfumers were trained in-house with companies such as Guerlain, while others learned the trade as apprentices to other perfumers. Perfume schools first came on the scene in the 1950s to meet ever-growing market demand. They were initially set up by industrialists, the main one being the Roure school, founded by Jean Carles in Grasse in 1946. The Givaudan school was opened in 1968 in Geneva and in 1974, the ISIPCA (International School for Postgraduate Studies in Perfume, Cosmetics and Food Flavour) was founded in Versailles. Finally, the École Supérieure du Parfum opened its doors in Paris and Grasse in 2011 as a graduate school offering training in perfume creation and management.

THE OLFACTORY TREE

A classification of the natural olfactory raw materials, International Perfume Museum, Grasse, France.

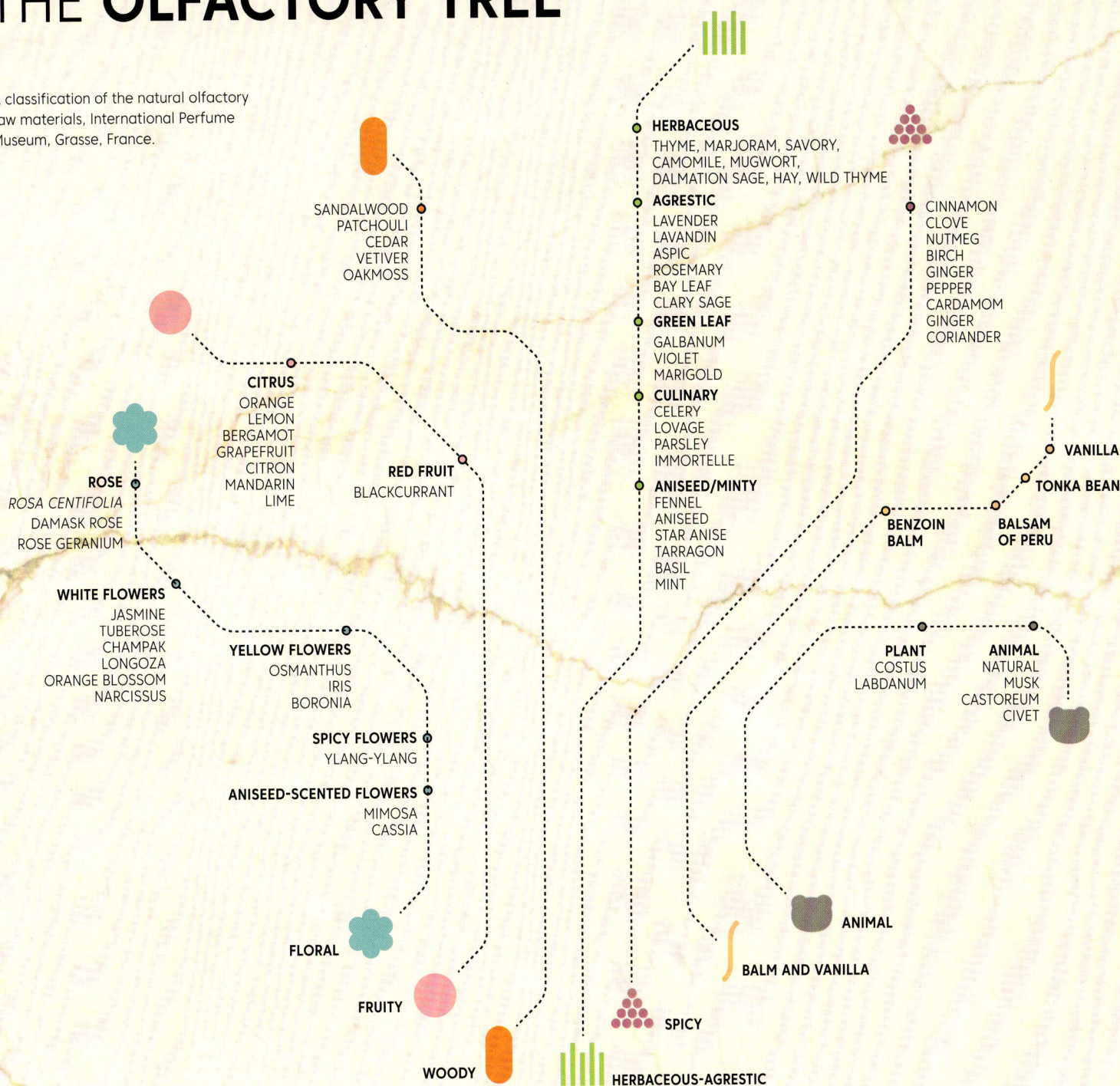

SANDALWOOD
PATCHOULI
CEDAR
VETIVER
OAKMOSS

HERBACEOUS
THYME, MARJORAM, SAVORY,
CAMOMILE, MUGWORT,
DALMATION SAGE, HAY, WILD THYME

AGRESTIC
LAVENDER
LAVANDIN
ASPIC
ROSEMARY
BAY LEAF
CLARY SAGE

GREEN LEAF
GALBANUM
VIOLET
MARIGOLD

CULINARY
CELERY
LOVAGE
PARSLEY
IMMORTELLE

ANISEED/MINTY
FENNEL
ANISEED
STAR ANISE
TARRAGON
BASIL
MINT

CINNAMON
CLOVE
NUTMEG
BIRCH
GINGER
PEPPER
CARDAMOM
GINGER
CORIANDER

VANILLA

TONKA BEAN

BENZOIN BALM

BALSAM OF PERU

CITRUS
ORANGE
LEMON
BERGAMOT
GRAPEFRUIT
CITRON
MANDARIN
LIME

RED FRUIT
BLACKCURRANT

ROSE
ROSA CENTIFOLIA
DAMASK ROSE
ROSE GERANIUM

WHITE FLOWERS
JASMINE
TUBEROSE
CHAMPAK
LONGOZA
ORANGE BLOSSOM
NARCISSUS

YELLOW FLOWERS
OSMANTHUS
IRIS
BORONIA

SPICY FLOWERS
YLANG-YLANG

ANISEED-SCENTED FLOWERS
MIMOSA
CASSIA

PLANT
COSTUS
LABDANUM

ANIMAL
NATURAL
MUSK
CASTOREUM
CIVET

FLORAL

FRUITY

WOODY

SPICY

HERBACEOUS-AGRESTIC

BALM AND VANILLA

ANIMAL

THE PERFUME PYRAMID

The balance of a perfume depends on the volatility, intensity and tenacity of its raw materials. The fragrance molecules are alive and interact continuously, sometimes coming together to form a harmonious whole and at other times stifling each other. Our sense of smell cannot take in all these aromas at once, but detects them individually as they evaporate. To reflect this, they are classified in a perfume pyramid. The top notes are the ones we notice immediately. They are the most volatile and are generally citrus, aromatic or marine accords. The middle notes are more marked. These are the floral, green and fruity aromas that come through after the top notes have disappeared. Finally, the base notes are the ones you can smell for hours after you have sprayed your perfume. They are voluptuous, long-lasting, ambers, spices, woods, enticing and oriental. Together, as if by magic, they form the perfume and the scent it leaves in its wake, known as the *sillage*.

THE PERFUMES THAT HAVE MADE HISTORY

WHICH PERFUMES HAVE LEFT THEIR MARK ON HISTORY? THERE ARE SO MANY IT IS DIFFICULT TO SINGLE THEM OUT. THERE ARE, HOWEVER, SOME ICONIC ONES, SUCH AS CHANEL NO. 5 AND GUERLAIN'S SHALIMAR, WHICH DISTIL SUBCONSCIOUS POWERS, AROUSE PASSIONS AND FORGE INTRIGUING CONNECTIONS. THESE PERFUMES HAVE THEIR OWN RITUALS AND UNIVERSAL LANGUAGE. THEY ARE TRUE WORKS OF ART.

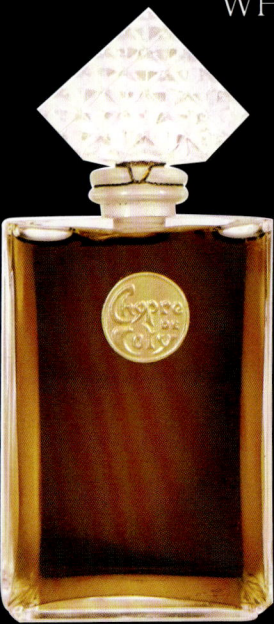

CHYPRE, COTY (1917)

The chypre accord was the epitome of unisex fragrance. The name (French for Cyprus) and concept came from Coty's 1917 perfume Chypre, a bergamot, oakmoss, cistus labdanum and patchouli blend inspired by a fragrant water, Eau de Chypre, that was made in the Middle Ages by perfumers on the island of Cyprus. Little by little, French perfumers got to know the formula and put several incarnations of Eau de Chypre on the market. It was more popular with men due to its rather dry top note, but in 1917 François Coty brought out a feminine version of this truly elegant perfume family. The scent was joyful and light but also elegant and sensual, like a voyage to a far-off dream island at the ancient crossroads of the perfume route. Recalling the forest smells of his childhood, Coty worked on an oakmoss accord without the overly earthy moss notes of famous perfumes such as Chypre by Roger&Gallet (1890) and Guerlain's Chypre de Paris (1909). He tinkered with different formulations to obtain the perfect balance between the citrus notes and the depth of the oakmoss, which he said he gathered himself in Fontainebleau Forest. He concealed the earthiness with copious amounts of jasmine and expertly combined this with synthetic notes. His formula was so revolutionary that it paved the way for a new perfume family. The elegant, modern fragrance was a runaway success and especially popular in the 1950s. A little accompanying note read, 'Mysterious and captivating aromas to accentuate the charm of brunettes.'

FEMME, ROCHAS (1944)

Femme was made just after the liberation of Paris, when strict rationing was still in place. It was created by Edmond Roudnitska for a man in love, Marcel Rochas, who wanted to give a perfume to his future wife and believed it should be possible to smell a woman's scent before you even see her. Femme symbolized the first reassuring signs of a new-found peace and was a resounding success. It owed its seductive charm to plum, a note hitherto unused in perfume, elevated by oakmoss and peach. However, most surprising of all was the exceptional 'volume' of the fragrance, which had the power to fill a room. It was launched in 1944 in the sumptuously fragrant surroundings of avenue Matignon, presented in a limited-edition numbered Lalique bottle. Luxury, refinement and femininity seemed to be the order of the day. However, to meet the demands of mass production, the original bottle was replaced in 1945 by the classic amphora-shaped container it is still sold in today, modelled on the generous hips and tiny waist of the movie star Mae West.

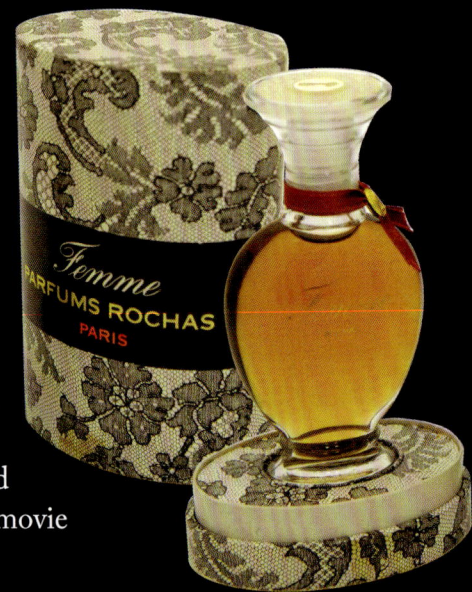

L'AIR DU TEMPS, NINA RICCI (1948)

L'Air du Temps, a poetic French expression used to describe the mood of the moment, encapsulates the subtle refinement of Nina Ricci in a perfume that has enchanted generations of women. Ricci's message to men was 'make love, not war' – a fragrant expression of 'Peace and Love' ahead of its time – which Francis Fabron translated into an extraordinary, spicy carnation and gardenia accord with a subtle bouquet of natural rose and jasmine. The fascinating thing about this perfume is that, on first smell, it is extremely simple, thanks to the natural ingredients, but as it develops, it becomes richer and more complex. Robert Ricci described it as delicate, young, romantic and sensual … a lively, well-balanced and harmonious perfume … which exudes a mysterious power of seduction.' The romantic bottle with its two intertwined doves came to symbolize peace, love and eternal youth. Sales took off rapidly in 1953 and, until the 1980s, one bottle of L'Air du Temps is said to have been sold every five seconds worldwide.

Copy of a sketch describing the olfactory composition of L'Air du Temps, created for the press kit for the 50th anniversary of the line in 1998, by Lionel Le Mehauté for Nina Ricci.

L'Air du Temps

Bergamote de Calabre
Jasmin de Grasse
Gardénia
Rose de Grasse, Œillet poivré
L'Air du Citron de Sicile
Famille Orientale
Santal des Indes Orientales,
Iris de Florence
Noix Muscade de Yougoslavie
Girofle de Zanzibar, Poivre noir de Madagascar

Soliflore · Œillet · Gardénia · Jasmin · Rose centifolia · Trisanthème

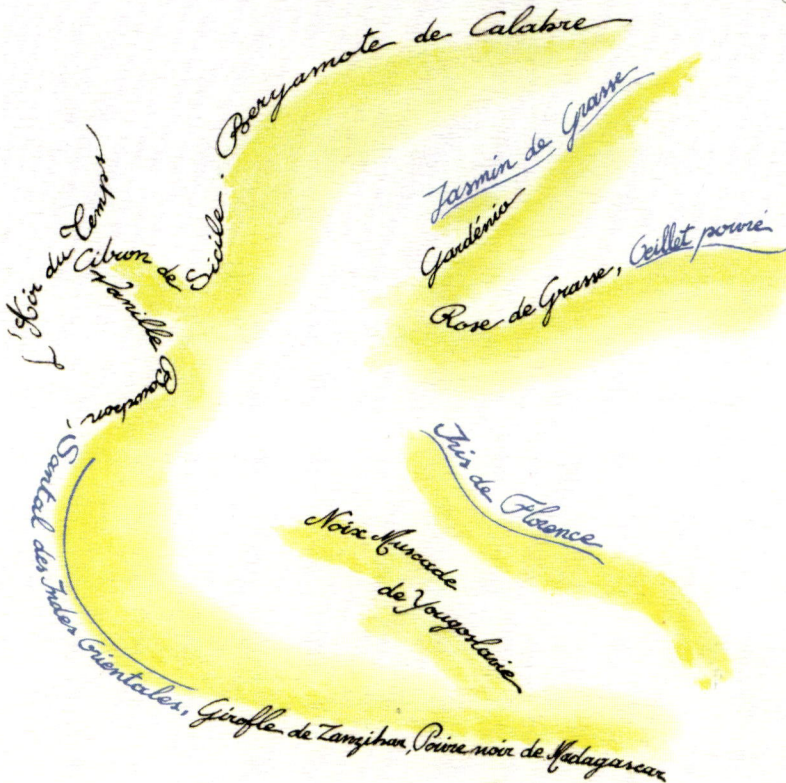

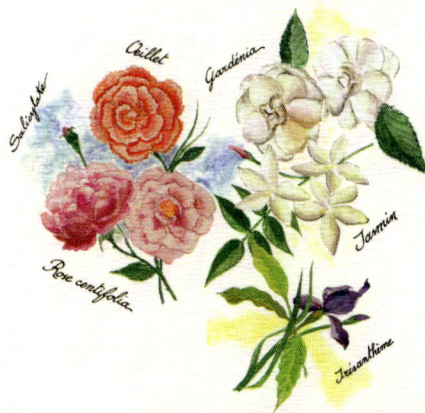

NINA RICCI
PARIS

YOUTH DEW, ESTÉE LAUDER (1953)

Youth Dew was launched at a time when the United States was forging its own style of perfume and was trying to reconquer the domestic market. Estée Lauder understood that the lifestyle of the American woman was radically different from that of her European counterpart. American women looked for French elegance in a perfume but, because of their more active lifestyle, only wanted to apply it once a day. They also liked powerful scents that turned heads. Youth Dew, a fragrant amber, incense, orange and benzoin oil composition that lasted all day long, fitted the bill, despite being a heady oriental at a time when florals and green or leathery fruity chypres were all the rage. For the modern woman consumer, Estée Lauder also made a perfumed bath oil with a record-breaking 70% concentration. The perfume not only sold extremely well worldwide but also unleashed the creative juices of the United States' perfume industry.

TRÉSOR, LANCÔME (1953, THEN 1990)

Armand Petitjean launched the first Lancôme perfume with this name in 1953. The artist Georges Delhomme, former creative director at Coty, had designed a solid cut-glass bottle faceted like a diamond and topped with a clip-on stopper with a roller, meaning it could be transported on a plane. In 1990, Sophia Grojsman updated Trésor, and the new version came in a Swarovski crystal inverted pyramid bottle designed by Lancôme and manufactured by Areca. It was a floral perfume with soft notes of peach, rose and apricot and comforting sandalwood, vanilla and amber, a joyful scent that was fully in keeping with a certain serene, romantic 1990s femininity that was rooted in the nostalgia of love and marriage. Confident, assertive and at ease with themselves, the women of the time bought into the power of this 'perfume for precious moments', as promised by the advertising campaign. The advert featured the iconic actress Isabella Rossellini filmed under the Louvre's inverted pyramid. She was later succeeded by Inès Sastre (1996), Kate Winslet (2007) and Penélope Cruz (2011) as faces of Trésor.

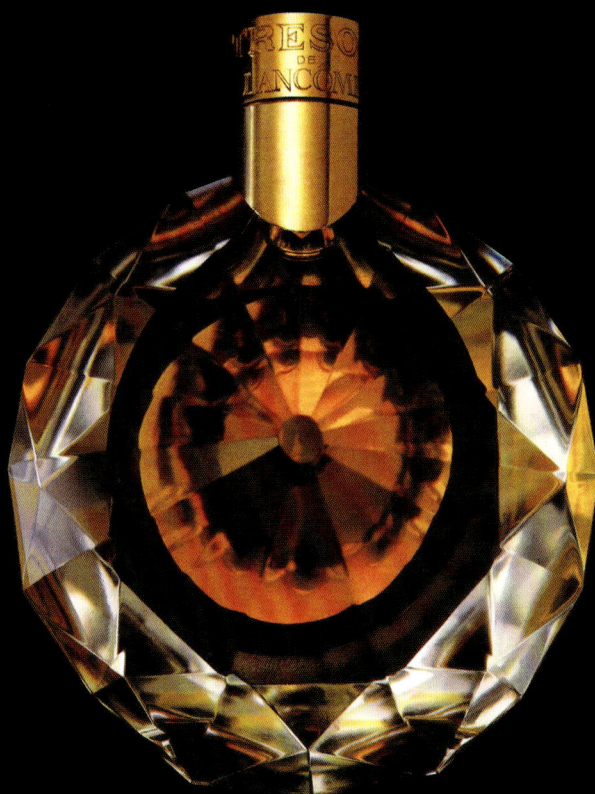

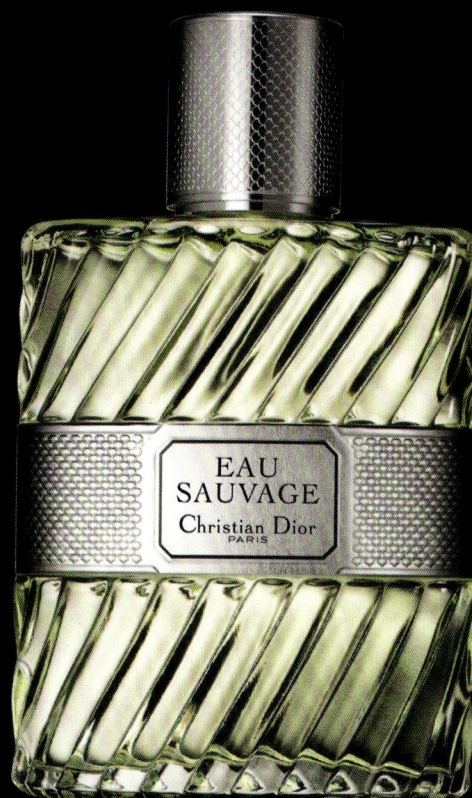

EAU SAUVAGE, DIOR (1966)

Dior's first perfume for men was created by Edmond Roudnitska and broke new ground in the history of male fragrance, introducing the idea of unisex perfumes. It was used by men as an aftershave but adopted by women because it had the lightness and transparency, that discreet but long-lasting scent they were looking for but could not find in female perfumes at the time. The composition was floral and, for the first time, the aldehyde hedione took centre stage, leaving a lingering fresh jasmine aroma in its wake. The opening citrusy petitgrain and lemon accord was sustained by basil and rosemary. The heart comprised floral notes of jasmine, rose, iris and carnation, another first for male perfumes, and the oakmoss, vetiver and musk base added a touch of warmth. Eau Sauvage was sporty, classic and elegant, as were the rounded curves of the glass, which gave the bottle a slightly softer feel than that of traditional male fragrances.

ANAÏS ANAÏS, CACHAREL (1978)

When Cacharel launched Anaïs Anaïs in 1978 it was something of a revolution, a social phenomenon. France's May 1968 riots, together with the civil unrest in different parts of the world during the 1960s, had changed the face of youth and their values forever. It was Cacharel founder Jean Bousquet's wish that the perfume be democratic, so it was launched in the French retail chain Monoprix and targeted at those who would buy it with their pocket money. These girls did not go to traditional perfume stores because they were looking for something new. They tended to shop in pharmacies, the antithesis of luxury perfume boutiques, where they bought their patchouli and vanilla essential oils and simple, light eaux de toilette. Cacharel positioned Anaïs Anaïs as a gentle, yet sexy, perfume for young women, with a slogan advertising it as 'le plus tendre des parfums' ('the most tender perfume'). The bottle, too, turned its back on conventional design with a return to a softer image merging past and present. Anaïs was a goddess of love and fertility in ancient Persia. It was one of many floral perfumes on the market at the time, but its team of perfumers created a bouquet of contrasts, fresh and soft, pure and intoxicating. The name was repeated to represent a woman of many facets, the innocent libertine character who gives its name to the novel by French author Colette, who sought adventure in the guise of love. In the space of five years, Anaïs Anaïs became the best-selling perfume on the French market and an international success, fuelled by a combination of its young style and affordable price, which was 30% lower than that of traditional perfumes.

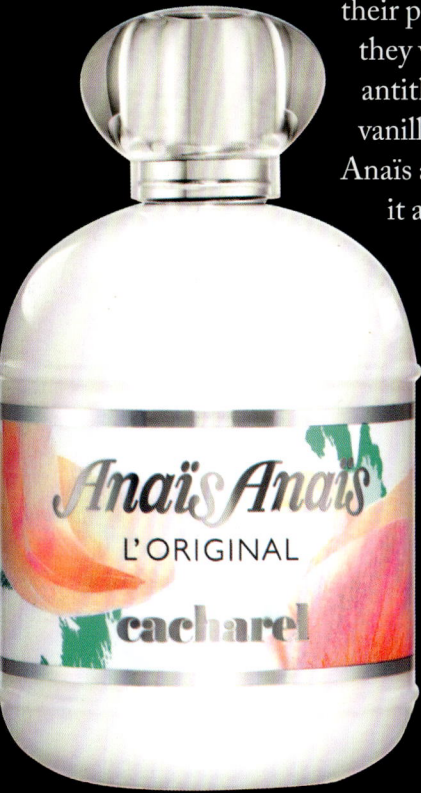

Anaïs Anaïs repackaged in 2014 on the release of Anaïs Anaïs Premier Délice.

COOL WATER, DAVIDOFF (1988)

Pierre Bourdon's Cool Water for Davidoff heralded the huge American fresh and clean trend of the 1990s with its predominant aquatic and marine notes. The aromatic fougère molecule dihydromyrcenol brought male perfumery into the modern era. In Cool Water, it was paired with lavender to produce a fresh sensation never before found in men's fragrances, and to achieve a palpable floral freshness without the use of marine notes. This clean edge, easy to detect in a male fragrance, dispelled the reductive stereotype of a virile hunk and the floral notes, rather than making it more 'feminine', combined with an amber and musk base to add sensuality. True to its name, a splash of this perfume was like diving into cool water, an image which worked well with the late 1980s masculine dynamic of freedom and escape.

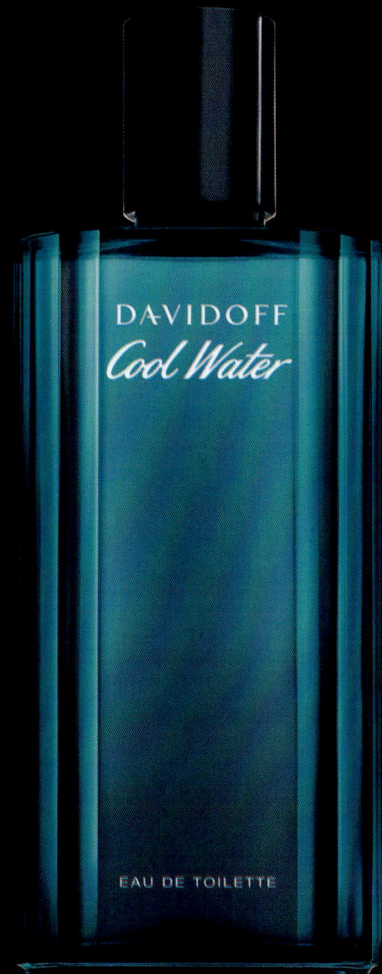

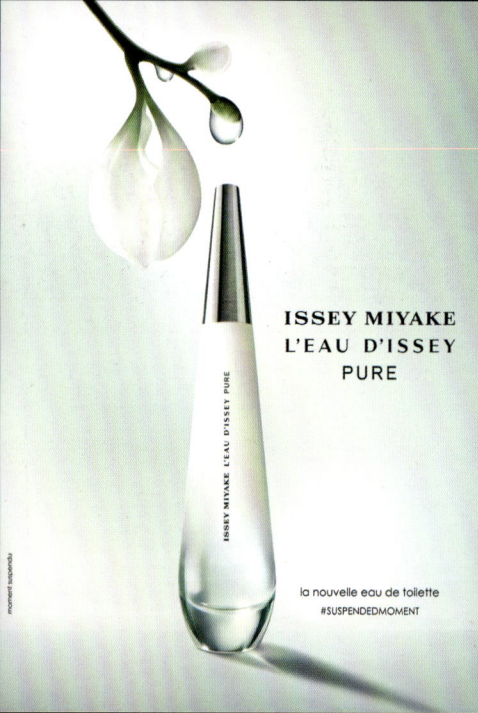

L'EAU D'ISSEY, ISSEY MIYAKE (1992)

Created in 1992 by Jacques Cavallier for the fashion designer Issey Miyake, L'Eau d'Issey is indicative of the aquatic trend, inspired by Japan and its mystical tradition, and has a high calone content. From rippling mountain streams to the ocean surrounding the archipelago, water is a vital element of Japanese life and a symbol of purity, because it reflects the soul of the Buddha. In the words of Issey Miyake, 'Nature is the greatest perfumer,' so he did not like manufactured scents. His inspiration was a childhood memory which he recounted to the perfumer: 'In Japan, the fifth of May is a festival for boys when people put iris leaves into the bath, giving the hot water a beautiful plant aroma. On other days, we added thick orange peel to the bathwater and the smell fused with that of the wooden bathtub.' Issey Miyake wanted a fragrance that smelled like water. So, Jacques Cavallier was given the not-inconsiderable task of recreating its scent, the smell of dew or falling rain on plants or of water caressing a woman.

ANGEL, THIERRY MUGLER (1992)

Thierry Mugler had been dressing women since 1978. As a trained dancer, he had a specific style which emphasized the shape of the body, working the Mugler magic to combine the formal and the sensual. In 1992, when the trend was for fresh and clean American-style fragrances and clear, transparent perfumes such as Bulgari's Eau Parfumée au Thé Vert and L'Eau d'Issey by Issey Miyake, Mugler created Angel, which defied cultural barriers to give women a modern fragrance with a touch of the ethereal. His inspiration was Guerlain's Shalimar, which his mother wore, and his vision was to make a perfume that a little boy would dream of giving to his own mother. Angel was a new take on the oriental accord with a hint of indulgent sweetness. It took Olivier Cresp 18 months to create the perfume, in which he sought voluptuous contrasts, fresh notes and sexy, gourmand aromas. But what really made Angel different was the combination of these with patchouli.

Angel was the brainchild of Thierry Mugler's imagination, conjuring up mythical characters, celestial symbols and infinite spaces. For him, the blue of the sky represented freedom. The star, his favourite symbol, was timeless and universal, and also the starting point of the Angel story.

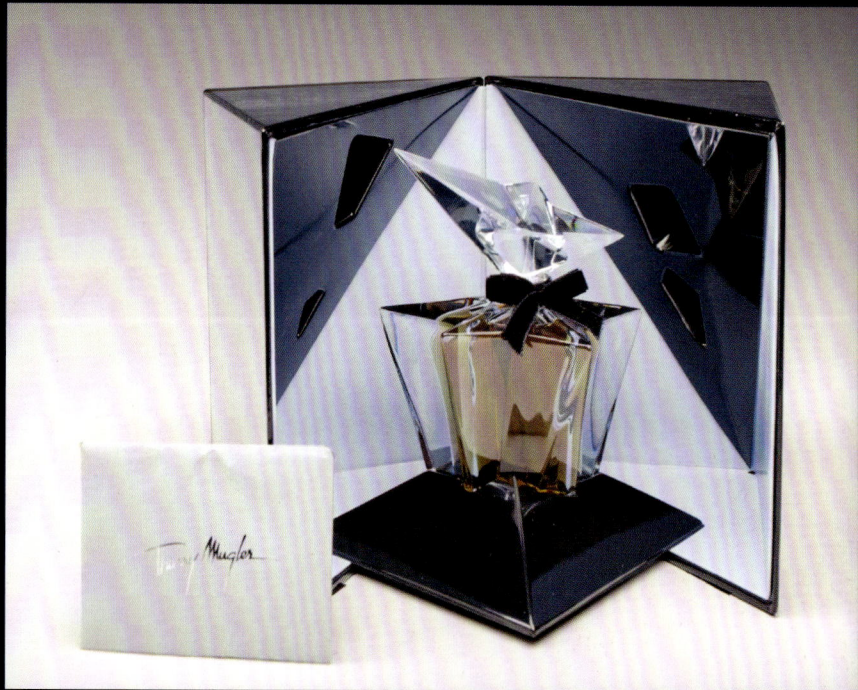

The perfume was innocent yet sensual, a warm fragrance in a glacial blue bottle, reflecting two sides of the female personality. The Angel woman was somewhere between a goddess and a girl, striving to balance glamour and charm in her multifaceted life. Mugler described Angel as a perfume so sensual that the person wearing it was almost good enough to eat but, here, to 'gourmandize' is not so much a guilty pleasure as the gift of a modern fairy.

CK ONE, CALVIN KLEIN (1994)

Calvin Klein's CK One, by Alberto Morillas, started the trend for unisex perfumes. Admittedly, two years earlier, Bulgari's Eau Parfumée au Thé Vert had taken us back to a time of non-gender-specific perfume inspired by Eau de Cologne, which was universal by nature, but it had been launched on the 1980s market, known for its excessive, highly individual fragrances. The breakthrough had to come from an affordable perfume that inspired confidence and was shared by all. So the first advertising campaign was all about friendship and synergy, embracing all genders, origins and sexual orientations in a concept that was revolutionary for its time and a rallying call for a generation that was hungry for connection and universality. The perfume itself fell into the American fresh and clean category and was aimed equally at men and women. It was simple and relaxed, with its signature green tea combining with bergamot, cardamom, pineapple and papaya on a heart of jasmine, violet and rose and a musk and amber base. What was surprising about this scent, however, was its truly natural feel, persistent freshness and sensual yet classic *sillage*. The frosted glass bottle had a simple aluminium cap and its eco-friendly, glue-free, recycled cardboard box was also ahead of its time. CK One was more than a fragrance; it was a brand with an identity that perfectly encapsulated the mood of a generation. It gave the icons of the time a run for their money and established itself as a long-standing leader.

LE MÂLE, JEAN PAUL GAULTIER (1995)

Right from his first collection of fragrances for men in 1983, Jean Paul Gaultier made it clear that the male perfume market should be on an equal footing with the female one, and men should have as much freedom and choice as women. In 1993, he released Classique in a bottle shaped like a corseted woman's bust – subversive for some, an expression of feminine strength for others – presented in a tin can. Male fragrance was becoming commonplace in the 1990s but, in 1995, Jean Paul Gaultier took it one step further with Le Mâle. Like its female counterparts Youth Dew and Opium, his composition was bursting with sensuality. Gaultier wanted it to embody the male personality, to be a bold, tongue-in-cheek, rebellious call to break with convention. Chantal Ross, the brand director, asked perfumer Christopher Sheldrake to help the young nose Francis Kurkdjian create the formula. Fougère reminded Jean Paul Gaultier of traditional shaving soap and the whole shaving ritual, but in Le Mâle it took on amber and oriental hues from the soft vanilla base notes. The bottle was modelled on the toned body of a tattooed sailor wearing a tight-fitting striped cotton top. It was presented in a simple tin can. The whole Le Mâle package had to be fun to tone down the male sensuality and sensitivity of the perfume itself. This male heartthrob was the alter ego of its female equivalent. Le Mâle was a light-hearted departure from social and perfume conventions. It became a form of manifesto, breaking new ground in the world of male fragrance.

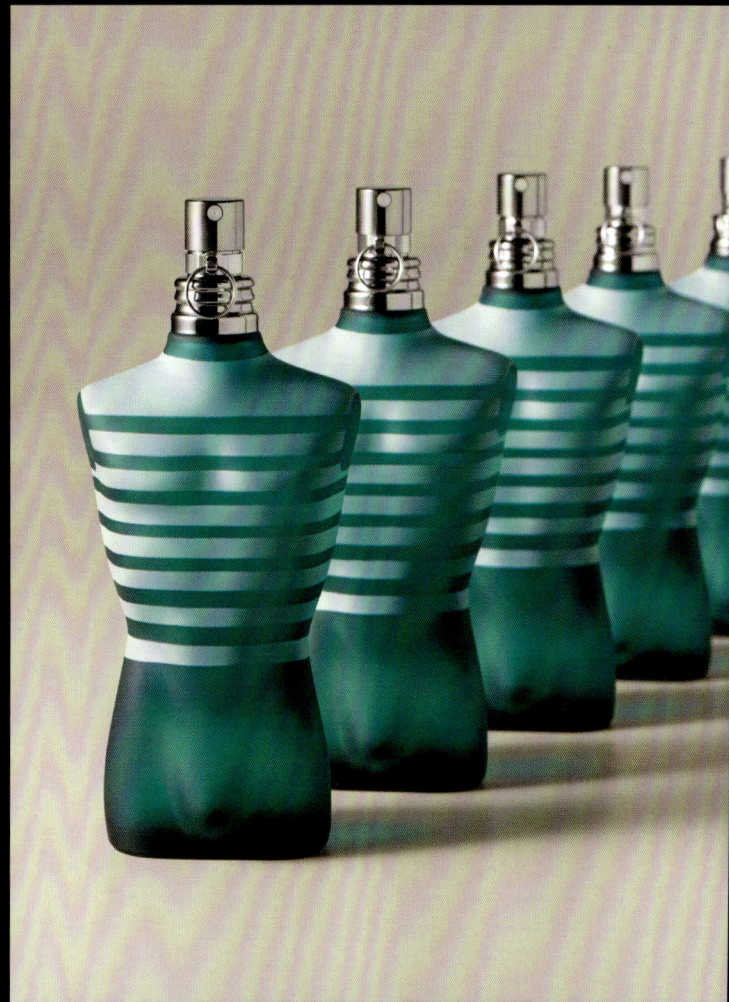

THE BOTTLES: COVETED BY COLLECTORS

LANCÔME'S ARTISTIC DIRECTOR GEORGES DELHOMME SAID IN 1935 THAT THE BOTTLE SHOULD 'BE A PORTRAIT' OF WHAT IT HOLDS. THE PROFESSION WORKS RELENTLESSLY ON THE PRESENTATION OF ITS PERFUMES IN A QUEST TO ACHIEVE ARTISTIC PERFECTION, AND THIS CAN ONLY BENEFIT THE COLLECTORS WHO PAY TRIBUTE TO THE KNOW-HOW AND EXPERTISE REQUIRED NOT ONLY OF PERFUMERS BUT ALSO ARTISTS, GLASSMAKERS AND BOX MANUFACTURERS.

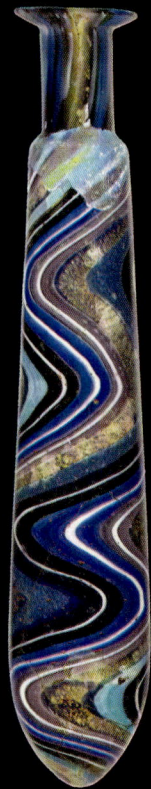

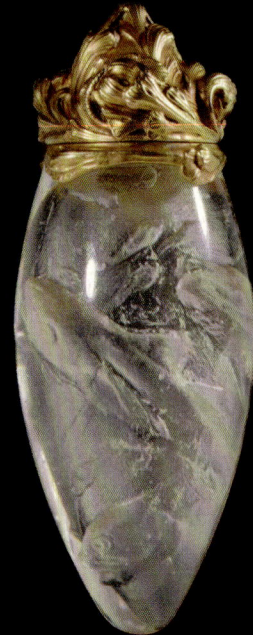

TREASURES OF ANCIENT TIMES

The Greeks, Romans and Egyptians preserved their fragrances in pots made of earthenware, terracotta and sometimes metal. Between the third and first centuries BCE, the Phoenicians and Babylonians invented blown glass, which would be adopted as the perfect material for perfume bottles. The Murano and Bohemian glassworks turned their hand to this new art, which fascinated the great Catherine de' Medici. She began to collect small bottles made from gold and precious stones. After her death, interest in these perfume bottles endured until the eighteenth century, when porcelain was introduced.

Above: Roman gilt and coloured glass perfume phial.

Top right: Scent bottle by Jules-René Lalique, 1902–05.

A VERY FRENCH FLAIR

Crystal was invented by chance in England in the seventeenth century, around 1627, and the result was a glass with exceptional light-reflecting and acoustic properties. In the eighteenth century, Bohemian crystal came into its own as a sturdy material with a beautiful sparkle, and replaced Venetian glass on royal tables. Crystal became hugely popular, especially in France, when the Baccarat factory opened in 1765 and the Saint-Louis factory began to specialize in the manufacture of perfume bottles. Gold- and silversmiths made chased gold and silver bottles combined with jasper and rock crystal. The once-popular Baroque lines were replaced by themes that were fashionable at the time: Rousseau's beloved return to nature, for instance, or chinoiserie. Chantilly porcelain was decorated with chinoiserie, while the Saint-Cloud factory was known for its gilt work and the Sèvres pottery produced pear-shaped bottles.

Porcelain Bottles Outside France

The Germans, Austrians and English had the monopoly on porcelain. Chelsea porcelain specialized in figurines with stopper heads. In Germany, Meissen was the first European manufacturer to make hard-paste porcelain and favoured rococo scenes, flowers, fruit and oriental motifs and battle scenes. The eighteenth century was the period of the vinaigrette, little cases containing bottles filled with fragrant essences.

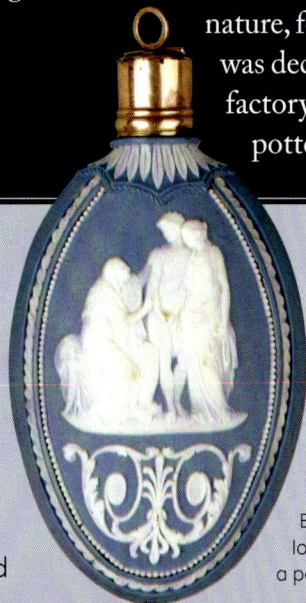

Earthenware bottle by Josiah Wedgwood, with a small loop attached to the metal stopper so it could be worn as a pendant, late eighteenth century.

THE NINETEENTH CENTURY: CHANGED PERCEPTIONS

In the nineteenth century, the bottle became a tangible way to attract customers and sell more perfume. As the houses grew, they put more and more products on the market and competition between the brands was fierce. They had to find new ways to make sure their products stood out, and branded bottles helped them make their mark. Bottle manufacturing was also caught up in the trend towards industrialization, but the change was gradual and quality was not compromised. Crystal was still very popular with Bohemia, France and Great Britain leading the way.

However, the most revolutionary invention was the spray bottle in 1870. By the late nineteenth century, perceptions of perfume had changed and, increasingly, bottle, packaging and advertising choices became as important as the fragrance itself. This led to perfumers joining forces with the biggest names in glass manufacture, Lalique, Baccarat and Saint-Louis to name but a few, and also graphic artists and advertisers. From 150 a day in 1897, bottle orders had reached 4,000 a day by 1907.

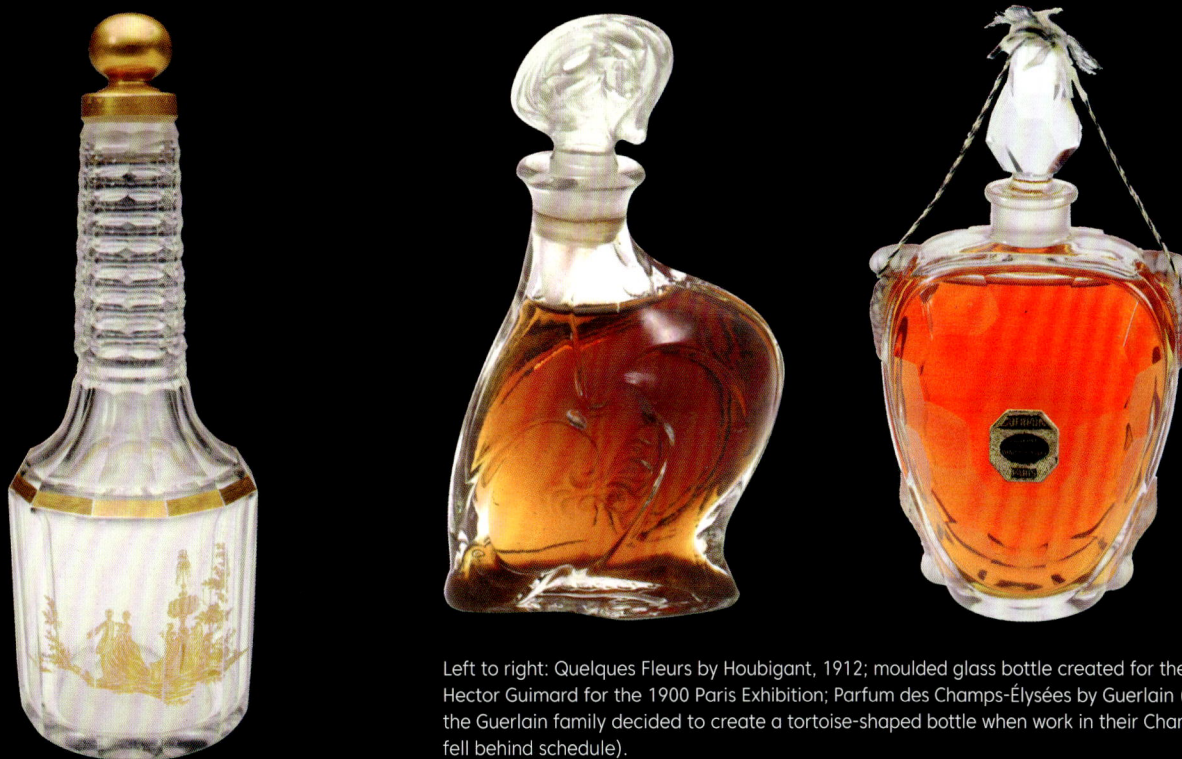

Left to right: Quelques Fleurs by Houbigant, 1912; moulded glass bottle created for the perfumer Millot by Hector Guimard for the 1900 Paris Exhibition; Parfum des Champs-Élysées by Guerlain (the story goes that the Guerlain family decided to create a tortoise-shaped bottle when work in their Champs-Élysées boutique fell behind schedule).

FROM ART NOUVEAU SCROLLS TO ART DECO GEOMETRICS

In the same way as Art Nouveau was intended to be a more democratic and mainstream art movement, perfume was set to become more accessible. For the 1900 Paris Exhibition, the great Art Nouveau designer and architect Hector Guimard created a moulded glass bottle with the archetypal sinuous lines of the movement for the perfumer Félix Millot (above, middle). In 1914, Guerlain launched its Parfum des Champs-Élysées perfume in a tortoise-shaped bottle (above, right). A masterpiece of Art Nouveau design, the flat facets of this animal-themed bottle did, however, herald the advent of the Art Deco movement. Most of

Guerlain's bottles were made by Baccarat, where the Art Deco maestro Georges Chevalier worked. His Djedi bottle (1926) in a poplar-wood box covered in green and gold leather was pure Art Deco. Liu (1927) was a black crystal version of the Chinese snuff box or tea caddy and bore the name (meaning 'secret') of the heroine of Puccini's grand opera *Turandot*. And so, from 1919 onwards, Art Deco took over from Art Nouveau. Bottles were increasingly geometric with straight and spherical forms and ornamental stoppers. Many beautiful art-inspired bottles were produced in the 1920s and 1930s.

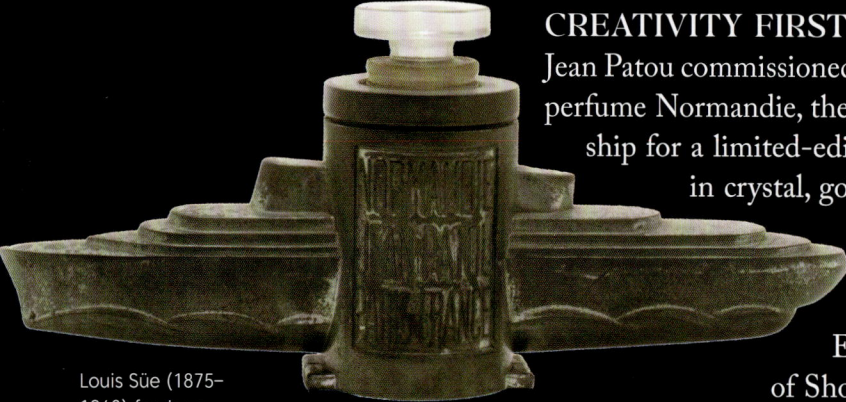

Louis Süe (1875–1968) for Jean Patou, Normandie, 1935. International Perfume Museum, Grasse, France.

CREATIVITY FIRST!

Jean Patou commissioned his bottles from Louis Süe and André Mare. For his perfume Normandie, they inserted a bottle inside a metal replica of a sailing ship for a limited-edition run of only 500. Caron perfumes were dressed in crystal, gold and silk by the self-taught Félicie Bergaud, who used the trimmings, lace and ribbons that reminded her of her former profession as a milliner. Crystal bottles were often covered in gold. The exuberant Elsa Schiaparelli used bright colours (the fuchsia pink of Shocking, for example; see page 126) and glass flowers, ribbons and Bohemian crystal. Her elegant, highly unusual creations included the tailor's dummy with its bouquet of blown-glass flowers for Shocking and the pipe-shaped bottle for Snuff.

see page 126

The Importance of the 1925 Paris Exhibition

This international exhibition, postponed due to World War I, finally took place from 28 April to 15 October 1925 in an area that stretched from the Esplanade des Invalides to the Grand Palais and Petit Palais. It was the birthplace of Art Deco, which broke away from the precepts of the nineteenth century. The perfume pavilion attracted the largest number of visitors. Art Deco style made an appearance here too, in many shapes and forms, from the most pared-back to the highly ornate, decorated with vibrant colours or black lacquer, in a similar way to the furniture of the period. In 1919, Henri Clouzot had commented that the artistic qualities of a perfume bottle enhanced the value of what was inside, calling upon glassmakers to seek out and create new models.

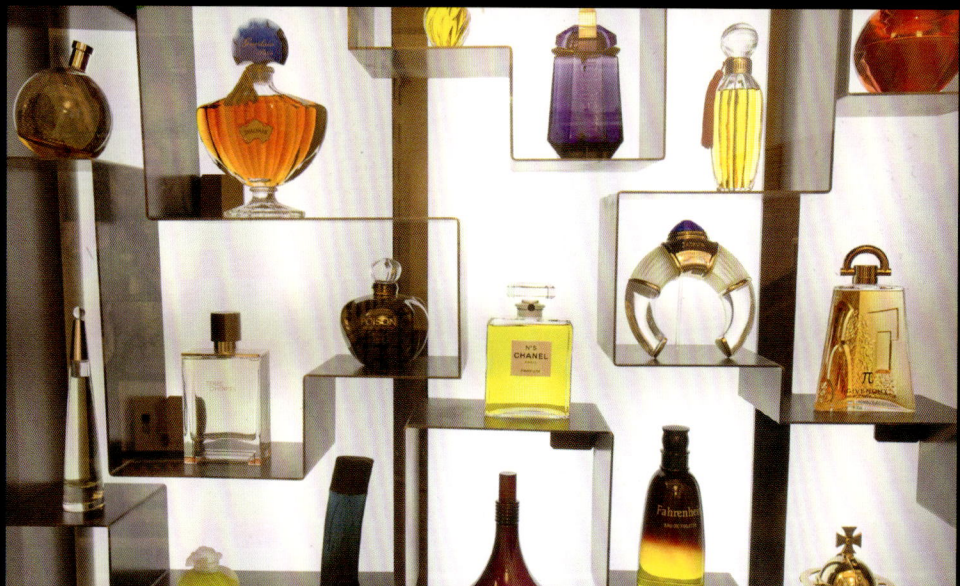

Perfume bottles on display at the International Perfume Museum in Grasse. The museum celebrates the global technical, aesthetic, social and cultural history of perfume use. It takes an anthropological approach, examining every aspect of the history of perfume, from raw materials to manufacture, industry, innovation, trade, design and customs, through objets d'art, decorative arts, textiles, archaeological evidence, unique creations and industrial shapes.

PERFUME HUNTERS

Until very recently, collecting perfume bottles was the preserve of those in the know. Today, these precious containers come up as auction lots at Drouot in Paris or at its American counterpart, Sotheby's. They can fetch astronomical prices so are within the grasp only of the privileged few or the big houses who, aware of the value of brand heritage, are increasingly keen to preserve pieces of their past. There are still some bottles hiding away in attics or waiting to be snapped up at car boot sales, and some experts and boutiques now specialize in sourcing perfume bottles and bottles of perfume. The difference between the two is that the perfume bottle is often unmarked and can date back to ancient times or the nineteenth century, sold empty to be filled with any fragrance. The bottle of perfume, on the other hand, generally carries the name of the perfumer and is filled with one of their compositions.

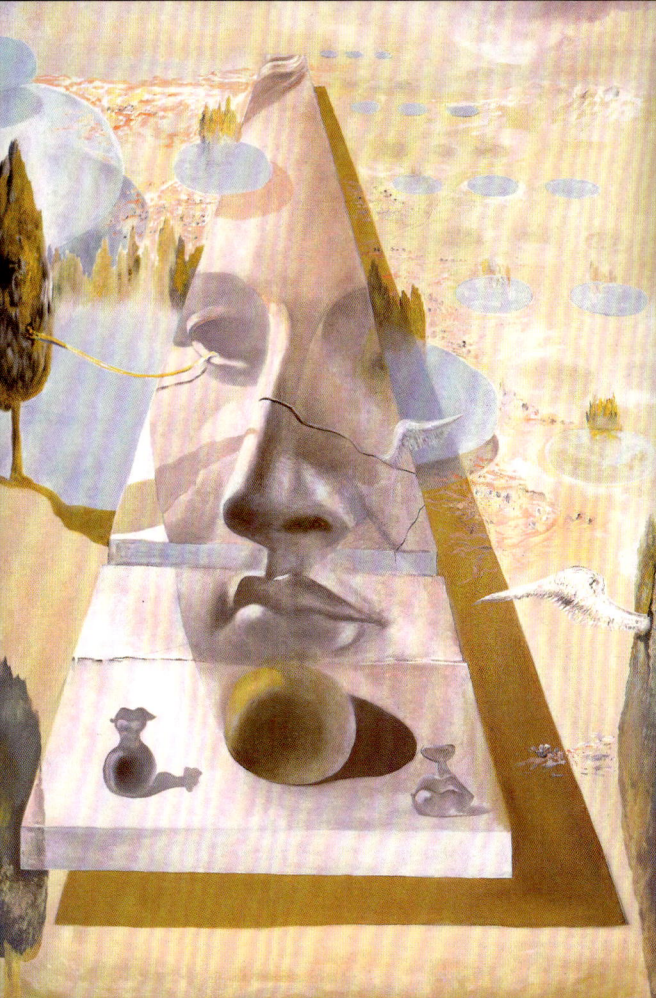

AN ARTIST'S CREATION

Salvador Dalí (1904–89) was an acclaimed and supremely versatile artist and iconic figure of the Surrealist movement, so it was only natural he should embrace perfume as another form of artistic expression. He once said that, 'Of the five senses, the sense of smell is incontestably the one that best conveys a sense of immortality.' In 1983, he created his first perfume as a tribute to his wife and muse, Gala, with whom he was madly in love. Dalí believed that perfume was the best 'messenger' of memories and moments of happiness. On completion of his painting *Apparition of the Face of Aphrodite of Knidos in a Landscape* in 1981, he sketched a bottle inspired by the sensual mouth and nose of the goddess of beauty and love. The limited-edition numbered crystal bottle for Dalí by Parfums Salvador Dalí, launched in 1983 at the Jacquemart-André Museum in Paris, was inspired by this sketch.

Left: *Apparition of the Face of Aphrodite of Knidos in a Landscape* by Salvador Dalí, 1981.

Right: Salvador Dalí's first perfume, launched as a limited, numbered edition in crystal bottles in 1983.

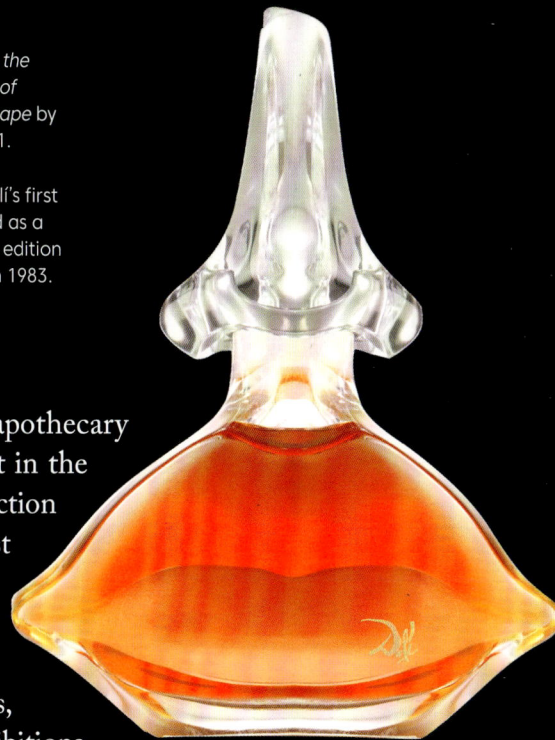

EXQUISITE COLLECTIONS

The private collection of the perfume company Drom began with apothecary bottles in 1911 and the founders, Bruno and Dora Storp, added to it in the 1920s. In 1967, Ursula Storp took over and completed the rare collection with bottles dating from antiquity to the present day. Numbering almost 3,000 items, it is now housed in a museum in Germany.

Léon Givaudan, co-founder with his brother Xavier of the company Givaudan, has a collection of over 100 extraordinary bottles, most of which date from the eighteenth century. Like all true aficionados, he was instinctively drawn to quality pieces, visiting museums and exhibitions and seeking out the best experts. The collection is still owned by Givaudan and is itself a work of art.

Jean-François Costa's bottle collection is also very famous. He was born into a family of Grasse perfumers and inherited the Fragonard perfume company, which was founded in 1926. He took over the helm in 1965 and, inspired by his uncle, the great collector Georges Fuchs, added a cultural dimension to the company when he opened his first perfume museum in Grasse and then a second near the Paris Opera. Jean-François Costa began acquiring perfume-related objets d'art in the 1950s and went on to make his name as one of the leading collectors with a collection that is remarkable in both diversity and quality. Epitomizing over 80 years of passion and retracing more than 3,000 years of the history of perfume, through objects such as medieval pomanders and Egyptian cosmetic spoons, it is on display in the company's museums. More than the perfume, it represents a whole way of life.

A WEAPON OF SEDUCTION

THROUGHOUT THE AGES, PERFUME HAS HAD A CLOSE
ASSOCIATION WITH SEDUCTION AND IT IS WITHOUT A
DOUBT THE OLDEST ALLY OF AMOROUS INFATUATION.
IT CAPTIVATES, SENDS A MESSAGE OF LOVE, LAUNCHES
AN ARMED OFFENSIVE ON POTENTIAL PARTNERS,
TACTICS THAT ARE ALL THE MORE SOPHISTICATED WHEN
APPLIED STRATEGICALLY TO SPECIFIC AREAS …

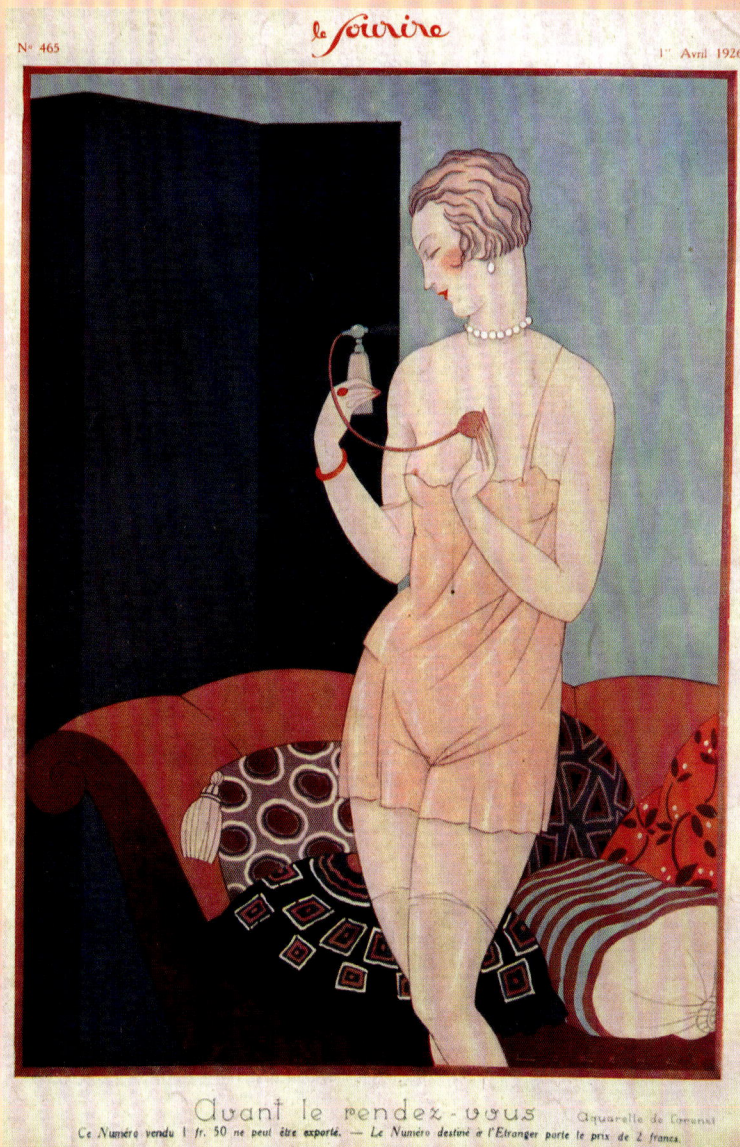

Avant le rendez-vous (Before the Meeting).
A woman in a slip applying perfume,
Lorenzi illustration from the April edition of
Le Sourire magazine, 1926.

IT'S ALL ABOUT THE RITUAL …

Perfume has always been a formidable weapon of seduction, signalling poise and self-control. It is applied precisely with a certain demeanour and an intimate gesture. A caress of oil over the skin, a spray onto fragrant flowing locks, a little dab in just the right spot behind the ear, on the pulse points of the wrist and behind the knees … it's all part of a serious game plan. The ritual is still sacrosanct and, it seems, capable of sending men and women into seventh heaven. Gabrielle Chanel summed it up nicely by telling women to apply perfume everywhere they wanted to be kissed.

… AND THE WEARER

Femininity possesses a power that lies not in brash self-assurance but in a furtive, inoffensive gesture when, believing herself to be alone, a woman reveals her natural grace with a slight tilt of her head or flick of her wrist. In the late nineteenth century, adverts depicted women sitting at their dressing table, applying perfume in the intimacy of their boudoir. Eveningwear became associated with this act and perfume was the finishing touch. The joy and pleasure of putting on perfume was palpable in these real-life scenarios – or phases of womanhood – which show well-dressed women of the time with a maid by their side, revealing their upper-class status. Even Eau de Cologne was no longer simply for personal care but used for beautification. The adverts were extremely sensual, offering a taste of the exquisite voluptuousness of a delicate scent that suffuses the whole body.

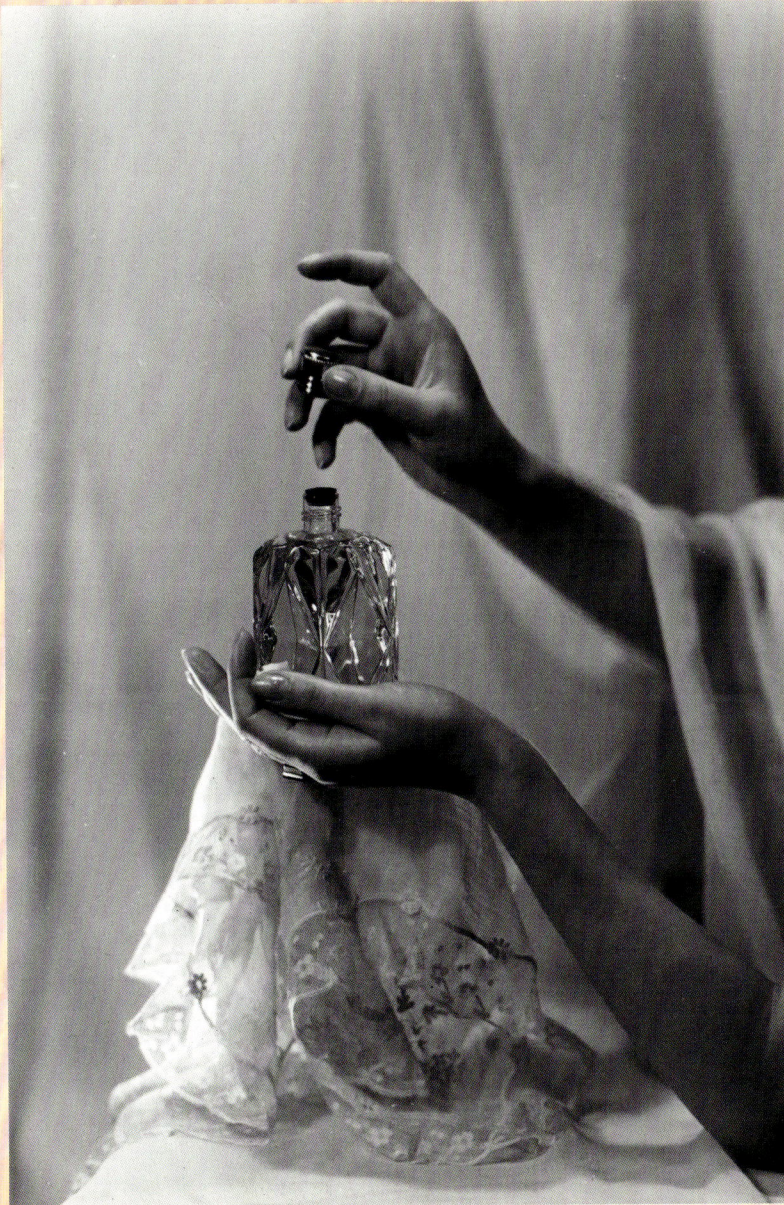

The act of applying perfume, photograph by Laure Albin Guillot, 1943.

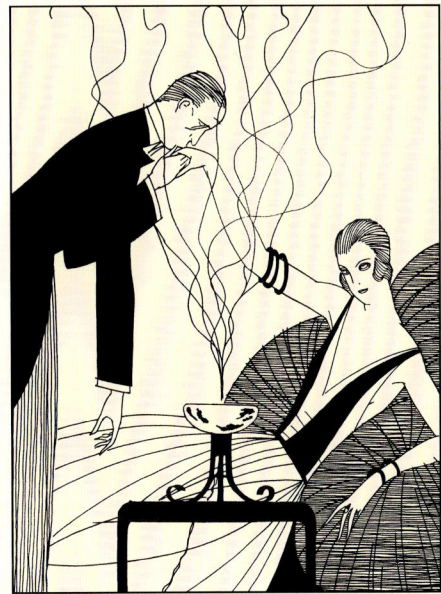

The right perfume in the right concentration

From the 1920s, alcohol-based perfumes were available in different concentrations. An elegant woman was still expected to change her outfit three times a day, in the morning, afternoon and evening. Daytime outfits were more subdued, and seductive attire was kept for eveningwear, so it was only natural that her perfume should reflect this. Extrait de Parfum, or pure perfume, which has a higher concentration of fragrance than eau de parfum, was reserved for special occasions.

Robj perfume burner, press advert by Hemjic, 1921.

SMELLING NICE FOR ONESELF AND OTHERS

The greatest seducers have never concealed the fact they used scent (and some even poison, the antithesis of perfume) to achieve their goal. Perfume is more than a simple pleasure. It is a love letter in a bottle, which legendary figures, from ancient times to the early twentieth century, have adapted to their own eras and shrouded in an aura of seduction. Since the time of the ancient Egyptians, perfume has played a very important role in sexual attraction. As the wise Ptahhotep wrote, 'Perfumes are the best way to care for the body.' Way back in time, the sense of smell – love incarnate – and perfumes were deemed animalistic, and decried because of their ability to ignite passion and lead to impulsive behaviour. Fuelled by fragrance, love could be fatal. Diametrically opposed to the Greek god Eros, Thanatos declared that perfume could also become demonic, intoxicating and narcotic, a 'poison of the heart'. The love potion thus took on connotations of witchcraft and evil. Perfumes have long been used to conceal poison, for instance during the Renaissance when perfume rings, as worn by the Medici family, and scented gloves were used to mask toxic odours. The Marquise of Montespan, one of the favourites of Louis XIV, was adept at using perfume, particularly tuberose, and poisons to thwart her rivals.

KING SOLOMON AND THE QUEEN OF SHEBA, AN EASTERN LOVE SONG, TENTH CENTURY BCE

'Pleasing is the fragrance of your perfumes; your name is like perfume poured out,' goes the erotic poem the Song of Songs (1:3), also known as the Song of Solomon. In it, in the Jewish tradition, the King of Israel, sage and poet, extols his burgeoning love for the Queen of Sheba, the 'dark-skinned beauty' whose kingdom extended from Eritrea to Yemen. The Horn of Africa was home to the most precious ingredients in perfumery – myrrh, frankincense, civet and ambergris – raw materials that were fragrant gifts exchanged between lovers and, when applied to their bodies, aroused intense passion. Solomon's love of beautiful smells is evident from his temple, built from fragrant juniper and Lebanese cedar wood, which serves as a magnificent backdrop to the Ark of the Covenant. A fourteenth-century Ethiopian tale, the Kebra Nagast (Glory of the Kings), tells the story of how Solomon and the Queen of Sheba got together. The queen refused his advances at first and the king accepted her rejection on the condition that she would covet nothing from his palace. Then, having been served a spicy meal, her mouth was burning, so she naively asked for water to cool it down. To satisfy her request, the course of a river was diverted. She was gently won over and lay down with the king. Their union resulted in a son named Menelik.

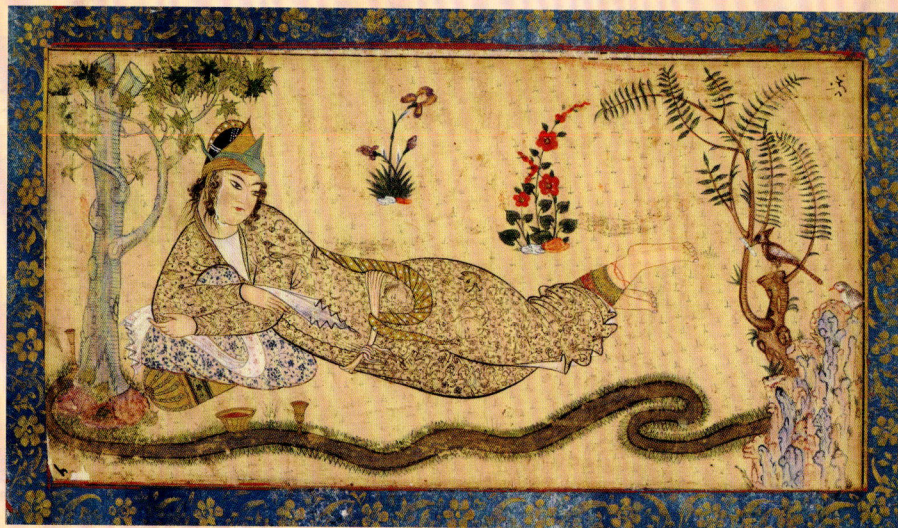

A recumbent Balqis, Queen of Sheba, holding a love letter intended for King Solomon, watercolour, circa 1590–1600.

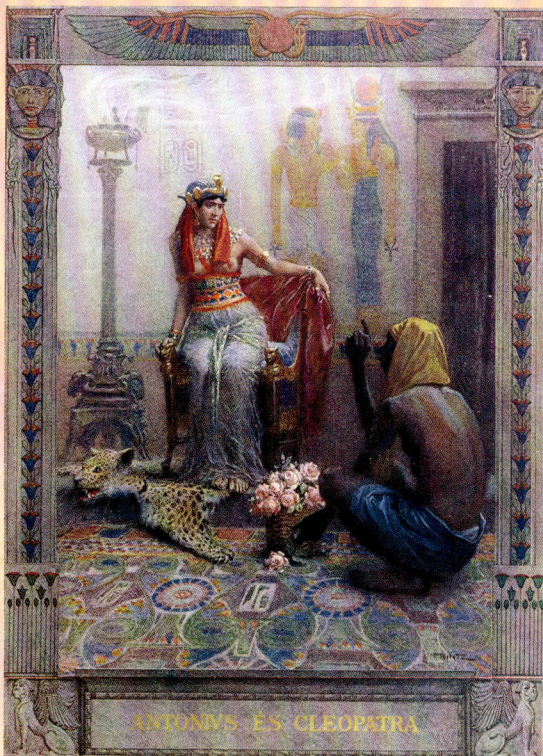

Above: Cleopatra in a scene from William Shakespeare's play *Antony and Cleopatra*, lithograph by Christian August Printz, nineteenth century.

Opposite: Mythological portrait of the members of Louis XIV's family in 1670, detail, by Jean Nocret, seventeenth century.

MARK ANTONY AND CLEOPATRA: FRAGRANCE UNITES ROME AND EGYPT, FIRST CENTURY BCE

Cleopatra was famous for her seductive long nose. French mathematician and philosopher Blaise Pascal said that if it had been shorter, 'the whole face of the earth would have changed'. However, her lovers' noses also played their part, because they were guided and drawn in by her intoxicating scents. The ambitious sovereign, devoted to restoring the grandeur of Egypt, did not think twice about using her charm to win over Julius Caesar and then Mark Antony. Dressed as Venus, she burned perfumes on the boat she used to go and meet the latter. Shakespeare's tragedy reads, 'Purple the sails, and so perfumed that / The winds were love-sick with them.' In keeping with Egyptian tradition, her body was oiled with a delicious fragrance, a sacred composition of myrrh, aromatics, citrus and flowers usually reserved for the gods and pharaohs. Mark Antony also underwent a beauty and fragrance ritual. Baths and fragrant preparations for the body were very important in Roman culture and the well-maintained bodies of the Empire's greatest dignitaries were embalmed with benzoin, aloe, saffron, musk and ambergris, each a scent associated with the gods of the Pantheon of Rome. The two lovers were united by a passion for fragrance even in death.

CATHERINE DE' MEDICI AND RENATO BIANCO BRING ITALIAN PERFUME TO FRANCE, SIXTEENTH CENTURY

When Catherine de' Medici arrived at the French court in 1533 to marry the future Henry II, she was accompanied by her favourite perfumer Renato Bianco, known in France as René le Florentin (René the Florentine). At the time, Florence was one of the capitals of perfume and its dispensary, Santa Maria Novella, was run by monks who supplied fragrant waters to major figures of the Italian elite. When she became Queen of France, Catherine very quickly established the fashion for Italian fragrances, perfumed gloves and little scent bottles that were slipped into garment pockets, reviving perfumery, which had fallen out of favour when steamrooms closed and bathhouses were abandoned. Festivities were a pretext for a profusion of scents. Floral waters were poured into the fountains, and fans, jewellery, masks and rare bird feathers were scented. This craze concealed another, less savoury, purpose of perfume. Court intrigues and intrigues of the heart led to the use and abuse of poisons, which were masked behind fragrant concoctions. Renato Bianco, who knew more than anybody how to exploit the ambivalent power of perfumes, was accused of making poisoned potions, sachets and gloves.

LOUIS XIV AND THE MARQUISE OF MONTESPAN, SEVENTEENTH CENTURY

During the reign of Louis XIV, the Court of Versailles became a model of refinement in which perfume played a vital part. For the courtiers, it was their accessory of choice to amplify their presence but also conceal unwanted body odours, which were inevitable when hygiene was still rudimentary. Louis XIV, nicknamed the Sun King, was successful in politics and love, bolstered by his fragrant allies of musk, civet, castoreum and, later, orange blossom. His favourite mistress, the extraordinarily beautiful and formidable Marquise of Montespan, reigned supreme at Versailles. When she lost the affection of her king, she took refuge in perfumes and love potions in a bid to lure him back. These spellbinding fragrances with a persistent, almost disturbing *sillage*, comprised the heady, spicy scents of lily, datura and tuberose, which were also excellent at masking poisons. Wrongly accused of having disposed of one of her rivals, she was banished from Versailles by the king. The remainder of Louis XIV's reign was more subdued. Tired of the heavy scents he had used and abused in his youth, he showed no favour towards any lady of the court who reeked of perfume. Even in the midst of winter, he would demand that windows be opened to ventilate a room if the air was saturated with fragrance.

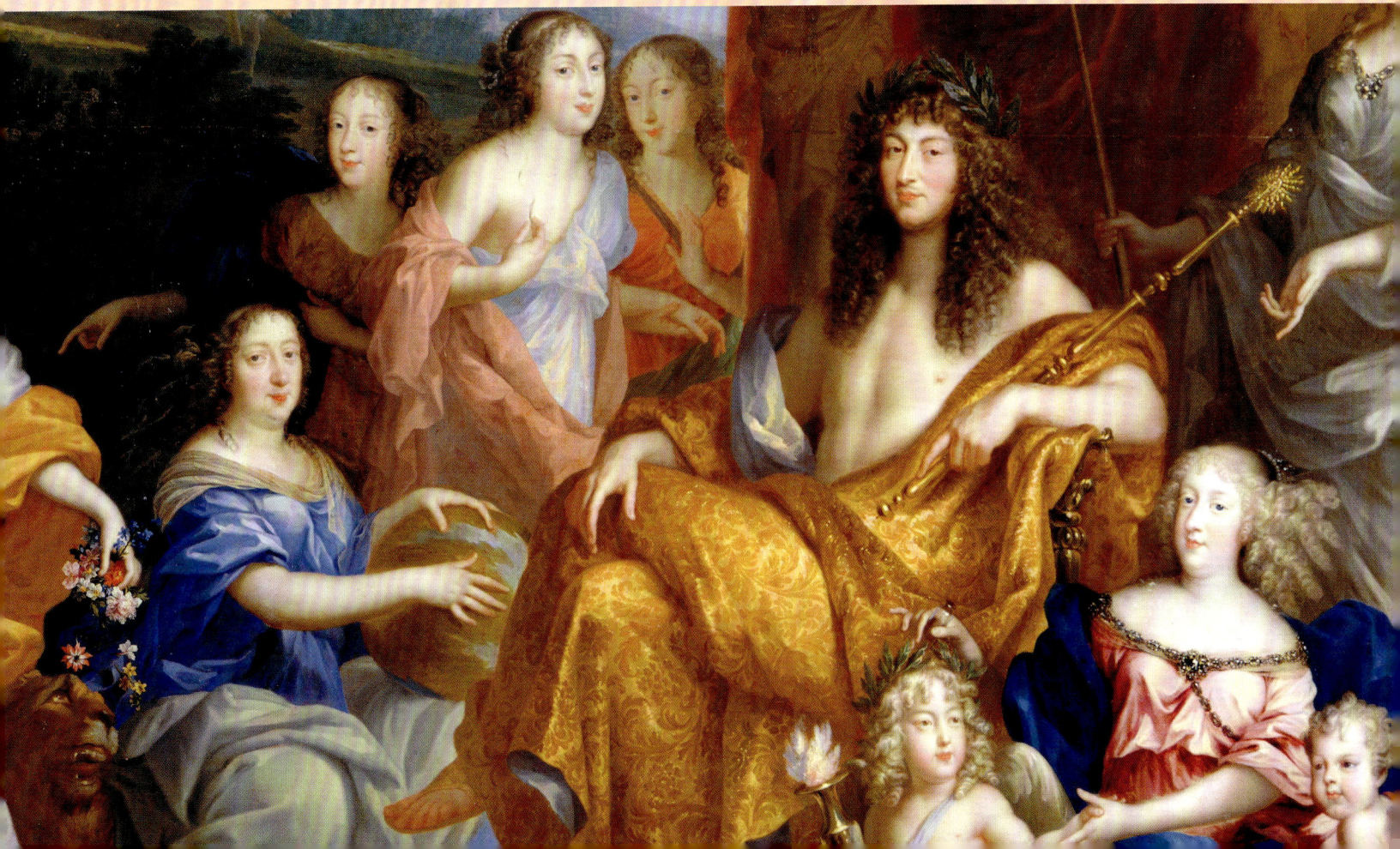

CASANOVA AND MARIE-ANTOINETTE: PERFUME IN THE ENLIGHTENMENT

Both Casanova and Queen Marie-Antoinette lived in the Age of Enlightenment, when life was good and perfume was more than ever a useful weapon in the arsenal of seduction. In his memoirs, the legendary libertine and inveterate womanizer Giacomo Casanova recounted 122 gallant adventures. He used perfume and its power of seduction to help him win over any woman he set his eyes on. A rosewater-scented handkerchief, iris or clove powder for his hair, sugared almonds flavoured with vanilla and amber ... his masterful use of scent conquered hearts. His name lives on as a character from history who left a lasting, fragrant impression as an elegant role model for all would-be Lotharios.

When Marie-Antoinette first arrived in France from Austria, she was warmly welcomed by the French people. She was famous for her youth, beauty, vivacity and trailblazing style. Her sumptuous gowns, light makeup and customized perfume compositions only served to widen her appeal. Royal perfumer Jean-Louis Fargeon took inspiration from the Trianon gardens at Versailles and their Viennese ambience for his personalized creations, aromatic bouquets of rose (Marie-Antoinette's flower), iris, musk, violet, tuberose and jasmine on a base of vanilla, wood and benzoin. A royal fragrance guaranteed to set heads spinning.

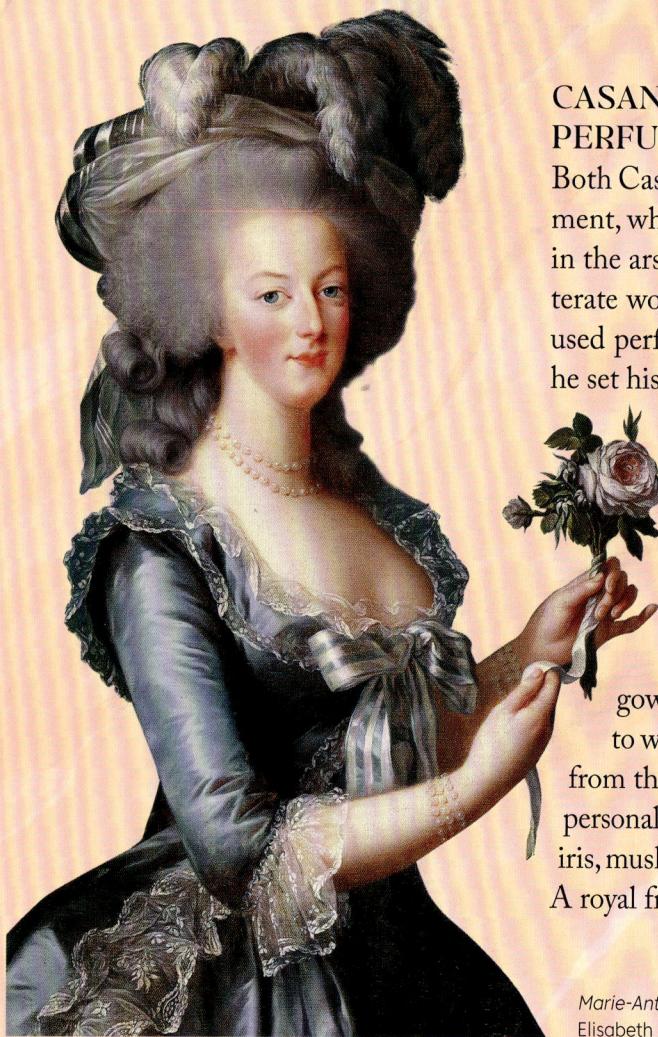

Marie-Antoinette, Queen of France, painting by Elisabeth Vigée-Lebrun, 1783.

THE HOUSE OF BONAPARTE, A FRAGRANT HISTORY

In the House of Bonaparte, the emperors and their wives all shared a love of fragrance. From Napoleon I to Empress Eugenie, the immoderate use of perfume was a mark of Imperial distinction. Napoleon I had his own signature Eau de Cologne, which he used each month. His appointed Parisian perfumers were Jean-Marie Farina, Gabriel-Gervais Chardin, Durochereau and J. Teissier. Napoleon had an acute sense of smell, so he was naturally drawn in by Josephine's heady, provocative aroma of musk and other scents. After he divorced her, and without waiting for the religious ceremony to celebrate his marriage to Marie-Louise of Austria in 1810, the emperor broke with royal protocol to join the future empress in her bedchamber,

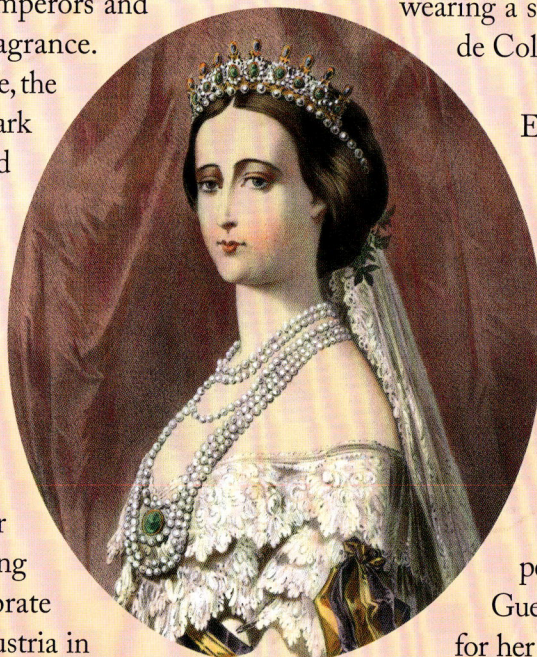

Engraving of Empress Eugenie.

wearing a simple nightgown – and also his Eau de Cologne.

The seductive, sophisticated Empress Eugenie made no secret of her love of luxury and encouraged her husband, Napoleon III, to take steps to stimulate the perfume industry. She loved scents, particularly patchouli, and used vast quantities of the cold cream that was all the rage in England at the time. Although sometimes considered frivolous, she was always admired for her elegance and exuded a fascinating, intoxicating aura. She became the perfumers' muse. Pierre François Pascal Guerlain created Eau de Cologne Impériale for her in 1853 and, in 1854, perfume house Creed opened a boutique in Paris and named its Jasmin Impératrice Eugénie in her honour.

LOUISE BROOKS AND THE FLAPPERS, THE SWEET SMELL OF FREEDOM

Mary Louise Brooks (1906–85) was the daughter of a staunch feminist who had passed on her independent spirit and need for freedom to her daughter. She made an impression at Paramount Pictures with her short hair and elfin face, and her flapper look and insouciance earned her roles as an independent woman, gangster's moll and dancer. Representing the entire, newly emancipated post-World War I generation, Louise Brooks became a fashion icon. She set the trend for shorter hemlines and haircuts. As always, perfume styles changed with the times and, in 1919, Caron launched Tabac Blond, a symbol of freedom and androgynous elegance, dedicated to the flappers and their beloved American cigarettes. In 1921, Gabrielle Chanel commissioned Ernest Beaux to create a 'perfume for women that smells like a woman' and not a bouquet of flowers. She wanted something abstract and that would be Chanel No. 5. Unfortunately, the Roaring Twenties suddenly gave way to the unprecedented Wall Street Crash and millions of Americans experienced financial ruin. Jean Patou's Joy, like a promise of reconstruction, offered up riches in a fragrance and Louise Brooks was its biggest fan.

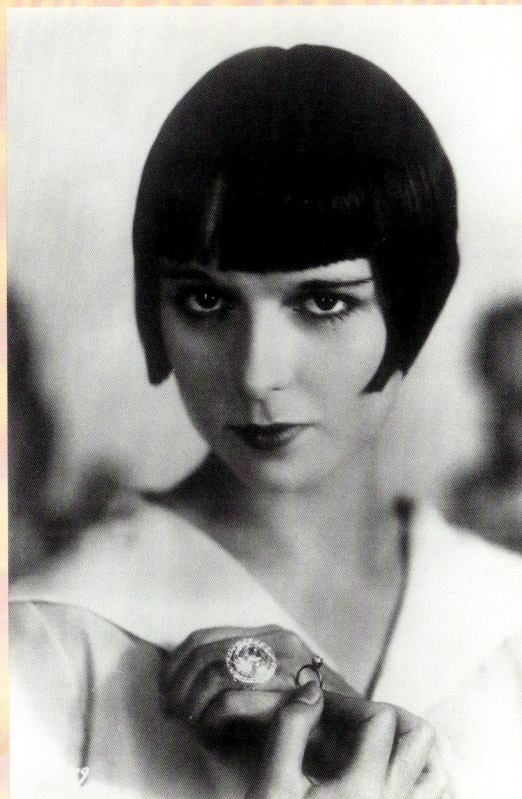

Right: American actress Louise Brooks in her role as Lucienne Garnier in Augusto Genina's movie *Beauty Prize*, 1930.

Below: Vaslav Nijinski and Ida Rubinstein in *Sheherazade*, by the illustrator George Barbier, 1913.

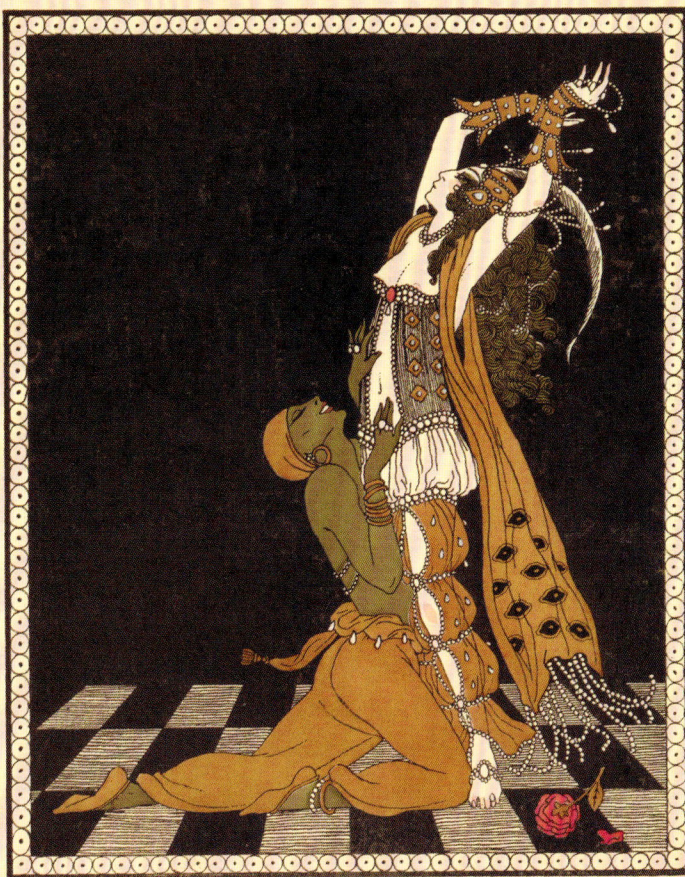

SERGEI DIAGHILEV AND THE BALLETS RUSSES: AN INFATUATION WITH THE EAST

Diaghilev was born into a noble family of musicians. He formed the Ballets Russes in 1907 and each of his shows was unique in its genre, involving dancers, poets, musicians and painters. They explored new themes, movements and sets and the Eastern-inspired productions by Léon Bakst were no exception. Male dancers came to the fore again and one of the most prominent performers, Vaslav Nijinsky, created a sensation with his interpretation of *Prelude to the Afternoon of a Fawn*, which was too erotic for some tastes. Before each performance, Diaghilev would spray the curtains of the Théâtre du Châtelet with Jacques Guerlain's 1919 Mitsouko, one of the first chypres, established as a perfume family in its own right in 1917 by Coty's Chypre.

Exoticism had taken on an oriental flavour with a general fascination with the fantasies of the Middle East, fuelled by legends of harems, or the sophisticated, mysterious Far East. Fashion designer Paul Poiret, who had established his own brand – Les Parfums de Rosine – in 1911, followed the trend with the launch of Aladin and Nuit de Chine. Perfume's infatuation with the Levant spearheaded what is known as the oriental family, characterized by soft, vanilla and amber notes.

THE PERFUME ROUTE IV

IN THE TWENTIETH CENTURY, SYNTHETIC MATERIALS BECAME AN INCREASINGLY IMPORTANT PART OF THE PERFUMER'S PALETTE, ACCOUNTING FOR AROUND 90%, BUT AFTER THE TURN OF THE CENTURY, NATURAL MATERIALS RETURNED TO FAVOUR. NEW ROUTES AND ENVIRONMENTALLY RESPONSIBLE, INTEGRATED SUPPLY CHAINS WERE CREATED ACROSS THE WORLD. AS THE THIRD MILLENNIUM DAWNED, NATURAL INGREDIENTS LOOKED LIKE THEY WERE HERE TO STAY, WITH RICH NEW SOURCES OF SUPPLY PROMISING A BRIGHT FUTURE.

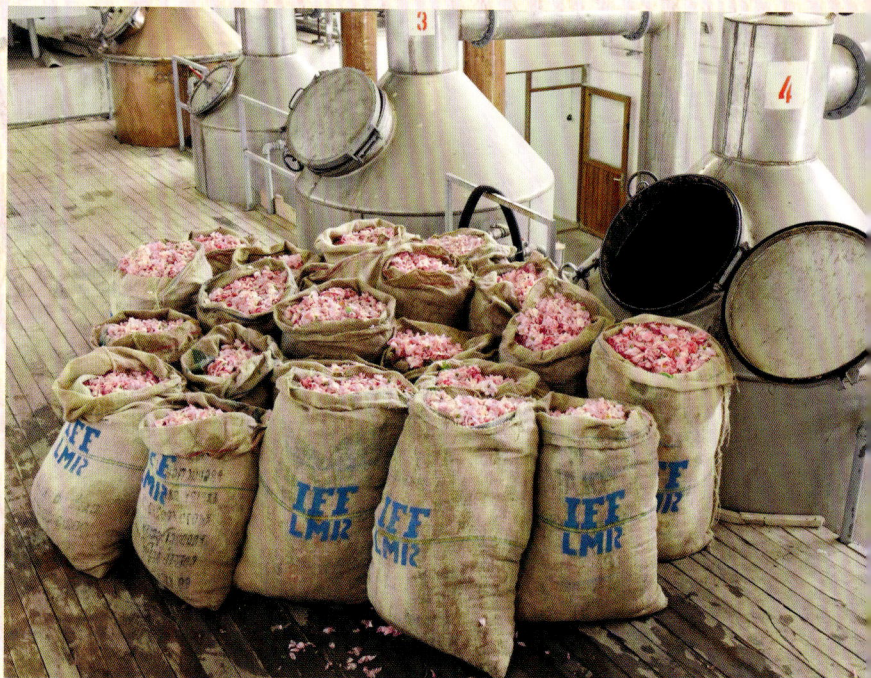

In a distillery, damask rose petals collected from a field owned by IFF-LMR in Turkey.

A CHANGE OF DIRECTION

When France went to war with Germany in 1939, the sources of raw materials declined. In August 1940, the Japanese occupied Indochina and, in late 1940, Thailand waged war on France to recover territories in Laos and Cambodia it had lost to the country in 1893, 1902 and 1907. France withdrew from Indochina in 1954, then Algeria became independent in the early 1960s. Many large-scale perfume manufacturers lost their factories. Between 1950 and 1970, the wars of independence disrupted perfume supply chains and many industrial sites, including the Domaine Sainte-Marguerite in Boufarik, Algeria, were nationalized. In the space of 10 years or so, many perfume manufacturers saw their factories in former colonies close.

DEFENDING A HERITAGE

Alongside this, industrialists in and around Grasse were facing stiff competition from large international groups. In the 1970s and 1980s, such groups bought a large share of the overall business in the perfume capital, which had been famous for supplying jasmine, rose, orange blossom, tuberose, violet and more to the world's greatest perfumers for 300 years. Cultivation of jasmine and Rose de Mai, also known as the Provence rose, in the Siagne valley, between the sea and the mountains, came under threat. Property speculation was rife, flower prices were volatile and labour costs high, which led to the slow and gradual disappearance of the land used to grow flowers for perfume, the closure of many production sites and fields being abandoned. From 5,000 in the 1930s, there remained a mere 20 sites covering some 50 hectares (124 acres). Jasmine growing moved to the Nile Delta in Egypt and later southern India. These two regions account for 90% of worldwide production today, split more or less 50:50 between them. Damask rose is increasingly grown in Turkey and Bulgaria. Orange blossom is in decline, but is gaining ground in Tunisia. Tuberose disappeared, only to reappear in India. Some violet production remains, but there is nascent competition from Egypt. It is the same story for mimosa, which gained momentum in Morocco and then India.

90,7%

D'INGRÉDIENTS D'ORIGINE NATURELLE

Pin essence

Citron essence

Mandarine essence

Orange essence

Géranium essence

Cardamone essence

Coriandre essence

Muscade essence

Palmarosa essence

Benjoin extrait

Sauge Sclarée extrait

Poivre rose Sfe

Thé noir Ceylan

Santal Australien essence

Vétiver essence

Cèdre essence

Copahu essence

Cypriol essence

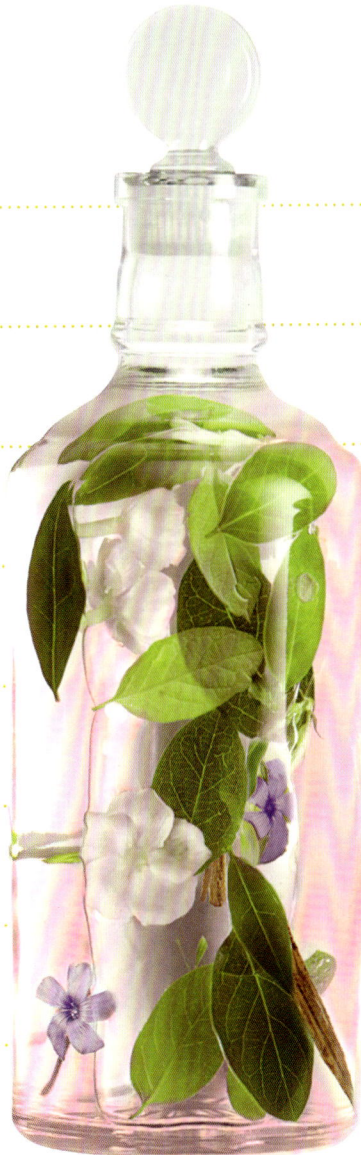

Ingredients in Extrait de Cologne Thé Fantaisie by Roger&Gallet, by the perfumer Alberto Morillas.

Map of the world showing the place of origin of the principal ingredients of perfume.
International Flavors & Fragrances, Inc. (IFF).

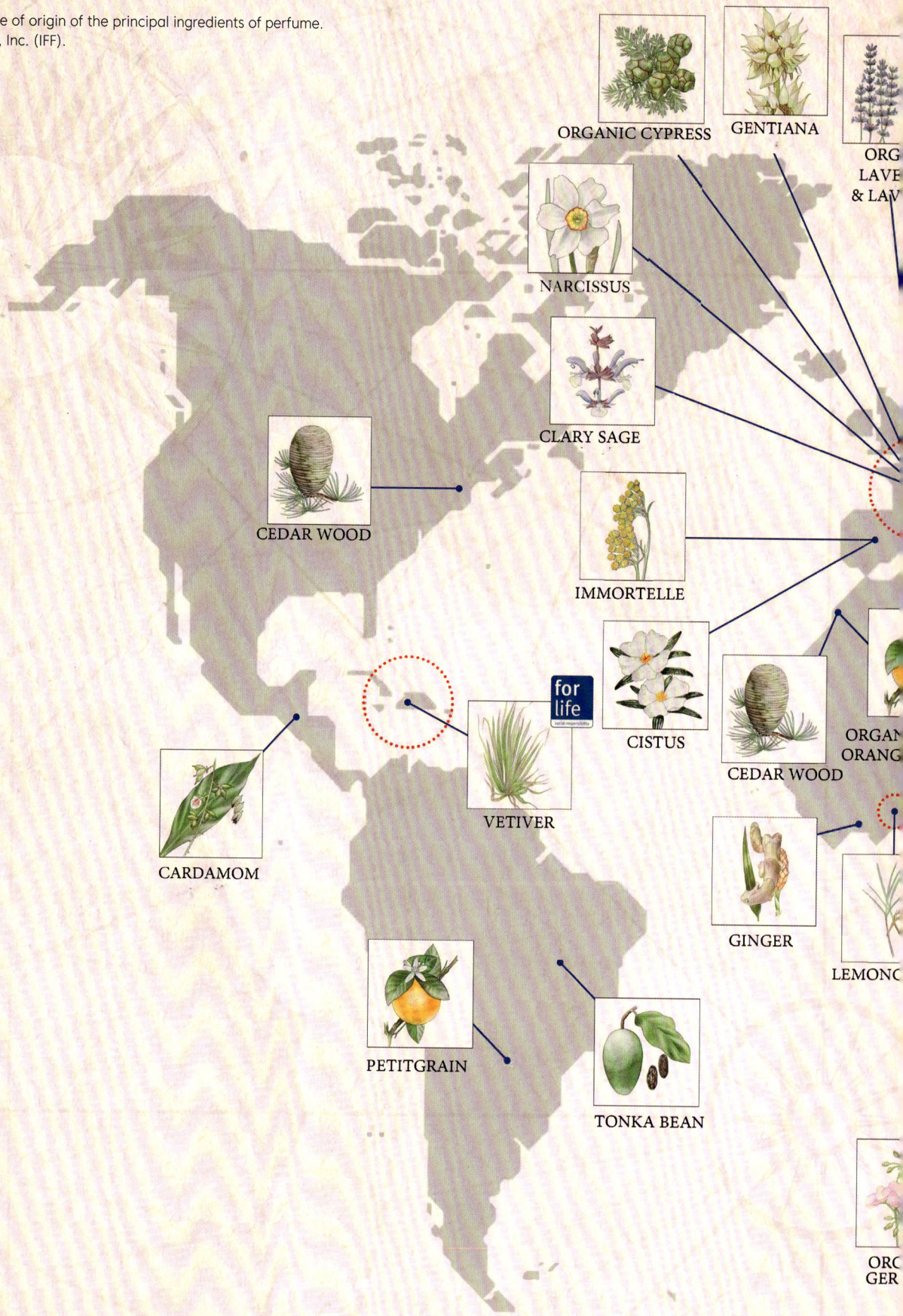

ORGANIC CYPRESS

GENTIANA

ORG
LAVE
& LAV

NARCISSUS

CLARY SAGE

CEDAR WOOD

IMMORTELLE

CISTUS

CEDAR WOOD

for life

VETIVER

ORGAN
ORANG

GINGER

CARDAMOM

LEMON

PETITGRAIN

TONKA BEAN

OR
GER

VERTICALLY INTEGRATED SUPPLY CHAIN
BENEFITTING FROM IFF–LMR EXPERTISE

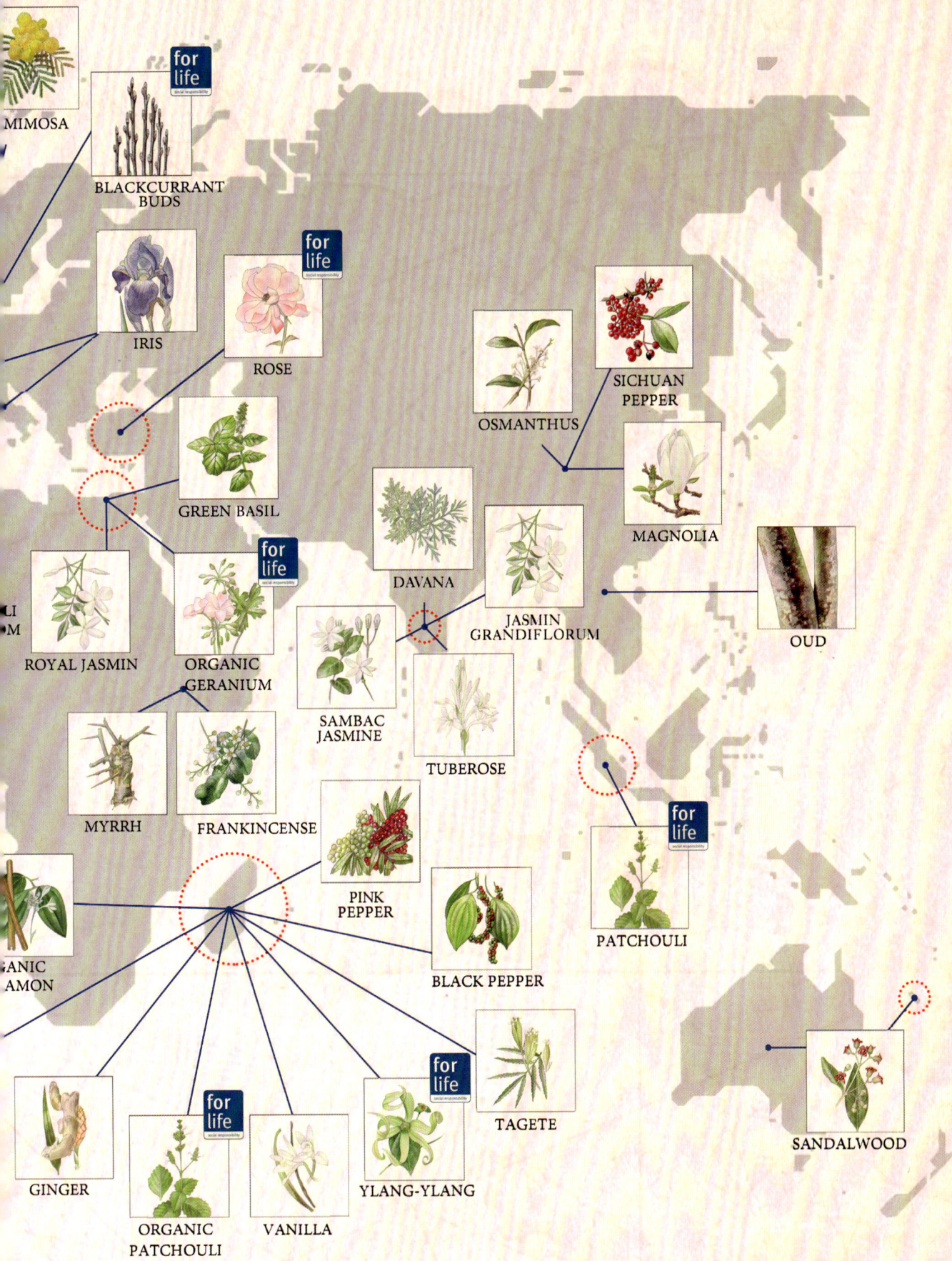

MIMOSA

BLACKCURRANT
BUDS

for
life

IRIS

ROSE

for
life

OSMANTHUS

SICHUAN
PEPPER

GREEN BASIL

MAGNOLIA

DAVANA

JASMIN
GRANDIFLORUM

OUD

ROYAL JASMIN

ORGANIC
GERANIUM

for
life

CI
)M

SAMBAC
JASMINE

MYRRH

FRANKINCENSE

TUBEROSE

PATCHOULI

for
life

PINK
PEPPER

BLACK PEPPER

GANIC
AMON

TAGETE

for
life

GINGER

ORGANIC
PATCHOULI

for
life

VANILLA

YLANG-YLANG

SANDALWOOD

153

87,8%
D'INGRÉDIENTS
D'ORIGINE
NATURELLE

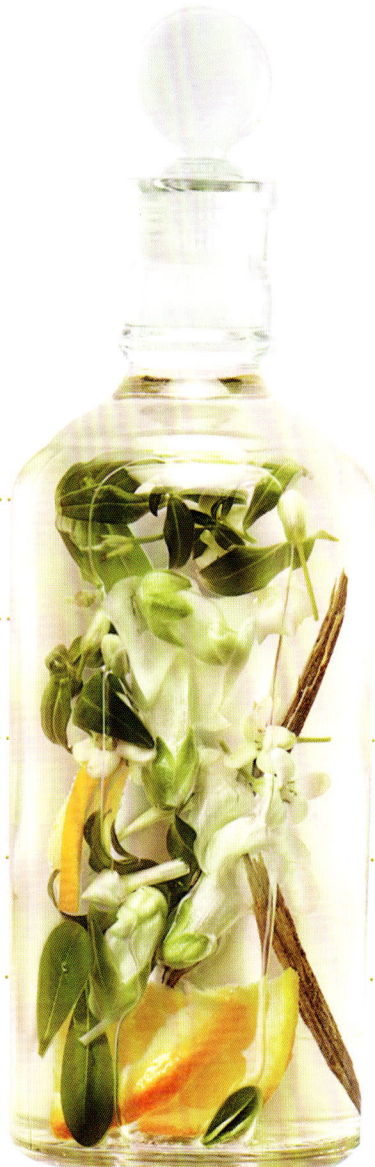

Néroli essence

Bergamote essence

Vétiver essence

absolu Fleur d'oranger

Graines d'Angélique extrait

Ylang Essence

absolu Jasmin Sambac

Mandarine Essence

Immortelle extrait

Petit grain
Bigarade essence

Bois de Cèdre essence

Ingredients in Extrait de Néroli Cologne by Roger & Gallet, by the perfumer Fabrice Pellegrin.

154

SECURING THE FUTURE

Sustainability first entered the equation in 1986, when raw material producers began to purchase organic plants. Today, however, plant biodiversity is more than ever under threat, so some perfume houses have adopted ethical procurement programmes to protect not only the plants but also know-how and expertise in the countries of origin. In these sustainable supply chains, many of which have Ecocert's Fair For Life certification, there are numerous challenges to overcome in order to establish long-term relations with perfume ingredient suppliers. The idea is to be able to make ethical and sustainable choices when sourcing the highest-quality raw materials. These supply sources, mostly located in Asia and the Indian Ocean with some in South America and other parts of the world, are protecting plant heritage by reintroducing old varieties and using native species. Sustainable programmes are shooting up all over the world. To cite some examples, the company International Flavors & Fragrances, Inc. (IFF) is working extensively on all its supply chains for rose in Turkey, iris, narcissus and black-currant bud in France, geranium in Egypt, vetiver in Haiti, cinnamon and ylang-ylang in Madagascar, patchouli in Indonesia and jasmine and tuberose in India. Chanel is protecting sandalwood in New Caledonia and ylang-ylang in the Comoros, Firmenich the green mandarin it sources from the Cai valley in Brazil, and Symrise cinnamon from Madagascar. In addition, some African countries undergoing political and economic stabilization are being encouraged by the World Trade Organization to invest in these raw materials, which promise great development potential. All these programmes safeguard production and encourage the younger generations. If perfume is to remain a luxury product, it is now more important than ever for the industry to wake up and embrace a more ethical way of operating.

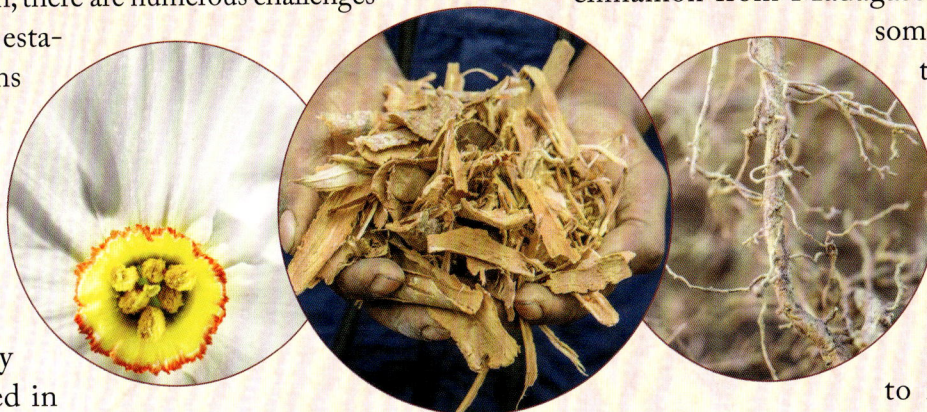

Above (left to right): International Flavors & Fragrances, Inc., and LMR Naturals' (IFF–LMR) narcissus from the Lozère region in France, cinnamon from Madagascar and vetiver from Haiti.

Grasse Fighting the Good Fight

Several producers have revived the tradition of flower cultivation in Grasse over the last decades. In 1983, Monique Rémy set up a company named LMR, for Laboratoire Monique Rémy (now owned by IFF), to promote the use of pure products and treasure florals. Being a great perfumer also means protecting the land and the associated know-how and expertise by growing biodynamically. Thus, because Rose de Mai and jasmine are vital ingredients in Chanel No. 5, in 1987 the company committed to working with local partners to ensure the long-term survival of these iconic flowers. The initiative was extended to include tuberose, iris, geranium and rose in 2016. Dior, for its part, has been forging exclusive partnerships with trusted suppliers since 2011 for the organic, small-scale production of its rose and jasmine and orange blossom. As for L'Oréal, in 2023 it announced a partnership with Cosmo International Fragrances to launch a revolutionary Green Sciences-based extraction process

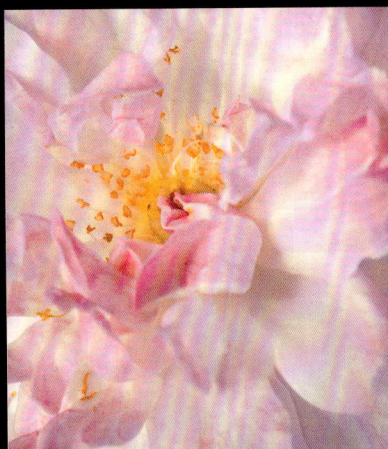

Rose de Mai grown for IFF-LMR.

INDEX

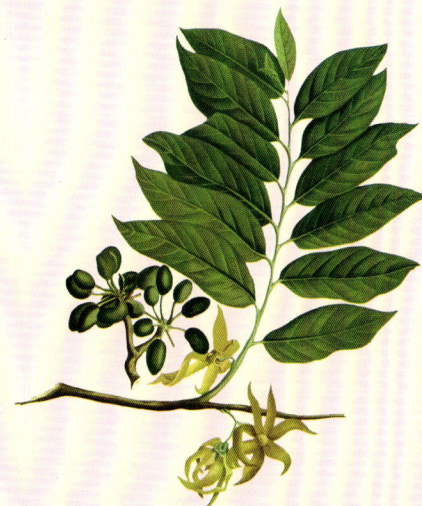

PICTURE CREDITS

p. 6 : Mazovian Museum, Plock, Poland. Ph. © Bridgeman Images; p. 7 t : Ph. © José Nicolas / Naturimages; p. 7 bm: Ph. © Museum of Fine Arts, Boston; p. 8 t r : Ph. © The Walters Art Museum; p. 8 bm: Ph. © Musée du Louvre, Dist. RMN-Grand Palais/Thierry Ollivier; p. 9: Ph. Coll. Archives Larbor; p. 10 t r : Musée National du Bardo, Tunis. Ph. © Valérie Perrin; p. 10 b: Ph. © The Metropolitan Museum of Art, New York; p. 11 t r : Ashmolean Museum, University of Oxford, UK. Ph. © Ashmolean Museum/HIP/Leemage; p. 11 bl : Ph. © Luisa Ricciarini/Leemage; p. 12 tl: © The Metropolitan Museum of Art, New York; p. 12 b: Ph. © Collection Dagli Orti / Jane Taylor / Aurimages; p. 13 t: Ph. Coll. Archives Larousse; p. 14-15: Ph. © Ragab Papyrus Institute, Caire/ G. Dagli Orti/ Aurimages; p. 15 br: Ph. Coll. Archives Larbor; p. 16 tr and contents page: Ph. © The New York Public Library; p. 16 ml: Ph. © François Guénet / akg-images; p. 17 tl: Ph. © De Agostini Picture Lib. / G. Dagli Orti / akg-images; p. 17 br: Ph. © Werner Forman / akg-images; p. 18: Ph. © The Cleveland Museum of Art; p. 19 tl: Ph. © Werner Forman Archive / Bridgeman Images; p. 19 b: Ph. © Getty Villa, Malibu; p. 20 tr: Ph. © The Metropolitan Museaum of Art, New York; p. 20 bl: Ph. Coll. Archives Larbor; p. 21 tl: Ph. © Erich Lessing / akg-images; p. 21 m: Ph. © The Metropolitan Museum of Art, New York; p. 21 m r: Ph. © The Metropolitan Museum of Art, New York; p. 22: Ph. © Wellcome Images; p. 23 tr: Museo Nazionale Romano delle Teme, Rome. Ph. © Nimatallah / akg-images ; p. 23 bl: Ph. © The New York Public Library, New York; p. 24: Ph. © Aisa/Leemage; p. 25 bl: Ph. © The Metropolitan Museum of Art, New York; p. 25 m: Ph. © Villa Getty, Malibu; p. 25 br: Ph. © Villa Getty, Malibu; p. 26 m: Museo Civico d'Arte, Palazzo dei Musei, Modène. Ph. © Deagostino/Leemage; p. 26 bl: Ph. Coll. Archives Larbor; p. 27 tr; Ph. © The New York Public Library; p. 27 m: Ph. Coll. Archives Larousse; p. 28: Musée du Louvre, Paris. Ph. © Werner Forman / akg-images; p. 29 tr: Ph. © Album / Prisma / akg-images; p. 29 b: Ph. Coll. Archives Larousse; p. 30 tr: Ph. © The Metropolitan Museum of Art, New York; p. 30 mr: Ph. © Wellcome collection; p. 31 m: Ph. © Wellcome Collection; p. 31 bl: Musée du Louvre, Paris. Ph. © RMN-Grand Palais / Franck Raux; p. 32: Ph. © Wellcome Collection; p. 33 m: Ph. © The Metropolitan Museum of Art, New York; p. 33 b: Ph. © Wellcome Collection; p. 34 tr: Ph. © The Metropolitan Museum of Art, New York; p. 34 bl: Ph. © British Library / akg-images ; p. 35: Ph. Coll. Archives Larbor; p. 36: Ph. © Biu Santé / res014582; p. 37: Ph. © Wellcome Collection: p. 38 tr: Musée du Louvre, Paris. Ph. © RMN-Grand Palais / Franck Raux; p. 38 b: Ph. © Rijksmuseum, Amsterdam; p. 39 t: Ph. © Library of Congress, Washington; p. 39 ml: Ph. © Wellcome Collection; p. 39 br: Ph. © The Holbarn Archive / Leemage; p. 40 tr: Ph. © Minneapolis Institute of Art; p. 40 bl: Ph. © Wellcome Collection; p. 41 tl: Ph. © Alix Marnat; p. 41 tr: Ph. © BIU Santé / res000033; p. 41 bl: Ph. © Wellcome Collection; p. 41 bm: Ph. © Bernard Bonnefon / akg-images; p. 42 tl: Ph. © Rijksmuseum, Amsterdam ; p. 42-43: 3-Ph. © BIU Santé / res39419; p. 44 tl: Ph. © The Metropolitan Museum of Art, New York; p. 44 br: Ph. © The Metropolitan Museum of Art, New York; p. 45 tl: Ph. © Roland et Sabrina Michaud / akg-images; p. 45 br: Ph. © The Metropolitan Museum of Art, New York; p. 46-47: Ph. © Rijksmuseum, Amsterdam; p. 48: Ph. © François Guénet / akg-images; p. 49 tr: Ph. © Carlo Barbiero, Coll. Musée International de la Parfumerie, Grasse-France; p. 49 m: Ph. © François Guénet / akg-images; p. 50 ml: Ph. © Archives Guerlain; p. 50 m: © Serge Lutens; p. 50 mr: Ph. © Archives Guerlain; p. 51 and 52: 2-© Yves Saint Laurent; p. 53 t: © Musée Yves Saint Laurent Paris / Sophie Carre (2018); p. 53 b: Ph. © The Metropolitan Museum of Art, New York; p. 54 tr: Château de Versaills. Ph. © RMN-Grand Palais / Franck Raux; p. 54 b: Ph. © Les Arts Décoratifs, Paris / Jean Tholance / akg-images; p. 55 t : Ph. © Heritage Images / Fine Art Images / akg-images ; p. 55 bl: Ph. © National Museum, Stockholm; p. 55 br: Ph. © The Metropolitan Museum of Art, New York; p. 56 tr: Ph. © Musée Carnavalet / Roger-Violle ; p. 56 m: Ph. © Christie's Images / Bridgeman Images; p. 56 b: Ph. H. Josse © Archives Larbor; p. 57 tr: Ph. © Christie's Images / Bridgeman Images; p. 57 b: Ph. © Houbigant Paris; p. 58 tr: Ph. © Roger-Viollet; p. 58 b: Ph. © Cleveland Museum of Art; p. 59: 2- Ph. © The Cleveland Museum of Art; p. 60: Ph. © Archives Municipales, Lyon (6FI129); p. 61 t: Ph. © The Metropolitan Museum of Art, New York; p. 61 b: Ph. © Rijkmuseum, Amsterdam; p. 62: Ph. © akg-images; p. 63: Ph. © BIU Santé / res008536; p. 64 t: Ph. © Patrimoine Roger&Gallet; p. 64 b d: Ph. © BIUSanté / dos000342; p. 65: Musée du Louvre, Paris. Ph. © RMN-Grand Palais / Jean-Gilles Berizzi; p. 66 tr: Ph. © FineArtImages /Leemage; p. 66 bl: Ph. © Bibliothèque Villa Saint-Hilaire, Grasse; p. 67 td: Ph. © DR; p. 67 b: Ph. © DR; p. 68 t: Ph. BIU Santé / P15260 ; p. 68 bl: Ph. © François Guénet / akg-images; p. 68 br: Ph. © Archives Guerlain; p. 69 tr: Ph. © BIU Santé / Res008536; p. 69 bl: Ph. © Archives Guerlain; p. 70 tr: Ph. © François Guénet / akg-images; p. 70 bl: Ph. © Collection IM / Kharbine Tapabor; p. 71: Ph. © Archives Charmet / Bridgeman; p. 72 tl: Ph. © Collection IM / Kharbine Tapabor; p. 72 br: Ph. © François Guénet / akg-images ; p. 73: Ph. © BIU Santé / res008536; p. 74 m: Ph. © Coll. Musée International de la Parfumerie, Grasse, France; p. 75 t : Ph. © Archives Larousse; p. 75 bl: Ph. Coll. Archives Larousse; p. 75 br: Ph. © Coll. Musée International de la Parfumerie, Grasse, France ; p. 76: Ph. © Patrimoine Roger&Gallet; p. 77 and 78: 2-Ph. © Patrimoine Roger&Gallet; p. 79 t: Ph. © Patrimoine Roger&Gallet; p. 79 b: Ph. © Patrimoine Roger&Gallet ; p. 80 tl: Ph. © Imagno / Austrian Archives / akg-images; p. 80 b: Ph. © Association François Coty; p. 81 mr: Ph. © Association François Coty; p. 81 bl: Ph. © Musée Carnavalet / Roger-Viollet; p. 82 tl: Ph. © Coll. Musée International de la Parfumerie, Grasse, France. © ADAGP, Paris and DACS, London 2024; p. 82 b: PH. © Bonhams, London, UK / Bridgeman Images; p. 83 m: Ph. © Eric Maillet. © Lancôme; p. 83 mr: Ph. © Hondo Digital. © Lancôme; p. 84: Ph. © MP / Leemage; p. 85 tl: Ph. © Houbigant Paris; p. 85 tr: Ph. © Archives Guerlain; p. 85 b: Ph. © Dazy Rene / Bridgeman Images; p. 86 : Ph. © Bibliothèque des Arts Décoratifs, Paris / Archives Charmet / Bridgeman Images; p. 87 t: Ph. © Look and Learn / Bridgeman Images ; p. 87 b : Ph. © Look and Learn / Valerie Jackson Harris Collection / Bridgeman Images; p. 88-89: Ph. © Musée Carnavalet / Paris Musées; p. 90 : Ph. Coll. Archives Larousse; p. 91 tl: Ph. © Nyodo News / Getty Images; p. 91 b: Ph. © Alamy; p. 92: Ph. © Selva / Bridgeman Images; p. 93 t: Ph. © IM / Kharbine-Tapabor; p. 93 m d : Ph. © Association François Coty; p. 93b: Ph. © BIU Santé / P15270; p. 94: Ph. © BIU Santé res008536; p. 95 tr: Ph. © BIU Santé / res008536; p. 95 m © François Guénet / akg-images; p. 95 b: Bibliothèque Forney, Paris. © François Kollar / Roger-Viollet; p. 96: Ph. © Coll. Musée International de la Parfumerie, Grasse-France; p. 9: Ph. © Patrimoine Roger&Gallet; p. 98: Ph. © François Guénet / akg-images; p. 99: Ph. © Mucha Trust / akg-images; p. 100 t : Ph. Coll. Archives Larousse; p. 100 b: Ph. Nadar Coll. Archives Larbor; p. 101: Ph. © François Kollar © Ministère de la Culture - Médiathèque du Patrimoine, Dist. RMN; p. 102: Ph. © Ed Feingersh/ Michael Ochs Archives/ Getty Images; p. 103 t: © CHANEL Photo Patrick Demarchelier / Daniel Jouanneau; p. 103 b: Ph. © Jean-Marie Perrier / Photo 12; p. 104: Ph. © Baccarat. ©Salvador Dalí, Fundació Gala -Salvador Dalí / DACS 2024; p. 105 mr © Cristallerie de Saint-Louis ; p. 105 bl: © Cristallerie de Saint-Louis; p. 106: Ph. © Kai Jünemann ; p. 107 tl: Musée Calouste Gulbenkian, Lisbonne. Ph. Coll. Archives Larbor; p. 107 mr: Ph. © Patrimoine Roger&Gallet; p. 108 tr: Ph. Coll. Groupe Pochet; p. 108 ml: Ph. © Enguerran Ouvray. © Groupe Pochet; p. 109: Ph. © Christian Dior Parfums, Paris; p. 110: © Houbigant Paris; p. 111 tr: Ph. © Archives Larousse; p. 111 b: Ph. © PVDE / Bridgeman Images; p. 112: illustration de René Grau pour Eau Sauvage de Dior, 1972. © Société René Gruau - www.renegruau.com ; p. 113 t: Ph. © François Guénet / akg-images; p. 113 b: © Davidoff Parfums / Coty; p. 114: Ph. © Jean-Baptiste Mondino. Courtesy Jean Paul Gaultier / PUIG; p. 115: illustration de René Gruau pour Eau Sauvage de Dior, 1978. © Société René Gruau - www.renegruau.com; p. 116 tl: Ph. © Private Collection / Archives Charmet / Bridgeman Images; p. 116 b: Ph. © Boris Lipnitzki / Roger-Viollet; p. 117 t: Ph. Coll. Archives Larbor; p. 117 m Ph. © François Guénet / akg-images; p. 117 b: © Archives Larousse; p. 118 t: © Patrimoine Lanvin, Paris; p. 118 b g : © Patrimoine Lanvin, Paris; p. 118 br: © Patrimoine Lanvin, Paris; p. 119: Publicité pour les parfums Lanvin, 1927. © Patrimoine Lanvin,

ABOUT THE AUTHOR

Élisabeth de Feydeau has a PhD in the history of perfume from the University of Paris-Sorbonne and teaches at the ISIPCA (a post-graduate school that is part or the University Paris Seine). She previously worked at Chanel and Bourjois before becoming an independent cultural adviser to leading luxury brands including Christian Dior, Thierry Mugler, Chanel, Guerlain and Lancaster. She is the author of several books, including *The Herbarium of Marie Antoinette* and the novel *A Scented Palace*, both of which have been translated into several languages.

AUTHOR'S ACKNOWLEDGEMENTS

My sincere thanks go to all contributors to this work, in particular:
Sophie Descours and Françoise Mathay, for their trust and wonderful support from its inception.
Valérie Perrin and Flore Arce Ross for the excellent photos they provided to accompany my text.
Florence Le Maux for the beautiful book design.
Sterenn Le Maguer-Gillon, archaeologist and researcher at the 'Medieval Islam' Laboratory (CNRS, UMR 8167) for her attentive reading of the text.
Aliénor de Feydeau and Amélie Lavie for their help and advice.
I would also like to thank all those who facilitated my research for their contribution to the book.
For my family, I know how much I owe you and thank you for your love and patience.

PUBLISHER'S ACKNOWLEDGEMENTS

We would like to thank all the museums, brands and institutions that provided access to their archives, particularly: the Association François Coty, Baccarat, BIU Santé Paris, Cacharel, Chanel, Cofinluxe, Coty, Cristallerie Saint-Louis, Davidoff, Dior, Groupe Pochet, Guerlain, Houbigant, IFF, Issey Miyake, Jean Paul Gaultier, Lancôme, Lanvin, the International Perfume Museum in Grasse, the Yves Saint Laurent Museum in Paris, Nina Ricci, Roger&Gallet, Serge Lutens, Thierry Mugler and Yves Saint Laurent.